Clinical Immunology

Reginald Gorczynski, MD, PhD
Professor, Departments Surgery and Immunology
University of Toronto and The Toronto Hospital
Toronto, Canada

Jacqueline Stanley, PhD
Course Director and Professor of Immunology
St. George's University, School of Medicine
St. George's, Grenada

Austin, Texas
U.S.A.

VADEMECUM
Clinical Immunology
LANDES BIOSCIENCE
Austin

Copyright ©2001 Gorczynski/Stanley
All rights reserved.
No part of this book may be reproduced or transmitted in any form or by any means, electronic or mechanical, including photocopy, recording, or any information storage and retrieval system, without permission in writing from the authors.
Printed in the U.S.A.

Please address all inquiries to the Publisher:
Landes Bioscience, 810 S. Church Street, Georgetown, Texas, U.S.A. 78626
Phone: 512/ 863 7762; FAX: 512/ 863 0081

ISBN: 1-57059-625-5

Library of Congress Cataloging-in-Publication Data

Clinical immunology / Reginald Gorczynski, Jacqueline Stanley.
  p. cm.
"Vademecum"
Includes index.
ISBN 1-57059-625-5
  1. Clinical immunology. I. Stanley, Jacqueline. II. Title.
  [DNLM: 1. Immunity. 2. Immune System. QW 504 G6605c 1999]
RC582.G67 1999
616.07'9--dc21
    DNLM/DLC   99-34618
    for Library of Congress   CIP

While the authors, editors, sponsor and publisher believe that drug selection and dosage and the specifications and usage of equipment and devices, as set forth in this book, are in accord with current recommendations and practice at the time of publication, they make no warranty, expressed or implied, with respect to material described in this book. In view of the ongoing research, equipment development, changes in governmental regulations and the rapid accumulation of information relating to the biomedical sciences, the reader is urged to carefully review and evaluate the information provided herein.

Dedication

Pat, Christopher and Laura
Brian and David

Contents

Section I: Essential Immunobiological Concepts in Clinical Immunology 1

1. An Introduction: The Immune System 2
Objectives 2
The Immune System 3
General Features 3
Innate Immune Responses 4
Adaptive Immune Responses 6
Cells That Function in Innate Immune Responses 8
Cells That Function in Adaptive Immune Responses 11
Tissues of the Immune System: General Features 12
Tissues of the Immune System: Primary Lymphoid Organs 12
Tissues of the Immune System: Secondary Lymphoid Tissues 14
Soluble Mediators of the Immune System 20
Molecules That Activate Lymphocytes 22
Molecules That Activate Lymphocytes: Monoclonal Activators 22
Molecules That Activate Lymphocytes: Oligoclonal Activators 24
Molecules That Activate Lymphocytes: Polyclonal Activators 24
Summary 25
Clinical Cases and Discussion 26
Test Yourself 29

2. Innate Immune Responses to Pathogens 31
Objectives 31
Innate Immune Responses to Pathogens 32
General Features 32
Role of Complement 32
Phagocytosis 32
Genetic Defects in NADPH Oxidase: Chronic Granulomatous Disease .. 42
Natural Killer Cells 42
Eosinophils 45
Summary 45
Clinical Cases and Discussion 46
Test Yourself 49

3. Antigen Presenting Cells 51
Objectives 51
Antigen Presenting Cells 51
Antigen Presenting Molecules: General Features 55
Antigen Presenting Molecules: Class I MHC Molecules 56
Antigen Presenting Molecules: Class II MHC Molecules 61
Antigen Presenting Molecules: CD1 Molecules 64
Summary 64
Clinical Cases and Discussion 65
Test Yourself 67

4. Soluble Mediators of Immunity I: Antibodies 69
Objectives 69
Antibodies 69
General Features of Antibodies 69
Structure Function Relationship of Antibodies 71
Properties of Immunoglobulin Isotypes 72
Monoclonal Antibodies 77
Monoclonal Antibodies as Therapeutic Agents 78
Clinical Trials 79
Summary 80
Clinical Cases and Discussion 81
Test Yourself 84

5. Soluble Mediators of Immunity II: Complement 85
Objectives 85
Complement 86
Complement Pathways: General Features 86
Complement Biological Activities 93
Complement Regulation 95
Complement and Coagulation Pathways Are Linked via Kallikrein 99
Complement Genetic Deficiencies 99
Role of Complement in Medicine 103
Xenotransplantation: Complement Is Deleterious 103
Summary 104
Clinical Cases and Discussion 105
Test Yourself 108

6. Soluble Mediators of Immunity III: Cytokines 110
Objectives 110
Cytokines 111
General Features 111
Cytokine Receptors That Engage the JAK/STAT Pathway 111
Cytokine Receptors That Engage SMADs 117
Biological Activities of Cytokines That Signal
  via the JAK/STAT Pathway 117
Clinical Relevance of Cytokines 120
Chemokines 124
Summary 125
Clinical Cases and Discussion 125
Test Yourself 128

7. Cells of Adaptive Immunity 130
Objectives 130
B-lymphocyte Antigen-specific Receptor 130
Constructing an Immunoglobulin 131
B-cell Differentiation: Bone Marrow 134
Clinical Significance: B-cell Neoplasms 137
Summary 137
T-lymphocyte Antigen-specific Receptor 137
Differentiation of Lymphoid Progenitor Cells in the Thymus 140
Transport of Lymphocytes from Primary
to Secondary Lymphoid Tissues 146
Summary 146
Clinical Cases and Discussion 147
Test Yourself 152

8. Antigen Dependent B-cell Differentiation 153
Objectives 153
Antigen Dependent B-cell Differentiation 153
Fate of Activated B Cells in Germinal Centers 155
Primary versus Secondary Immune Responses 159
Clinical Significance 159
Models of Signal Transduction in B-cell Activation 160
Negative Signaling in B Cells 161
B-cell Responses to T-independent Antigens 163
Summary 164
Clinical Cases and Discussion 164
Test Yourself 166

9. T Lymphocytes 168
Objectives 168
CD4+ T cells: Antigen Induced Differentiation 168
Memory CD4+ T Cells 174
Clinical Relevance of Type 1 versus Type 2 Cytokines 175
CD8+ T Cells: Antigen Induced Differentiation 177
Memory CD8+ T Cells 179
Clinical Relevance CD8+ T Cells 179
Model of Signal Transduction in T-cell Activation 180
Negative Regulation of T-cell Signaling 182
Memory Lymphocytes in Immunosurveillance 182
Gamma/Delta T Cells 184
Summary 185
Clinical Cases and Discussion 186
Test Yourself 189

10. Inflammation 190
- Objectives 190
- Inflammation 191
- General Features 191
- Vasodilatation, Increased Vascular Permeability and Edema 191
- Recruitment of Neutrophils and Monocytes to the Site of Inflammation 195
- Adaptive Immune Responses in Inflammation 202
- Role of Innate and Adaptive Immunity in Inflammation 203
- Clinical Relevance 204
- Summary 204
- Clinical Cases and Discussion 205
- Test Yourself 209

11. Immunological Responses to Microbes 211
- Objectives 211
- Immunity to Microbes 212
- General Features 212
- Host Defenses to Extracellular Bacteria 212
- Resistance to Immunity: Extracellular Bacteria 217
- Host Defenses to Viruses 217
- Resistance to Immunity: HIV 222
- Host Defenses to Intracellular Bacteria 224
- Resistance to Immunity: Intracellular Bacteria 226
- Host Defenses to Fungi 227
- Resistance to Immunity: Fungi 229
- Summary 230
- Clinical Cases and Discussion 232
- Test Yourself 236

Section II: Clinical Immunology in Practice 239

12. Immunization 240
- Objectives 240
- Immunization 241
- Passive Immunization 242
- Active Immunization or "Vaccination" 244
- Forms of Vaccines 247
- Vaccine Efficacy and Safety 254
- Successful Application of Vaccine Technology 255
- Limited Use Vaccines and Experimental Vaccines 256
- Uses of Vaccines (for Other than Control of Infection) 258
- Summary 258
- Clinical Cases and Discussion 259
- Test Yourself 264

13. Hypersensitivity Reactions 266
Objectives 266
Hypersensitivity Reactions 267
General Features 267
Type I: Immediate Hypersensitivity Reactions 267
Type II: Antibody-mediated Hypersensitivity Reactions 272
Type III: Immune-complex Mediated Hypersensitivity 276
Type IV: Cell-mediated Hypersensitivity 278
Summary 282
Clinical Cases and Discussion 283
Test Yourself 287

14. Autoimmunity 289
Objectives 289
Autoimmunity 290
General Features 290
Tolerance Induction 290
Loss of Self Tolerance 293
Immunopathology of Autoimmune Disorders:
Autoreactive Antibodies 296
Immunopathology of Autoimmune Disorders:
Cell Mediated Immunity 299
Immunotherapy of Autoimmune Disease: Suppression 301
Immunotherapy of Autoimmune Disorders: Cytokine Modulation 306
Summary 307
Clinical Cases and Discussion 308
Test Yourself 312

15. Immunodeficiency Disorders 314
Objectives 314
Immunodeficiency Disorders 315
General Features 315
Primary Immunodeficiency Disorders 315
Primary Immunodeficiency Disorders: Progenitor Cells 315
Primary Immunodeficiency Disorders: T Cells 319
Primary Immunodeficiency Disorders: B Cells 320
Primary Immunodefieciency Disorders: Phagocytic 323
Primary Immunodeficiency Disorders: Other Leukocytes 323
Primary Immunodeficiency Disorders: Complement System 323
Secondary Immunodeficiency Disorders 327
Secondary Immunodeficiency Disorders: Acquired 329
Secondary Immunodeficiency Disorders: Abnormal Production
of Immune Components 330
Summary 330
Clinical Cases and Discussion 331
Test Yourself 335

16. Tumor Immunology 337
- Objectives 337
- Tumor Immunology 338
- General Features 338
- The Concept of Immunosurveillance 338
- Tumor Antigens 340
- Tumor Immunosurveillance 344
- Effector Mechanisms for Elimination of Tumors 345
- Evasion of Immune Surveillance 349
- Immunology in Diagnosis or in Monitoring Prognosis 354
- Novel Therapies: Enhancing Antigen Presentation by Dendritic Cells 355
- Novel Therapies: Cytokines and other Molecules Transfected into Tumor Cells Themselves 357
- Novel Therapies: Modification of CTL as a Strategy for Enhancing Tumor Immunity 359
- Novel Therapies: Monoclonal Antibodies and Immunotherapy 359
- Summary 360
- Clinical Cases and Discussion 361
- Test Yourself 366

17. Transplantation 367
- Objectives 367
- Transplantation 368
- General Features 368
- Classification of Grafts According to Their Source 368
- Classification of Graft Rejection 371
- Genetics of Transplantation 373
- Immunology of Graft Rejection 379
- Tissue Differences in Clinical Transplantation 387
- Graft Versus Host Disease 389
- Immunosuppression in Transplantation 389
- Summary 391
- Clinical Cases and Discussion 392
- Test Yourself 396

Index 398

Preface

The primary purposes of this book are first, to introduce the reader to the fundamental components of the immune system and the basic concepts involved in understanding how those components interact to achieve host defense, and second to highlight how that understanding proves invaluable to diagnosis and treatment of a wide variety of clinical disorders. In the introductory chapters attention is focused on the cells and factors which make up both the innate and acquired immune systems. While the innate system is often thought of as the "primitive" immune system, we will see that it is in many ways no less complex and wide-ranging, in its action than the acquired (adaptive) system. The acquired immune system is, itself, composed of a unique collection of specialized cells (lymphocytes) which have the remarkable capacity to undergo genomic DNA rearrangements to generate populations with a seemingly infinite capacity to recognize foreign (non-self) molecular determinants. As might be expected, development of such diversity necessarily brings with it the concomitant need to ensure that the self is still recognized as such (and thus protected from whatever host defense mechanisms are brought to bear upon "foreign", non-self, material (or organisms). Understanding how self:nonself discrimination occurs naturally, how and why it sometimes fails, and how it may be controlled exogenously, remain some of the key problems in contemporary immunology and clinical immunology.

In order to maintain the reader's interest in the clinical perspective behind the immunology discussed, we have highlighted clinical cases at the end of each chapter, which pinpoint some of the issues discussed in the preceding pages. However, in the second half of this book, with the reader now armed with the necessary basic immunological tools and concepts, several topics of clinical importance are discussed in considerably more detail. While each of these chapters can be read in isolation, the novice to immunology as a discipline will generally find it useful to have read Chapter 1, which gives a broad overview of the field of immunology, before consideration of any of the other chapters in the book. In addition, it will be beneficial to all readers of these more clinical chapters to make liberal cross-reference to preceding chapters in the earlier portions of the text. The clinical problems which follow each of these latter chapters are presented in a slightly different format, with more attention now paid to the clinical aspects of the immunological problems, and generally less detail being provided to the basic immunological components. We have made every effort in these sections to be as contemporary as possible, and references are frequently given to ongoing clinical trials of the numerous novel therapies which are underway to test our current growing understanding of the immunobiology of human diseases.

It is our hope that all readers of this book, whether they be basic immunology students, medical students, clinicians or teachers, will find it to be a valuable resource. As a resource book, it provides the essential immunological facts needed to understand clinical problems, and affords an understanding of frequently encountered clinical problems so that they become easier to comprehend at the level of basic immunobiology. If, after finishing the book, the reader is also stimulated to pursue a greater in depth understanding of any of the problems we discuss, we will have achieved our objectives.

Reginald Gorczynski
Jacqueline Stanley

ICONS

 Natural Killer cell
 Monocyte
 Macrophage
 Neutrophil
 Dendritic cell

 B cell
 Plasma cell
 Monomeric Ig / Dimeric IgA
 Pentameric IgM

 Mast cell or Basophil
 Intraepithelial T cell
 M cell
 Columnar epithelial cell
 Follicular dendritic cell

 Thp
 Th0
 Th1
 Th2
 pCTL
 CTL / γ/δ T cell intrathymic maturation / γ/δ T cell extrathymic maturation

Section I

Essential Immunobiological Concepts In Clinical Immunology

In the Section I chapters we have developed a broad overview of the workings of the mammalian immune system and highlighted the multiple regulatory mechanisms which exist within these interacting populations of cells. By judicious use of some clinical case discussions at the end of each chapter we have attempted to guide the reader to understand the relevance, for the practicing clinician, of the basic science we have presented in each section. In contemporary internal medicine however, the clinical immunologist deals predominantly with a number of key conditions, and these are certainly worthy of highlighting unto themselves.

1 An Introduction: The Immune System

Objectives	2
The Immune System	3
General Features	3
Innate Immune Responses	4
Adaptive Immune Responses	6
Cells That Function in Innate Immune Responses	8
Cells That Function in Adaptive Immune Responses	11
Tissues of the Immune System: General Features	12
Tissues of the Immune System: Primary Lymphoid Organs	12
Tissues of the Immune System: Secondary Lymphoid Tissues	14
Soluble Mediators of the Immune System	20
Molecules That Activate Lymphocytes	22
Molecules That Activate Lymphocytes: Monoclonal Activators	22
Molecules That Activate Lymphocytes: Oligoclonal Activators	24
Molecules That Activate Lymphocytes: Polyclonal Activators	24
Summary	25
Clinical Cases and Discussion	26
Test Yourself	29

Objectives

At the conclusion to this chapter, the reader will have a firm understanding of the fundamental components of the immune system, and how they interact in achieving defense against environmental pathogens and/or foreign substances (antigens). Host defense has been classically subdivided into the two categories **innate immunity** and **adaptive immunity**. The innate immune system, which functions as a "first-line" of defense to invading pathogens (antigens), is composed of cells and molecules that provide rapid host protection without memory or specificity for the responses in which they engage. The principal cell types in innate immunity are **phagocytes** (**macrophages and neutrophils**) and **natural killer (NK) cells**. A system of serum proteins, the complement system, is also intimately involved in innate immunity.

In marked contrast to the rapidity with which the innate immune system is activated, naive cells engaged in adaptive immune responses require several days to develop their effector function. Moreover, the cells (**lymphocytes**), characteristic of adaptive immune responses, are restricted in their recognition repertoire in that each cell recognizes only one antigen. As a result, following initial encounter with antigen, adaptive immune responses are dependent upon mechanism(s) that ensure clonal expansion of the activated cells. Adaptivity and specificity, which are hallmarks of lymphocyte-mediated immune responses, refer to the pre-exist-

---

Clinical Immunology, by Reginald Gorczynski and Jacqueline Stanley. 2001 Landes Bioscience

ing "infinite" array of cells each with a unique receptor, such that this pool of cells provides immunity to all conceivable antigens. Another feature of the adaptive immune response is that, following initial antigen encounter, the immune system retains a supply of **memory cells,** which can respond more quickly to rechallenge with the same antigen than the naive (uneducated) immune system. Soluble molecules produced by activated lymphocytes include **antibodies, cytokines,** and **chemokines.**

The immune system is further subdivided according to the tissues involved in differentiation/maturation of immune responses. Development of lymphocytes takes place in **primary immune tissues** (bone marrow/spleen/thymus), while activation of lymphocytes takes place in **secondary immune tissues** (lymph nodes, tonsils and adenoids, spleen, and mucosa-associated lymphoid tissues (MALT)). The two classes of lymphocytes, B and T cells, are found in discrete areas of these secondary tissues. In addition, other cells implicated in the development of acquired immune reactions, such as dendritic cells and macrophages, are also found in distinct areas of the lymphoid organs.

Finally, we need to consider classification of adaptive immune reactions in terms of the stimulus that induces immunity. Molecules that activate a single (antigen-specific) clone of responding cells are called monoclonal activators, while those stimulating multiple clones (mitogens) are called polyclonal activators. Small molecules are often nonimmunogenic until coupled to larger molecules. In this scenario, the small molecule is called a **hapten,** and the larger one a **carrier.** When B cells are activated to produce antibodies, they may need "help" from T cells (**T-dependent antigen responses**), or activation may occur independently of this help (**T-independent antigens**). Immune responses to antigens (especially T-dependent ones) are often enhanced by **adjuvants.**

THE IMMUNE SYSTEM

General Features

Our ability to coexist with the vast array of microbes present in our environment is a measure of the efficacy of various defense systems to monitor *insults* to the internal cellular environment from the extracellular world. Arguably the most important of these defense systems is the immune system. In essence the immune system is the instrument by which the body discriminates **self** from **nonself,** and destroys nonself. Important functional elements of the immune system include several cell types, tissues, serum proteins, and small peptides such as chemokines and cytokines. While components of the immune system interact with one another, detailed discussion is simplified by classification into two categories, innate immunity and adaptive immunity.

The innate immune system is made up of cells and molecules that function early in the protective response to a foreign substance (antigen), using primitive receptors found also within the invertebrate world to distinguish *self* from *nonself*. There is no unique antigenic specificity that triggers the elements of the innate immune system, which, we shall see later, makes this system quite different from the "more developed" adaptive immune system (dependent upon lymphocytes). Furthermore, these innate responses do not confer any host advantage upon subsequent exposure to the same microbe. In other words, innate immunity does not lead to immunological memory; again this is in sharp contrast to lymphocyte-mediated immune function.

From a phylogenetic point of view, the adaptive immune response is a more recent development than innate immunity. However, various components of each system have been co-opted into use by the other system. Thus, recruitment of cells during adaptive immune responses, and their activation, is often contingent upon the action of cytokines generated during innate immunity. Adaptive immune responses, in turn, lead to the production, by specific cells, of effector molecules including cytokines, and other serum proteins called antibodies. Antibodies and cytokines, themselves, often contribute to the effector function of cells functioning within innate and/or adaptive immune processes. In contrast to the quick response time for innate immune processes, naive cells that mediate adaptive immunity require several days to become formidable effectors. Lymphocytes are restricted in their recognition repertoire, with each cell responding only to one unique portion (**epitope**) of an antigen.

Hence, while the immune system is conveniently considered to provide two modes of host defense, in reality innate and adaptive immune responses act in concert, but differ with respect to: (i) specificity; (ii) immunological memory, i.e., the ability to "recall" previous exposure to antigen; and (iii) constancy of response time and magnitude of the response (Table 1.1).

INNATE IMMUNE RESPONSES

Our first lines of defense against infectious agents are the natural physical and chemical barriers that prevent microbes from invading our bodies. Intact skin and mucosal linings are effective physical barriers unless they are compromised. Chemical barriers also serve as deterrents to infectious agents. As example, **lysozyme** present in secretions splits the cell walls of gram positive bacteria; **spermine** (in semen) prevents the growth of gram positive bacteria; the acid pH of the

Table 1.1. Characteristics of the innate and the adaptive immune system

Characteristic	Immune System	
	Innate Immune System	Adaptive Immune System
Immunological Memory	—	+
Specificity	—	+
Response Time Constancy	+	—

stomach prevents colonization of most bacteria. Once infectious agents have penetrated these physical and chemical barriers, nonspecific mechanisms of host defense are induced in an attempt to eliminate the intruders. Phagocytes, natural killer cells, inflammatory cells, and antigen presenting cells are the principal cells that function in innate immunity (Fig. 1.1).

In addition to the induction of cellular aspects of innate immunity, a system of serum proteins, the complement system, is intimately involved in this form of immunity. Following the deposition of a spontaneously generated fragment of a serum complement protein onto a microbial membrane, particularly bacterial cell membranes, the complement system is activated. Triggering complement activation signals a cascade of activation of complement component proteins, leading to the generation of various protein fragments with distinct biological activities that contribute to host defense. In addition, cytokines released during induction of cellular immunity, in conjunction with antigen presentation by antigen presenting cells, recruit the adaptive immune system, which enhances host defense. The innate immune system, therefore, is characterized by responses that lack memory and specificity, but display constancy with respect to magnitude and rate of the response to antigen.

ADAPTIVE IMMUNE RESPONSES

Adaptive immune responses (also known as acquired immune responses) are mediated by lymphocytes (Fig. 1.2). The system is "adaptive" in that, even before exposure to the pathogen, lymphocytes have been developed that recognize an infinite array of antigens. While there are millions of each lymphocyte type (T and B) present, each antigen is recognized by only a few (in the limit one) cells. In fact, each lymphocyte responds to only one unique portion (**epitope**) of an antigen. Effective immunity following exposure to a pathogen requires multiple copies of the lymphocytes recognizing the pathogen. As a result, specific lymphocytes undergo binary division (proliferation) that leads to the generation of numerous progeny specific for an epitope on the pathogen. Because the progeny respond to the same antigenic epitope as that of the parent, the parent and the progeny constitute what is termed a **clone** (Fig. 1.3). **Clonal expansion is crucial to generate effective immunity against pathogens during first exposure (primary response)**, thus ensuring that a sufficient number of lymphocytes specific for that pathogen are available. After the pathogen is cleared not all of the cells that encountered antigen die. Rather the immune system retains a supply of *memory cells*, which can respond much more quickly to rechallenge (**secondary response**) with the same antigen that induced the clonal expansion. This constitutes the process of antigen-specific immunological memory.

Adaptive immune responses, in turn, lead to the production of effector molecules including cytokines, and other serum proteins, called antibodies or immunoglobulins, by specific cells. These effector molecules themselves often contribute to innate and/or adaptive immune processes. As an example, particular antibodies complexed with antigen can trigger the activation of the complement system.

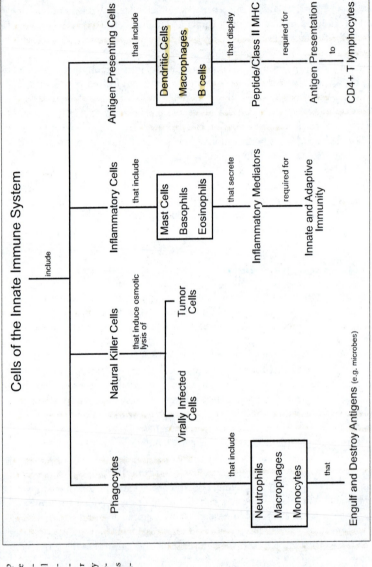

Fig. 1.1. Concept map depicting cells of the innate immune system. The main cell types in innate immunity are phagocytes, natural killer cells, inflammatory cells, and antigen presenting cells. Each has a particular role in innate immunity.

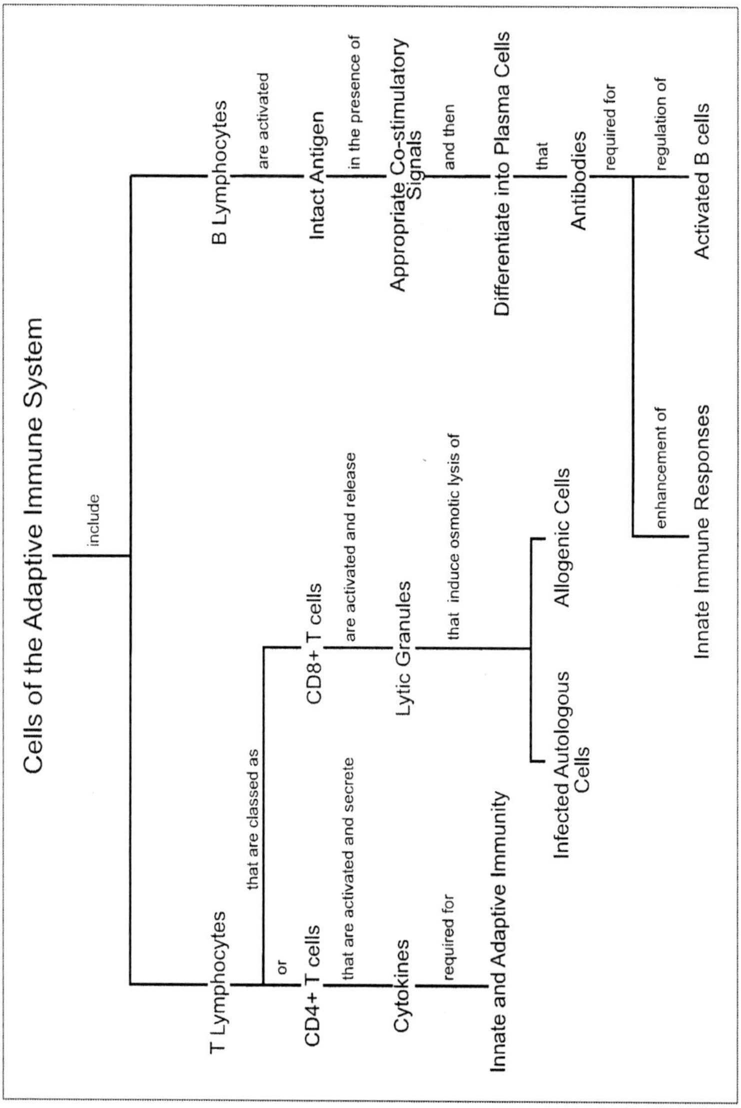

An Introduction to the Immune System 7

Cells of the Adaptive Immune System

- **include**
  - **T Lymphocytes**
    - *that are classed as*
      - **CD4+ T cells**
        - *that are activated and secrete*
          - **Cytokines**
            - *required for*
              - **Innate and Adaptive Immunity**
      - *or*
      - **CD8+ T cells**
        - *are activated and release*
          - **Lytic Granules**
            - *that induce osmotic lysis of*
              - **Infected Autologous Cells**
              - **Allogenic Cells**
  - **B Lymphocytes**
    - *are activated*
      - **Intact Antigen**
        - *in the presence of*
          - **Appropriate Co-stimulatory Signals**
            - *and then*
              - **Differentiate into Plasma Cells**
                - *that*
                  - **Antibodies**
                    - *required for*
                      - *enhancement of*
                        - **Innate Immune Responses**
                      - *regulation of*
                        - **Activated B cells**

Fig. 1.2. Concept map depicting cells of the adaptive immune system. There are two broad classes of lymphocytes, B lymphocytes and T lymphocytes, each with a specific role in the immune response.

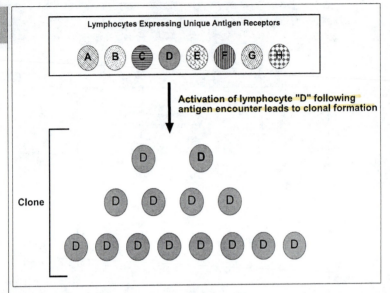

Fig. 1.3. Activation of a lymphocyte leads to clonal formation. Specific lymphocytes undergo binary division (proliferation) that leads to the generation of numerous progeny (clone) specific for an epitope on the pathogen.

While the early stages in complement activation by antibody/antigen complexes differ from that described earlier for innate immunity, activation by either route eventually yields the same biological mediators due to convergence of the two pathways to a common pathway. The adaptive immune system, therefore, is characterized by responses that show memory and specificity, but are variable with respect to magnitude and rate of the response to antigen.

CELLS THAT FUNCTION IN INNATE IMMUNE RESPONSES

The principle cell types in innate immunity are phagocytes (macrophages and neutrophils) that engulf and destroy foreign substances, and natural killer (NK) cells, whose main role is to destroy infected host (**autologous**) cells (Figs. 1.1, 1.4). Activation of either cell type is accompanied by secretion of many molecules including cytokines that enhance innate immunity, either directly or indirectly via adaptive immunity. Antigen presenting cells represent another group of cells classed with innate immunity. These cells deliver antigen to distinct lymphocytes, a process termed antigen presentation. For effective presentation by antigen presenting cells (APC), antigen fragments must be expressed on the APC surface, cradled within the groove of special molecules termed major histocompatibility proteins. Another class of cell, the inflammatory cells, facilitates both innate and adaptive immune responses through the inflammatory products secreted following their activation.

An Introduction to the Immune System

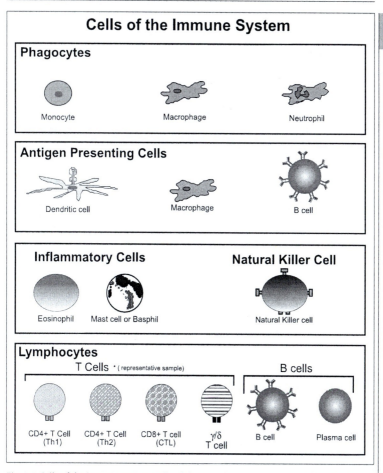

Fig. 1.4. Cells of the immune system. Cells of the innate immune system and the adaptive immune system are illustrated. Note that there are several types of cells in the various categories.

Phagocytes

Phagocytes are cells whose function is primarily phagocytosis. **Phagocytosis is a defense mechanism by which microorganisms, especially bacteria and other extracellular microbes are engulfed and destroyed by phagocytes**. Predominant phagocytes include **neutrophils** and **monocytes/macrophages** (Figs. 1.1, 1.4). The **neutrophil** is the dominant type of circulating polymorphonuclear granulocyte. The term **monocyte** refers to immature macrophages. Monocytes are typically found in circulation and have a limited capacity for phagocytosis. When monocytes migrate to different tissues, they mature into macrophages. Mature **macrophages** exist in tissues and are named according to the particular area of the body in which they reside (Table 1.2). In addition to its role in phagocytosis, the **macrophage serves as a link between innate and adaptive immunity** by delivering antigen to distinct lymphocytes, a process termed antigen presentation (see below).

Antigen presenting cells
Antigen presenting cells (APC) are cells that endocytose antigen, process it into fragments (peptides), and then display various fragments on the cell surface. For effective presentation antigen fragments must be expressed on the APC surface, cradled within the groove of special molecules termed, **class II major histocompatibility proteins** (class II MHC). These cell surface complexes of peptide/class II MHC represent the form of antigen that is recognized by a subset of lymphocytes, T lymphocytes. Antigen presenting cells include dendritic cells, macrophages, and B cells (Figs. 1.1, 1.4). B cells are lymphocytes that function as antigen presenting cells in addition to their role in adaptive immunity.

Natural killer cells
The main role of **natural killer (NK) cells** is destruction of virally infected autologous (self) cells. There is evidence that natural killer cells also destroy some tumor cells (Figs. 1.1, 1.4). Exposure to certain small molecules termed **cytokines** (e.g., interleukin-2 and interleukin-12), enhances the ability of NK cells to kill their targets. In the presence of high concentrations of interleukin-2, NK cells differentiate to lymphokine activated killer cells (LAK cells). LAK cells are cytotoxic and are more potent killers than the NK cells.

Inflammatory cells
Inflammatory cells include **mast cells, basophils, and eosinophils** (Figs. 1.1, 1.4). Basophils are the circulating counterpart of the tissue mast cells. Eosinophils are found primarily in tissues, and in smaller numbers, in the circulation. These inflammatory cells play a role in the development and/or maintenance of the inflammatory response, which is an integral part of immunity.

Mast cells are present in gut, lung, and in most tissues (including connective tissue) adjoining blood cells. Mast cells express high affinity receptors for differ-

Table 1.2 Phagocytic cell nomenclature

Tissue	Phagocytic Cell Nomenclature
Blood	Monocyte
Bone Marrow	Monoblasts
Central Nervous System	Microglial Cells
Liver	Kupffer Cells
Synovium	Synoviocytes
Lung	Alveolar Macrophages
Lymph Node and Spleen	Macrophages

ent molecules, all of which (when crosslinked) can trigger the degranulation of mast cells and release of inflammatory mediators present in the granules. The granules contain **histamine**, and the **leukotrienes LTC4, LTD4, and LTE4, eosinophil chemotactic factor of anaphylaxis (ECF-A)** and **platelet activating factor (PAF)**. The leukotrienes, LTC4, LTD4, and LTE4 were previously collectively referred to as slow releasing substance of anaphylaxis (SRS-A). Because mast cells are present in tissues they are activated early in the response. Some of the molecules secreted at the site of tissue injury serve as chemotactic factors for other cells, including basophils and eosinophils. Molecules secreted by eosinophils include **major basic protein (MBP)**, and **eosinophil cationic protein (ECP)**, both of which play a role in the destruction of some parasites (e.g., helminths).

CELLS THAT FUNCTION IN ADAPTIVE IMMUNE RESPONSES

Cells that function in adaptive immunity are **lymphocytes** (Figs. 1.2, 1.4). There are two broad classes of lymphocytes, **B lymphocytes** and **T lymphocytes**. Each cell type has a distinct function and mode of activation. In addition, subsets of cells within each class of lymphocytes have distinct roles. Lymphocytes possess unique antigen recognizing receptors, which endows them with the ability to interact with one antigen, but not another.

B lymphocytes

B lymphocytes express cell surface antigen receptors termed **antibodies** or **immunoglobulins**. These cell surface antibodies are the instruments by which B cells recognize and interact with antigen. In the presence of specific antigen, and appropriate costimulatory molecules, B cells will clonally expand and differentiate into antibody secreting **plasma cells**. For protein antigens, B-cell differentiation requires stimulation with cytokines secreted by T cells, as well as cognate interaction with a subset of T lymphocytes.

T lymphocytes

T lymphocytes are cells that express antigen recognizing receptors termed **T cell receptors**. T cells express one of two types of T-cell receptors, alpha/beta receptors or gamma/delta receptors. This designation refers to the polypeptides that make up the receptor. Most of the T cells in the body express alpha/beta receptors. Unless otherwise specified, the term T cell in this book refers to T cells expressing alpha/beta T-cell receptors. Alpha/beta T-cell receptors recognize, and interact with, antigen fragments that are displayed in the groove of proteins expressed on the surface of cells. The proteins that display antigen fragments are termed either class I MHC or class II MHC.

There are two major subsets of T lymphocytes, defined by the presence of protein markers, **CD4 and CD8**, on the cell surface. The CD4+ subset of T cells recognize antigen fragments presented in association with class II MHC expressed on the surface of antigen presenting cells. T cells expressing the CD4 marker are also referred to as **T helper (Th) cells**, because they secrete cytokines required for both innate and adaptive immunity. Th cell subsets secrete distinct patterns of cytokines which can be used to define the subsets, Th1 and Th2. Th1 cells secrete Type 1 cytokines; Th2 cells secrete Type 2 cytokines. The activities of different components of the immune system are altered in the presence of Type 1 or Type 2 cytokines.

T cells expressing the CD8 marker are termed **CD8+ T cells** or **cytotoxic T cells** (CTL). Cytotoxic T cells are capable of destroying autologous cells expressing an antigen fragment in the groove of a class I MHC molecule. These autologous cells are commonly referred to as **target cells** (not antigen presenting cells). CD8+ T cells are also capable of destroying allogenic cells, as occurs in the context of tissue and/or organ transplantation.

TISSUES OF THE IMMUNE SYSTEM: GENERAL FEATURES

Immune tissues are broadly classed according to their roles in the immune system. Tissues that serve as developmental sites for lymphocytes are termed **primary immune tissues,** while those tissues that serve as activation sites are termed **secondary immune tissues.** Primary immune tissues include the bone marrow and thymus. Although there is evidence for the development of lymphocytes outside these primary tissues, the sites have not been identified. Secondary immune tissues include the lymph nodes, tonsils and adenoids, spleen, and mucosa-associated lymphoid tissue. The bone marrow and liver (the latter particularly in conditions of lympho-hematopoietic stress) can also be considered secondary lymphoid tissue.

TISSUES OF THE IMMUNE SYSTEM: PRIMARY LYMPHOID ORGANS

Bone marrow
In the early stage of embryogenesis, blood cells arise from the yolk sac, and later from the liver and spleen. During the later stages of embryogenesis, and after birth, the bone marrow is the hematopoietic tissue that gives rise to most mature nonlymphoid blood cells including monocytes, granulocytes, eosinophils, basophils, erythrocytes, and platelets. These blood cells have a relatively short life span and are replaced continuously by progeny of self-renewing **pluripotent stem cells**, a process termed **hematopoiesis**. Under the influence of cytokines, and other factors produced by bone marrow stromal cells, blood cells go through distinct stages of differentiation and maturation before being released into the blood. Soluble mediators that have been shown to play a role in hematopoiesis include c-kit ligand, interleukin-3 (IL-3), interleukin-7 (IL-7), and the colony stimulating growth factors (CSF): G-CSF, M-CSF, and GM-CSF (G = granulocyte, M= monocyte).

Pluripotent stem cells also give rise to precursor lymphoid cells. Under the influence of the local microenvironment some of the lymphoid precursors will give rise to mature B cells, while other precursors will leave the bone marrow and migrate to the thymus. The bone marrow is, therefore, the site of B-cell development and maturation. B-cell development occurs prior to antigen exposure and is often referred to as **antigen-independent B-cell maturation**. B-cell maturation was initially shown to occur in the chicken's *Bursa of Fabricius*, and the human site of B-cell maturation is often referred to as the "bursa equivalent". The fundamental event of B-cell development is the expression of a unique B-cell antigen receptor (antibody) on its cell surface. This receptor is the instrument by which B cells will recognize antigen. Expression of any given B-cell antigen receptor is a random event, and some of the receptors expressed on B cells will recognize self-proteins and be potentially autoreactive. The cells expressing receptors that recognize self-molecules undergo **tolerance induction,** a process in which potentially autoreactive cells are deleted or inactivated (anergized). B-cell maturation is also characterized by the expression of cell surface proteins that play a role in subsequent B-cell activation, while other expressed proteins serve as phenotypic B-cell markers. These mature naive B cells leave the bone marrow and seed the periphery.

Thymus

The thymus is the site of T-cell maturation. At puberty the thymus weighs 30-40 grams. Thereafter, it undergoes progressive involution and extensive fatty infiltration. Whether the remaining thymic rudiment is responsible for adult T-cell maturation and selection, or whether an extra thymic source exists for these adult functions, is not known. The thymus is a bi-lobed organ, with each lobe further subdivided into lobules. Each lobule has a cortex and a medulla (Fig. 1.5). A blood-thymus barrier prevents the passage of molecules from the blood to the thymic cortex. In contrast, the blood vessels of the thymic medulla have no such barrier.

By analogy with B cells, the most significant event of T-cell maturation is the cell surface expression of a unique antigen receptor, the T-cell receptor. Expression of a specific T-cell receptor is a random event, which results in the expression of some T-cell receptors that are of no value to the host, as well as some which are potentially autoreactive. During thymic maturation, processes termed respectively

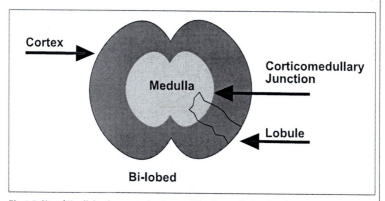

Fig. 1.5. Site of T-cell development: the thymus. The thymus is the site of T-cell maturation. It is a bi-lobed organ, with each lobe being divided into lobules. Each lobule has a cortex and a medulla. T-cell maturation occurs primarily in the cortex, while the medulla serves as a site for final screening, and elimination of autoreactive cells.

death by neglect and **negative selection** delete these two types of T cells. Approximately 50 million precursor cells enter the thymus daily with only approximately one million surviving the selection process. T cells that survive the selection process are said to have been **positively selected** and will undergo lineage commitment. Lineage commitment refers to a phenotypic change such that either a CD4 or a CD8 molecule is on the cell surface (not both). Because the expression of CD4 or CD8 determines the role of the T cell in the periphery, lineage commitment determines the biological function of the T cell. Thymocytes migrate from the cortex to the medulla where they undergo a second screening process to further ensure that self reactive T cells are destroyed before leaving the thymus.

TISSUES OF THE IMMUNE SYSTEM: SECONDARY LYMPHOID TISSUES

Secondary lymphoid tissues include the lymph nodes, tonsils and adenoids, spleen, and mucosa-associated lymphoid tissues (MALT). These tissues are the major sites of adaptive immune responses, though the actual site where the initial immune response occurs is determined by the mode of antigen entry (Fig. 1.6). If antigen is carried via the lymphatics, the initial site of the adaptive immune response is the lymph node; if antigens are blood-borne, the initial site of the adaptive immune response is the spleen; and if antigens enter via mucosal tissue, MALT serves as the initial site of the adaptive immune response.

Lymph nodes

Lymph nodes are encapsulated organs strategically located along lymphatic channels throughout the body. Afferent lymphatics penetrate the connective tissue that encapsulates the lymph node (Fig. 1.7) and empty their contents into the subcapsular sinuses. The sinuses are lined with tiny apertures that allow lymph

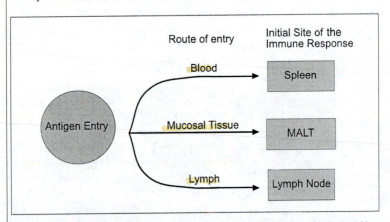

Fig. 1.6. Site of initial immune response depends on the route of antigen entry. The initial immune response is determined by the mode of antigen entry. The lymph node, spleen, and MALT serve as the initial site of the immune response for antigen that enters via the lymphatics, the blood, or the mucosal tissues, respectively.

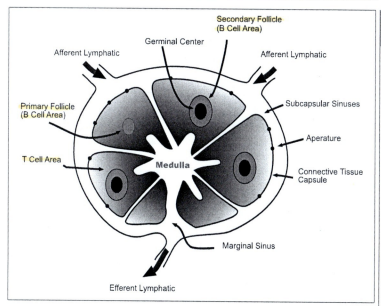

Fig. 1.7. Schematic illustration of a lymph node. Lymph nodes are encapsulated organs with both afferent and efferent lymphatics. The sinuses are lined with tiny apertures that allow lymph and its contents to seep through the lymph node and come into contact with lymphocytes. Different cells of the immune system predominate in the primary follicles, secondary follicles, interfollicular regions, and the medulla.

and its contents to seep through the lymph node and come into contact with lymphocytes. In addition, the sinuses have extensions that protrude through to the central portion of the lymph node allowing lymph to reach the medullary region and access the efferent lymphatics. The nodes consist of an outer cortex, a paracortex, and the medulla.

The outer cortex of lymph nodes is the region where follicles, primary and secondary, are located. Follicles are termed primary or secondary based on the absence or presence of germinal centers. Both types of follicles contain B cells, as well as macrophages, dendritic cells, and follicular dendritic cells. However, **primary follicles** contain predominantly mature resting B cells and no germinal centers, whereas **secondary follicles** contain **germinal centers**, of antigen-activated B cells. The regions between the follicles contain predominantly T cells interspersed with dendritic cells. The medulla contains macrophages, dendritic cells, and plasma cells. Plasma cells are differentiated B cells that secrete antibodies. The plasma cells reside in the medulla and secrete antibodies into circulation.

Antigen, dendritic cells and circulating lymphocytes gain entry into lymph nodes via afferent lymphatics. As the lymph percolates through the sinuses (cortical and medullary), the majority of antigen is removed by phagocytic cells lining the sinuses or present in the medulla. Lymph also percolates through the sinus lining apertures. These small apertures provide access to and between the follicles for lymph and antigens, as well as dendritic cells carrying antigen. Consequently, lymphocytes present in the lymph nodes are exposed to lymph borne antigens.

Spleen

The **spleen** is an encapsulated secondary lymphoid organ containing two major types of tissues, red pulp and **white pulp** (Fig. 1.8). The white pulp is the region of the spleen that functions as a secondary lymphoid tissue because it contains the majority of lymphoid cells. The predominant T-cell region, the area surrounding the central arteries and arterioles, is termed the **periarteriolar lymphatic sheath** (PALS). The predominant B-cell regions are the primary and secondary follicles that exist as outgrowths of the PALS.

The marginal zone contains primarily dendritic cells and macrophages. However, some T and B cells can be identified in this region, likely reflecting their site of entry into the white pulp. Because the marginal zone contains many macrophages and dendritic cells, both of which are antigen presenting cells, antigen can be trapped and presented to T cells homing from the circulation to the white pulp. In addition, antigen presenting cells can migrate to the white pulp region and present antigen to the resident T cells.

The spleen has no afferent lymphatic vessels; however, efferent lymphatic vessels originate in the spleen and serve as exit routes for antibodies and some circu-

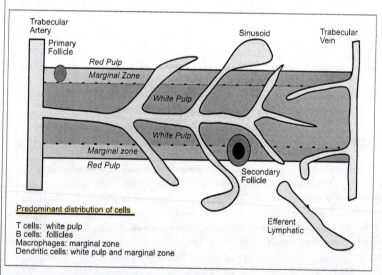

Fig. 1.8. Schematic representation of the spleen. The white pulp is the region of the spleen that functions as a secondary lymphoid tissue because it contains the majority of lymphoid cells. The predominant T-cell region, the area surrounding the central arteries and arterioles, is called the periarteriolar lymphatic sheath (PALS). The predominant B-cell regions are the primary and secondary follicles that exist as outgrowths of the PALS. The marginal zone contains primarily dendritic cells and macrophages.

lating cells. Structurally, there are many sinuses within the marginal region. These structures "link" the arteriole and the venous circulation. They differ from common capillaries in that their endothelial cell lining is discontinuous. Spaces between the sinus endothelial cells permit the entry of circulating cells, and bloodborne antigen, into the spleen.

Mucosa-associated lymphoid tissue

The human body is in constant contact with microorganisms, most of which never penetrate the internal milieu due to the presence of intact skin, or mucosal surfaces. Mucus forms a protective surface in the respiratory, genitourinary, and gastrointestinal tracts, as well as in the buccal cavity and on adenoids and tonsils (Fig. 1.9). Although intact skin is essentially impenetrable, the mucus covering is neither as impervious nor as continuous. This discontinuous nature of mucus provides cellular areas where microorganisms can gain access into the body.

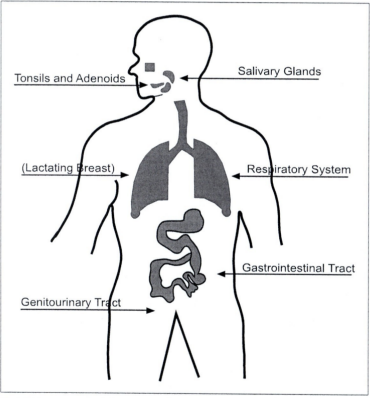

Fig. 1.9. Mucosa-associated tissues. Mucus forms a protective surface over the respiratory, genitourinary, and gastrointestinal tracts, as well as in the buccal cavity and on adenoids and tonsils. Underlying the epithelial cells of these tissues is the lamina propria, which contains the cells that comprise mucosal immunity.

The term, mucosa-associated lymphoid tissue (MALT) is a general term for the unencapsulated lymphoid tissues present in regions underlying the mucosal areas. Some MALT regions are more precisely defined. These include the gastrointestinal (gut) associated lymphoid tissue (GALT); bronchus associated lymphoid tissue (BALT); and the lymphoid tissue found within the buccal cavity in tonsillar tissue, salivary glands etc. With few exceptions, the lymphoid components of MALT, regardless of localization, are essentially alike, and analogous to those described above for the spleen and lymph nodes. Because lymphoid components in MALT are unencapsulated, they are more diffuse. In some regions lymphoid cells are organized into discrete aggregates of follicles surrounded by other lymphoid cells; in other areas follicles are sparse and scattered. Organized aggregates of follicles present in the GALT are termed Peyer's patches. Microbes generally enter mucosa-associated lymphoid tissue via specialized epithelial cells, M cells, present in the mucosal lumenal lining, to reach the underlying lamina propria, which is the site containing follicles and immune cells including phagocytic cells, dendritic cells, and lymphocytes.

Gut-associated lymphoid tissue

Gut-associated lymphoid tissue (GALT) is a MALT region that has been well described. In general, columnar epithelial cells, interspersed with goblet cells and intraepithelial T cells (gamma/delta and alpha/beta) constitute the lining of the small intestine (Fig. 1.10). The mucus secreting goblet cells deposit a protective layer of mucus that separates and protects the cells of the lumenal lining from the lumenal contents. In those regions where there are no goblet cells the mucus layer is sparse or absent, and this is referred to as the **follicle associated epithelium (FAE)**. In the FAE a specialized cell, the M cell, serves as a port of entry for microbes into the lamina propria. Intracellularly, M cells have very few lysosomes typical of phagocytic cells, suggesting that phagocytosis is not their role. However, numerous cytoplasmic vesicles, characteristic of transport sacs, are present implying that microorganisms are engulfed by the M cell, and transported from the lumenal surface to the basolateral surface via vesicles. The basolateral surface is characterized by irregular invaginations that form pockets large enough to accommodate lymphocytes, dendritic cells, or phagocytes. Microorganisms that reach the lamina propria via M cells encounter host defense mechanisms present there. The organized aggregates of follicles are termed Peyer's patches, and in humans these are more abundant in the ileum than in the jejunum.

Several organisms are pathogenic because they have evolved ways to subvert GALT mechanisms. As an example, some viruses and bacteria are able to replicate in M cells after their uptake, and they then disseminate to peripheral tissues when they are exocytosed at the M cell basolateral face. Infection with a strain of Shigella leads to productive infection because Shigella escapes from the M cell vacuole and spreads laterally, thereby infecting adjacent cells in the lumenal lining. Invasion of M cells by some Salmonella species leads to destruction of the M cells. This results in a discontinuity in the cellular lining of the intestine, invasion of bacteria, dissemination, and bacteremia.

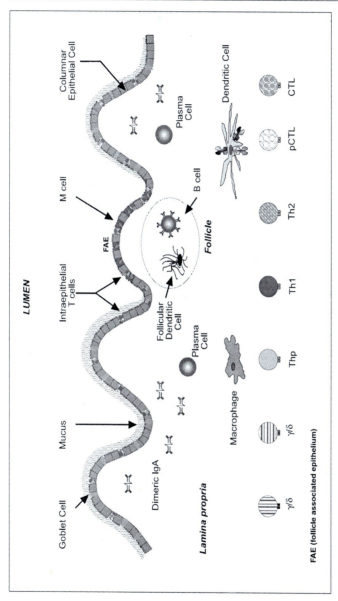

Fig. 1.10. Gut-associated MALT: structural organization. The lamina propria, which underlies the cells lining the gut epithelium, contains cells of both innate and adaptive immunity. These cells are activated when pathogens enter into this region, generally using the M cell as a port of entry. M cells do not have a mucus covering and so pathogens can bind to these cells and transcytose into the lamina propria.

Soluble Mediators of the Immune System

Soluble mediators of the immune system include antibodies, complement proteins, small peptides such as cytokines and chemokines (Fig. 1.11). These effector molecules contribute to both innate and adaptive immune processes. Furthermore, the presence or absence of these soluble mediators determines the course of the immune response to a pathogen.

Antibodies

Antibodies, also known as **immunoglobulins (Igs)**, are bifunctional molecules whose polypeptide chains define an antigen binding site and a site that carries out the biological activity of the molecule. The polypeptide chain of the antibody that determines biological activity also defines its isotype. The antibody isotypes IgM, IgD, IgG, IgE, and IgA correspond to the μ, δ, γ, ε, and α polypeptides, respectively. Hence, biological activity and antibody isotype are closely related. Antibodies are expressed on the cell surface of B cells. When these cells are stimulated (e.g., by antigen) they differentiate into antibody secreting plasma cells. These secreted antibodies serve as effector molecules for cells functioning in the innate and/or adaptive immune systems. As example, particular antibodies trigger the activation of the classic complement pathway (see below).

Complement

Complement is a term used to describe a family of proteins that facilitate elimination of microorganisms, particularly extracellular bacteria. The complement system is composed of numerous (~30) activation and regulatory proteins synthesized mainly by the liver. Many of these proteins circulate as dormant enzymes serving as substrates for other complement proteins that have, themselves, been sequentially activated. This mode of sequential activation gives rise to the expression, *complement pathway*. There are two pathways of complement activation, the **alternative pathway** of activation and the **classical pathway**, each converging into a **common/terminal pathway**. The initiating stimulus for activation of the alternative pathway of complement (innate immunity) is the deposition of spontaneously generated fragments onto a microbial cell surface. The initiating stimulus for activation of the classical pathway of complement (adaptive immunity) is either IgM or IgG bound to antigen. Activation of complement by either pathway generates protein fragments, all of which have distinct biological activities that contribute to host defense.

Cytokines

Cytokines are small peptides secreted mainly by activated leukocytes. Different cytokines may trigger the same biological responses, a characteristic termed *functional redundancy*. Additionally, cytokines are pleiotropic, with each cytokine

Fig. 1.11. (opposite) Concept map depicting soluble mediators of the innate immune system. Soluble mediators include antibodies, cytokines, chemokines, and complement. These molecules function in both the innate and adaptive immune systems.

An Introduction to the Immune System

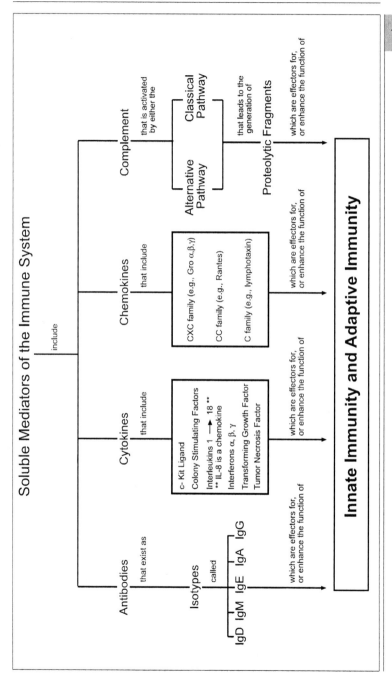

mediating numerous, apparently unrelated biological effects. Cytokine secretion is the primary role of CD4+ T cells. Other cell types, including activated macrophages, dendritic cells, natural killer cells, (and others) can also secrete cytokines, though this does not seem to be their primary role. Secreted cytokines influence the course of both innate and adaptive immune responses (Fig. 1.11).

Chemokines

Chemokines are molecules that were first identified by nature of their ability to induce leukocyte accumulation in tissue sites of inflammation. Interest has focused on the role of chemokine production in clinical diseases. Chemokines have been subdivided into four classes based on the position of invariant cysteine residues in their amino acid sequence. Most prominent amongst these classes are the so-called CC and CXC chemokines, members of which include monocyte chemoattractant protein-1 (MCP-1), macrophage inflammatory protein 1α (MIP-1α), and RANTES (regulated on activation, normal T cell expressed and secreted cytokine); and IL-8, IFN inducible protein 10 (IP-10), and cytokine induced neutrophil chemoattractants (CINC, GRO) respectively (Fig. 1.11).

MOLECULES THAT ACTIVATE LYMPHOCYTES

There are three general classes of molecules that activate lymphocytes, (i) those that activate a single clone (monoclonal activators); (ii) those that activate most or all clones (polyclonal activators); and (iii) those that activate more than one clone, but not all clones (Fig. 1.12) (oligoclonal activators).

MOLECULES THAT ACTIVATE LYMPHOCYTES: MONOCLONAL ACTIVATORS

Antigens

An **antigen** is a substance that is recognized by lymphocytes. Historically, antigens were defined as molecules that induce an immune response. More recently, the term **immunogen** has been designated to refer to molecules that induce the activation of T cells or B cells in the presence of appropriate costimulatory molecules. Although not technically correct, the term antigen is still commonly used to refer to substances that induce an immune response. In this book, we use the historical definition of the term antigen, in place of the term immunogen. Although antigens induce immune responses, the B cells and T-cell antigen receptors recognize a unique region of the antigen (epitope). Other terms, interchangeable for epitope, are **determinant group**, or **antigenic determinant**. Complex antigens contain several different epitopes. For some antigens, particularly protein antigens, B-cell activation occurs only in the presence of T-cell cytokines, and cognate interaction with activated T cells. Consequently, these antigens are termed T-dependent antigens.

Properties of immunogenicity for monoclonal activators

Not all molecules are antigenic (immunogenic). Potent antigens are characterized by: (i) complexity; (ii) high molecular weight (> 5 kd); and (iii) foreignness.

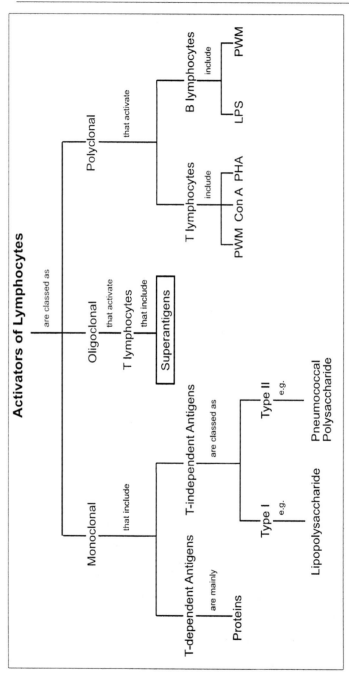

Fig. 1.12. Concept map depicting monoclonal, oligoclonal, and polyclonal activators. There are three general classes of molecules that activate lymphocytes; those that activate a single clone (monoclonal activators); those that activate all clones (polyclonal activators); and those that activate several, but not all clones (oligoclonal activators).

Proteins are more immunogenic than polysaccharides, which are more immunogenic than nucleic acids or lipids. When nucleic acids or lipids are coupled to proteins, they become immunogenic. Although polysaccharides are not very immunogenic, the A, B, O blood group antigens and the Rh antigens are clinically relevant immunogens. Small molecules, less than 5 kd, become immunogenic when coupled to large proteins. In this procedure, the small molecule is termed a **hapten**, and the larger molecule a **carrier**. The phenomenon is termed, the **carrier effect**.

T-independent antigens

Polysaccharide molecules can activate B cells in the absence of T cell help. (T cells do not recognize polysaccharides). These antigens are termed **T-independent antigens**. T-independent antigens are divided into two categories, Type I and Type II. The prototypic **Type II T-independent antigen** is pneumococcal polysaccharide, a component of the capsule surrounding *Streptococcus pneumoniae*. Pneumococcal polysaccharide does not possess mitogenic activity. It only stimulates activation of mature B cells that express receptors specific for **pneumococcal polysaccharide**. The prototypic **Type I T-independent antigen** is lipopolysaccharide, a cell wall component of gram negative bacteria. At high concentrations, **lipopolysaccharide** is mitogenic (see below). However at low concentrations it activates only B cells that express receptors specific for lipopolysaccharide.

Enhancing immunogenicity of monoclonal activators

The immune response to an antigen can be enhanced in the presence of **adjuvants**. This is important for immunization when administering vaccines. Alum precipitate, a suspension of aluminum hydroxide mixed with antigen, is used in human vaccines to enhance immunogenicity. Alum is thought to slow the release of antigen, such that presentation of antigen to T cells is prolonged. A common adjuvant used in studies with laboratory animals is Freund's complete adjuvant (a water in oil emulsion with killed *Mycobacterium tuberculae*).

MOLECULES THAT ACTIVATE LYMPHOCYTES: OLIGOCLONAL ACTIVATORS

Superantigens activate subsets of T cells. These superantigens, often bacterial products, act in a nonantigen specific and oligoclonal fashion on T cells. They bind specifically to regions of the T-cell receptor termed Vβ. In the entire T-cell repertoire there are approximately 200 Vβ shared by the entire T-cell population. As a result, triggering the activation of all the clones that express any given Vβ leads to the clonal expansion of many, but not all, clones (oligoclonal).

MOLECULES THAT ACTIVATE LYMPHOCYTES: POLYCLONAL ACTIVATORS

Mitogens are naturally occurring molecules with the capacity to bind to, and trigger proliferation of, many clones of lymphocytes. B-cell mitogens include pokeweed mitogen (PWM) and high concentrations of **lipopolysaccharide**. T cell mitogens include **concanavalin A** (Con A), **phytohemagglutinin** (PHA), and **pokeweed mitogen**. Con A and PHA are plant glycoproteins, more commonly called lectins.

SUMMARY

Important functional elements of the immune system include several tissues, cell types, serum proteins, and small peptides, called cytokines. While components of the immune system interact with one another, detailed discussion is simplified by classification into two categories, innate immunity and adaptive immunity. In reality, innate and adaptive immune responses act in concert. The innate immune system is made up of cells and molecules that function very early in the protective response to a foreign substance. The principal cell types in innate immunity are phagocytes (macrophages and neutrophils) that engulf and destroy foreign substances, and natural killer (NK) cells, whose main role is to destroy virally infected autologous (host) cells. Antigen presenting cells and inflammatory cells are classified with innate immunity. However, they are required for adaptive immune responses. In addition to the induction of cellular aspects of innate immunity, a system of serum proteins, the complement system, is intimately involved in this form of immunity. The innate immune system is characterized by responses that lack memory and specificity, but display constancy with respect to magnitude and rate of the response to antigen.

In contrast to the rapid response time for innate immune processes, cells that mediate adaptive immunity require several days to become formidable effectors. Resting lymphocytes are restricted in their recognition repertoire, with each cell responding only to one unique portion (epitope) of an antigen. While there are millions of each cell type (T and B) present, each antigen is recognized by only a few (in the limit one) cells. Thus, there must occur further massive clonal expansion of the specifically activated T or B cells after initial encounter with antigen to generate sufficient numbers of antigen specific lymphocytes that will protect against the invading pathogen. After the pathogen is cleared not all of the cells which encountered antigen die. The immune system retains a supply of *memory cells*, which can respond much more quickly to rechallenge with the same antigen than did the naive cells. This constitutes the process of antigen-specific immunological memory. The adaptive immune system, therefore, is characterized by responses that show memory and specificity, but are variable with respect to magnitude and rate of the response to antigen.

Immune tissues are broadly classed according to their role in the immune system. Tissues that serve as developmental sites for lymphocytes are termed primary immune tissues, while those tissues that serve as activation sites are termed secondary immune tissues. The bone marrow is the site of B-cell development and maturation, while the thymus is the site of T-cell maturation. Secondary lymphoid tissues include the lymph nodes, tonsils and adenoids, spleen, and mucosa-associated lymphoid tissues (MALT). Soluble mediators are effectors of both the innate and adaptive immune responses. Antibodies, complement proteins, and small peptides called cytokines serve in this capacity. The presence, or absence, of these soluble mediators determines the course of the immune response to a pathogen.

There are two general classes of molecules that activate lymphocytes, those that activate a single clone (monoclonal activators) and those that are polyclonal activators (mitogens). Small molecules, less than 5kd, become immunogenic when coupled to large proteins. In this procedure, the small molecule is termed a hapten and the larger molecule a carrier. The phenomenon is termed the carrier effect. B cell activation in response to protein antigens occurs only in the presence of T cell cytokines and cognate interaction with activated T cells. Consequently, these proteins are termed T-dependent antigens. In contrast, polysaccharide molecules can activate B cells in the absence of T cell help. These antigens are termed T-independent antigens. The immune response to an antigen can be enhanced in the presence of adjuvants. Alum precipitate, a suspension of aluminum hydroxide mixed with antigen, is used in human vaccines to enhance immunogenicity.

CLINICAL CASES AND DISCUSSION

Clinical Case #1
You are coordinating a community-clinic-based program which has just started testing a novel antibiotic that offers promise for treating community-acquired pneumonia. After 200 patients have been treated successfully with no apparent adverse effects, you discover that two of the newer patients enrolled in the trial have developed anemia after taking the drug for seven days. What are possible explanations for these results, and how would you proceed to confirm them? What actions would you take next?

Discussion Case #1
Background
One of the first things to consider is that you might be dealing with a drug toxicity reaction that has been missed before, or for some reason (perhaps related to peculiar metabolism of drug in these individuals) has only shown up in these particular cases. There are certainly instances where this has proven to be the case. Much more commonly, however, we would be concerned about an autoimmune hemolytic anemia being responsible. The mechanism by which this develops is, in general, the following.
   a. Drug binds to red cell membranes (nonspecific, noncovalent binding; occasionally the drug binds covalently following chemical interaction with red cell membrane proteins/lipids).
   b. The red cell then acts as a "carrier" for this novel "hapten" (the drug) which elicits an antibody reaction. There are insufficient epitopes on the drug to be recognized by both T cells (seeing the carrier portion) and B cells (seeing the hapten portion), so in the absence of this interaction with carrier red cells, autoimmune reactivity does not occur.

An Introduction to the Immune System

c. After carrier:hapten interaction, the B cell becomes activated, produces antibody to the drug (hapten), and these antibodies bind to the hapten-coupled red cells. In the presence of complement, red cell lysis occurs.

d. Alternatively, cells bearing Fc receptors can phagocytose or opsonize the Ig-coated red cells, leading to their removal from the circulation. In either case, red cell depletion is seen as a drug-induced anemia.

Tests

Evidence for these reactions can be obtained using the so-called Coomb's test, either a direct or an indirect test. The indirect test looks for evidence for reactive antibody in the serum that can lyse red cells in a test tube. Without using hapten-coupled red cells in vitro, this test is unlikely to work. However, the direct Coomb's test examines evidence for antibody already deposited on the red cell surface. Red cells taken from the patient are treated with anti-Ig coupled to an immunofluorescent dye. If there is antibody on the surface of the red cells, they fluoresce in this test.

Treatment (Procedure)

Drug-induced autoimmune hemolytic anemias are common. With evidence for such a reaction, your subsequent course of action must include the following. **First, stop treating these individuals with the drug!** Second, alert other physicians who are using this reagent to this significant side-effect. Finally, you must decide (with others) whether the risk-benefit ratio is in favor of continuing with its usage.

Clinical Case #2

A patient is suffering from a profound bacteremia caused by an unidentified pathogen. While the antibiotics you are using seem to be effectively eradicating the organism, the patient does not seem to be improving. A colleague suggests you may be dealing with adverse effects associated with bacterial toxins, mitogens or superantigens. How would you determine which is the likely culprit? What other effects do these agents have?

Discussion Case #2

Background

Bacterial toxins can have pleiomorphic effects, ranging from altering cell membrane ion exchange (e.g., those causing enteric dysentery) to direct toxicity to cells by virtue of interfering with specific cell functions. As an example, tetanus toxin blocks signaling at neuromuscular junctions; pertussis toxin interferes with G-coupled receptor signaling and thus immune and other physiological functions. Without some starting point it is difficult to devise a strategy to test for bacterial toxin mediated effects.

Bacterial mitogens are classified according to the cell populations they activate. Those acting as B-cell mitogens cause polyclonal activation of B cells, regardless of their antigen specificity. The mitogen binds to a discrete receptor (not the Ig receptor) on target B cells. For lipopolysaccharide, the prototypic B-cell mitogen, this receptor has been characterized as the CD14 molecule. These activated B cells differentiate to antibody secreting plasma cells (generally low affinity IgM), and evidence for existence of the bacterial mitogen can often be recognized by this polyclonal B-cell activation in vivo.

Lipopolysaccharides, however, often cause activation of other cells of the immune system (especially macrophages and monocytes), leading to production of inflammatory cytokines, including interleukin-1 (IL-1), interleukin-6 (IL-6), and tumor necrosis factor (TNF). Often over-production of the cytokines causes pathology, and could certainly explain this patient's findings. This would best be investigated by analyzing, in vitro, evidence for B-cell mitogenesis. B cells could be stimulated in vitro with material from the patient's serum or a culture supernatant of the organism, and the observations in vivo (e.g., serum cytokine, Ig levels) are compared with the in vitro findings.

Bacterial T-cell mitogens, as the name implies, cause polyclonal T-cell activation and cytokine production. In this case, T-cell activation results in the expansion of all T cells and production of T cell derived cytokines such as interleukin-2 (IL-2), interleukin-4 (IL-4), and interferon gamma (IFNγ), etc. The mitogen binds to a non-T-cell receptor site to induce these changes. Pathology can be associated with the cytokines produced. As an example, IL-2 can cause the so-called capillary-leak syndrome, associated with increased permeability of capillary endothelium. Once again, the optimal approach to identifying a possible T-cell mitogen effect would be to assess evidence for this in vitro with purified T cells and attempt to correlate in vitro findings with those in vivo.

Finally, bacterial superantigens are an interesting family of molecules that act in a nonantigen specific but nonpolyclonal (**oligoclonal**) fashion on T cells. These molecules bind to regions of the T-cell receptor termed Vβ regions. These regions are NOT those normally used by T cells for interacting with antigen. Each superantigen stimulates expansion of different subsets of T-cell receptors that share a particular Vβ region. This is in contrast to mitogens that induce division of all T cells, not just a subset. The superantigens can often be identified by the particular Vβ subset that the proliferating T-cell receptors express.

Many bacterial toxins have been found to be superantigens, and are believed to cause pathology by virtue of this property. Following an initial hyperproliferation, the expanded T cells expressing the particular Vβ region eventually undergo apoptosis (cell death), resulting in depletion of cells expressing T-cell receptors with that particular Vβ region. Identification of superantigen reactivity depends upon these properties. One could look for either expansion of unique TCR Vβ subsets (early), or deletion of the same (late), in the infected individual.

Tests

I   Polyclonal B-cell activation in response to lipopolysaccharide results in an increased number of B cells expressing CD14. To measure an increase in the number of CD14+ B cells, peripheral blood cells are reacted with a

fluorescein tagged anti-CD14 antibody. Counting is performed by fluorescence activated cell sorting (FACS). Similarly, increases in IgM can be measured and counted using fluorescein tagged anti-IgM antibodies.
II Macrophages and monocytes secrete cytokines (IL-1, IL-6, and TNF) in response to lipopolysaccharide. To test for the presence of these cytokines the patient's serum is absorbed onto plates coated with anti-IL-1, anti-IL-6, or anti-TNF antibodies in an ELISA (enzyme linked immunoadsorbent assay) reaction. To examine evidence for bound cytokine, a second anti-cytokine antibody is added, covalently linked to an enzyme (e.g., horse radish peroxidase coupled anti-IL-6), followed by addition of enzyme substrate. We then measure the colorimetric change following enzymatic digestion of substrate.
III In response to T-cell mitogens, T cells secrete IL-2 and IL-4. To test for a possible T-cell mitogen effect, purified T cells are isolated from peripheral blood cells and cultured. Culture supernatants are analyzed for IL-2 and IL-4 using ELISA assays as in (II). Serum levels of IL-2 and IL-4 can also be determined by ELISA.
IV To test for a superantigen effect, peripheral blood cells are reacted with fluorescein-tagged antibodies specific for a particular Vβ region of the T-cell receptor (anti-Vβ antibodies). Analysis is performed by FACS. The timing of the test, with respect to the course of the infection, will influence interpretation of the results. If the test is performed early in the course of an infection, evidence for a superantigen-induced proliferation of a T-cell population is manifest as an increase in the number of T cells expressing receptors with a particular Vβ region. In contrast, if the test is performed late in the course of infection, superantigen effects are manifest as a deletion of the same population of T cells.

Treatment
Treatment is symptomatic. That is, treat low blood pressure with fluids, and fever with acetaminophen etc. Newer treatments focus on the potential use of anti-cytokine antibodies, arguing that many of the changes seen in these patients are due to nonspecific inflammation from a cytokine "storm".

TEST YOURSELF

Multiple Choice Questions
1. Antigen presenting cells display antigen fragments in association with class II MHC molecules. Which one of the following cells does not function as an antigen presenting cell?
   a. B cells
   b. Dendritic cells
   c. Neutrophils
   d. Macrophages

2. In the spleen the lymphoid tissues are mainly located in the
   a. white pulp
   b. marginal zone
   c. red pulp
   d. sinusoids
3. Microbes gain access to the lamina propria of the gut associated MALT, via
   a. intraepithelial T cells
   b. goblet cells
   c. M cells
   d. columnar epithelial cells
4. Polyclonal activators of T cells include all the following EXCEPT
   a. PWM
   b. LPS
   c. Con A
   d. PHA
5. The prototypic T-independent antigen, Type 1, is
   a. pneumococcal polysaccharide
   b. lipopolysaccharide
   c. concanavalin A
   d. phytohemagglutinin

Answers 1. (c) 2. (a) 3. (c) 4. (b) 5. (b)

Short Answer Questions

1. Differentiate between innate and adaptive immunity. List the cell types that function in each system.
2. List the physical and chemical barriers that microbes must breach to enter the body.
3. Identify the classes of soluble mediators that function in immunity.
4. List five antibody isotypes.
5. Differentiate between T-dependent and T-independent antigens. Give examples. List mitogens that activate B cells and those that activate T cells.

Innate Immune Responses to Pathogens

Objectives	31
Innate Immune Responses to Pathogens	32
General Features	32
Role of Complement	32
Phagocytosis	32
Genetic Defects in NADPH Oxidase: Chronic Granulomatous Disease	42
Natural Killer Cells	42
Eosinophils	45
Summary	45
Clinical Cases and Discussion	46
Test Yourself	49

OBJECTIVES

This chapter introduces the **innate immune system**, along with the effector molecules and cells that participate in innate host defense. These cells and molecules function early following host challenge by pathogens. The innate system shows significant conservation in evolutionary terms. Cell-bound receptors present on cells of the innate defense system are conserved across evolution (so-called **primitive pattern recognition receptors, PPRR**), recognizing common (lipid and carbohydrate) motifs on the pathogen. Molecules of the **complement system**, along with other inflammatory cell products, including **chemokines** and **cytokines** function in innate immunity. From a cellular point of view, neutrophils and macrophages are the principal effectors of nonspecific host defense, and, when activated, trigger intracellular enzyme cascades that kill the engulfed microorganisms, particularly bacteria.

Innate defense mechanisms against viral infections, unlike bacterial infections, are a function of cells capable of recognizing and destroying infected cells before significant replication of virus occurs. These killer cells, foremost amongst which are so-called **natural killer (NK) cells**, also express primitive receptors on the surface. An added complexity to NK cell action is the coexistence of other cell surface receptors that can turn off the killing action of the NK cell when they recognize host cells. Finally, eosinophils also play a major role in host immunity, particularly in host resistance to intestinal parasites.

Clinical Immunology, by Reginald Gorczynski and Jacqueline Stanley. 2001 Landes Bioscience

INNATE IMMUNE RESPONSES TO PATHOGENS

General Features

The innate immune system is made up of cells and molecules that function early in the protective immune response to pathogens. Cells of the innate immune system distinguish pathogens from *self* using primitive receptors that have a broad specificity. The innate immune system is mobilized once natural physical and chemical barriers, that normally prevent microbes from entering our bodies, have been penetrated. Complement activation, phagocytosis, and cell-mediated cytotoxicity are the principal means of innate host defense. Inflammatory cell products, chemokines, and cytokines all contribute to the enhancement of innate immunity.

Role of Complement

A system of serum proteins, the so-called **alternative pathway** of the **complement system**, is intimately involved in innate immunity. One of the proteins of the complement system (C3) is spontaneously hydrolyzed to produce the fragment, C3b and a smaller fragment. C3b is produced in low concentrations, and is normally quickly inactivated. However, when C3b deposits onto a microbial surface, activation of the complement cascade is triggered, generating various protein fragments with distinct biological activities that contribute to host defense (Fig. 2.1). In particular C3b production is amplified, and it serves as an opsonin for phagocytic cells when deposited on microbial cell surfaces. Some of the C3b molecules generated form a component of an enzyme complex that triggers events leading to the formation of the membrane attack complex (MAC). The insertion of MAC into a cell membrane induces osmotic lysis of the cells, or bacteria, into which it inserts. Finally, some of the protein fragments generated in the complement activation cascade are **anaphylatoxins** (C3a, C5a). These anaphylatoxins bind to cognate receptors on **mast cells** and **basophils**, inducing their degranulation and associated release of histamine and other inflammatory mediators. **Histamine** acts on endothelial cells causing them to contract, and in so doing, vascular permeability is increased. This increase in vascular cell permeability is required for phagocytes, and other circulating leukocytes, to gain entry to the infected tissues.

Phagocytosis

Phagocytic cells

Phagocytosis, the process by which organisms are engulfed and destroyed by phagocytic cells, is a major defense mechanism for eradication of invading microorganisms. **Neutrophils** and **macrophages** are the predominant phagocytes. Neutrophils comprise some 60% of the circulating leukocytes in peripheral blood. Neutrophils mature from precursor cells in the bone marrow with more than a billion cells being generated daily. Only a small percentage of these cells is stored

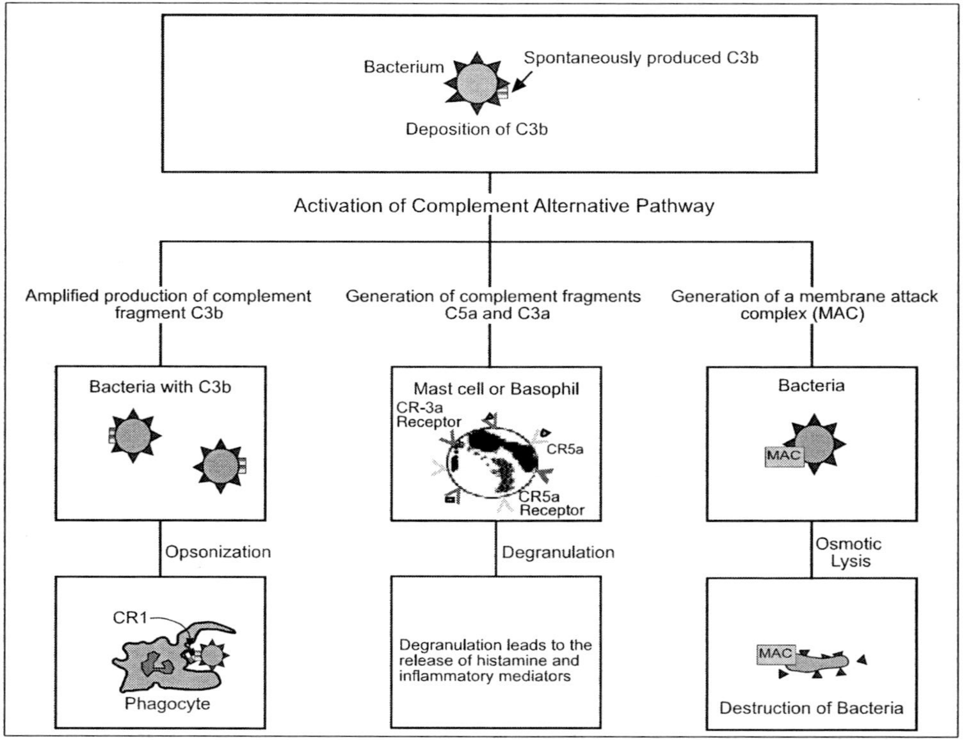

Innate Immune Responses to Pathogens

Fig. 2.1. Activation of the alternative pathway of complement enhances innate immunity. The deposition of a spontaneously generated fragment, (C3b), of serum complement proteins onto a microbial membrane triggers activation of the complement cascade. Various protein fragments with distinct biological activities are generated that enhance innate immunity.

in the bone marrow, with the majority being released into circulation. Once neutrophils are released into circulation they have a half-life of 8 hours. A number of inflammatory cytokines generated in the early phase of an immune response enhance release of neutrophils from the bone marrow. Monocytes are blood borne cells derived from bone marrow progenitors. These cells comprise only about four percent of circulating leukocytes, and when recruited into tissues, they differentiate into macrophages. Macrophages are more effective at phagocytosis than monocytes, have a much longer half-life than neutrophils, and can serve as antigen presenting cells for CD4+ T-cell activation.

Recruitment of phagocytes into infected tissues

Circulating neutrophils and monocytes are attracted to sites of infection by **chemotactic molecules** derived from complement activation, as well as by **chemokines** secreted by activated endothelial cells and other cells. Under inflammatory conditions, neutrophils and monocytes **marginate** along, and attach to, the lumenal surface of activated vascular endothelial cells via **adhesion molecules**. These phagocytes secrete enzymes that break the integrity of the local vascular basement membrane, already exposed following histamine action. These openings in the basement membrane serve as portals of entry for phagocytes and other leukocytes into the infected tissue, a process referred to as **diapedesis** (Fig. 2.2). In tissues, monocytes differentiate into macrophages. Mature macrophages and neutrophils phagocytose and destroy invading microbes. Secretion of inflammatory mediators and cytokines accompanies the phagocytic process, and leads to an enhancement of the inflammatory response, as well as recruitment of more cells to the site of infection.

Recognition of pathogens: direct or opsonin-mediated

Recognition of pathogens by phagocytes may be direct or opsonin-mediated. Direct recognition of pathogens occurs via primitive receptors (so-called **primitive pattern recognition receptors, PPRR**), found also within the invertebrate world, which distinguish pathogens from *self*. Phagocytes also recognize pathogens INDIRECTLY using cell surface receptors that recognize molecules that have bound to, or been deposited on, the pathogen cell surface. The molecules that have attached to the pathogen are termed **opsonins** (Fig. 2.3). Recognition and phagocytosis is then **opsonin-mediated**. Opsonins are the products of: (i) complement activation (C3b); (ii) B-cell activation (IgG); and (iii) cytokine mediated activation of hepatocytes (C-reactive protein, CRP). Interaction of any of these pathogen-bound opsonins triggers the process of phagocytosis (Fig. 2.4).

Regardless of the mechanism by which pathogens are recognized and bound, the process of internalization and degradation is similar. Recognition and binding of the pathogen is followed by its ingestion as a portion of the plasma membrane extends outward and surrounds the microbe, forming a phagocytic vacuole termed a **phagosome**. In general, this phagocytic vacuole serves as the "battlefield" where microorganisms are subsequently destroyed by phagocytic "weapons" including: (i) **lysosomal enzymes**; (ii) **reactive oxygen intermediates**; and (iii) **reactive nitrogen intermediates**.

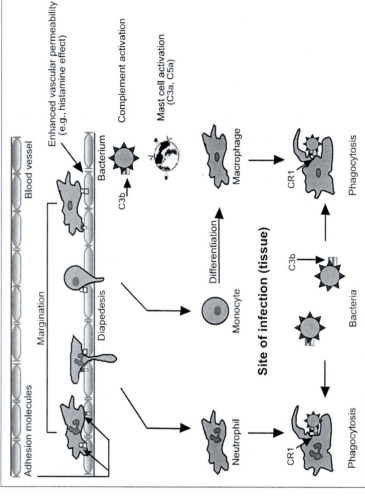

Fig. 2.2. **Diapedesis of neutrophils and monocytes to the site of infection.** At sites of infection, neutrophils and monocytes marginate and attach to the lumenal surface of activated vascular endothelial cells via adhesion molecules. These phagocytes secrete enzymes that create holes in the basement membrane, serving as portals of entry for phagocytes and other leukocytes into the infected tissue, a process known as diapedesis.

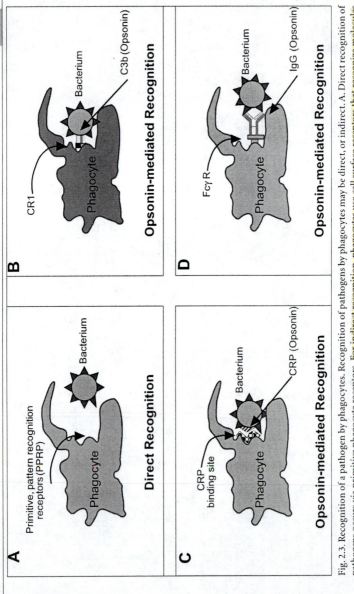

Fig. 2.3. Recognition of a pathogen by phagocytes. Recognition of pathogens by phagocytes may be direct, or indirect. A. Direct recognition of pathogens occurs via primitive phagocyte receptors. For indirect recognition, phagocytes use cell surface receptors that recognize molecules (opsonins) that have bound to, or have been deposited on, the pathogen cell surface. B. complement fragment C3b). C. heat shock protein, CRP, (C-reactive protein) D. IgG produced in adaptive immunity.

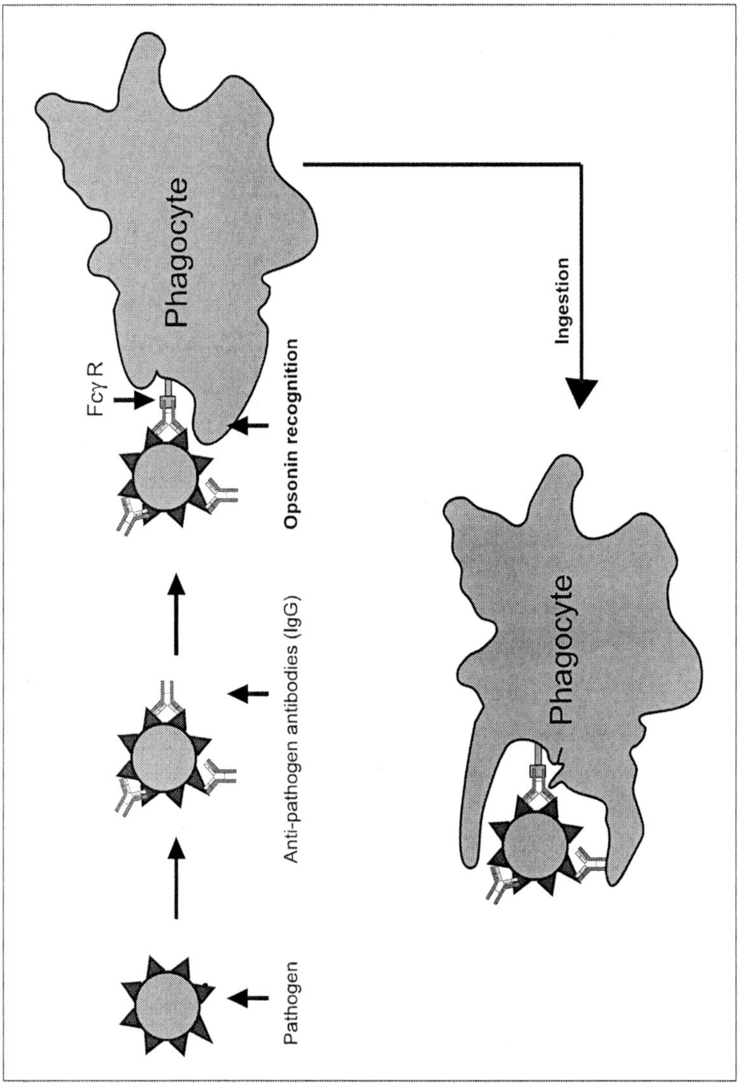

Fig. 2.4. Opsonin-mediated (IgG) recognition by FcγR on the phagocyte is followed by ingestion of the pathogen. The innate and adaptive immune systems act in concert. Antibodies produced in adaptive immunity facilitate phagocytosis because phagocytes express receptors (FcγR) that bind antibodies that are bound to the pathogen, triggering ingestion of the pathogen.

Phagosomes and phagolysosomes

Recognition and binding of microorganisms triggers the assembly of the enzymatic complex, **NADPH oxidase** and formation of the **phagocytic vacuole**, the **phagosome**. Recognition and binding of microorganisms is also accompanied by mobilization of glycogen stores. The glucose so derived is metabolized via the pentose phosphate pathway to generate NADPH, which is required for the function of the NADPH oxidase complex (below). **Phagosomes** are vesicles that contain the engulfed pathogen. **Lysosomes** present in the cytosol fuse with the phagosome to form a fusion product, the phagolysosome, into which lysosomal granules are discharged (Fig. 2.5). Lysosomal granules contain many enzymes (including lactoferrin, lysozyme, and defensins) that are cytostatic/cytotoxic to microorganisms. These molecules play a role in host immunity as follows: (i) lactoferrin binds iron, thereby removing an essential ingredient for microbial growth; (ii) lysozyme destroys muramic acid in bacterial cell walls; (iii) defensins permeabilize bacterial and fungal membranes. Lysosomal granules also release myeloperoxidase, an enzyme required to generate hypochlorite, a potent antimicrobial agent that mediates its function by halogenating bacterial cell walls.

Activation of NADPH oxidase generates reactive oxygen intermediates

NADPH oxidase is a multisubunit enzyme complex whose components, in the resting phagocyte, are distributed in both the plasma membrane and the cytosol. Phagocytosis triggers its assembly on the phagocytic vacuole. Phagocytosis is accompanied by a respiratory burst (an increase in oxygen consumption), attributable to the activation of **NADPH oxidase** that uses oxygen, in the presence of cytosolic NADPH, to generate superoxide anion. Superoxide anion is a **reactive oxygen intermediate (ROI)**. This is the initiating step for the generation of the other ROIs: hydrogen peroxide, hydroxyl radical, and hydroxyl ion (Fig. 2.6). Hypochlorite, a potent antimicrobial agent is formed in the presence of hydrogen peroxide and chloride ion, when the lysosomal enzyme myeloperoxidase is available.

$$Oxygen + NADPH \rightarrow Superoxide + Proton + NADP+$$

The superoxide, so formed, spontaneously forms hydrogen peroxide in the reaction:

$$Superoxide + Protons \rightarrow Hydrogen\ Peroxide + Oxygen\ (O_2)$$

Superoxide and hydrogen peroxide serve as substrates for the iron-catalyzed Haber Weiss reaction:

$$Superoxide + Hydrogen\ Peroxide \rightarrow Hydroxyl\ Radical + Hydroxyl\ Ion + O_2$$

In the presence of chloride ion and hydrogen peroxide, myeloperoxidase catalyzes the reaction:

$$Hydrogen\ Peroxide + Chloride\ Ion + Proton \rightarrow Hypochlorite\ and\ Water$$

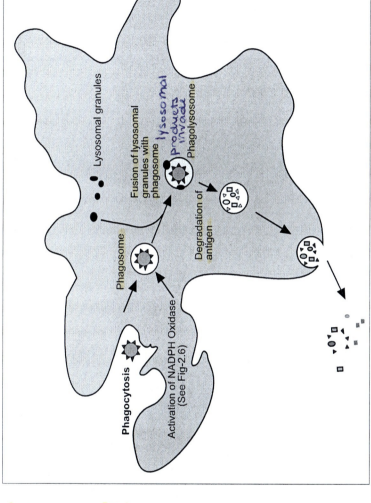

Fig. 2.5. Phagocytosis of an antigen and its degradation. Recognition and binding of microorganisms is followed by ingestion of the pathogen as the invaginating plasma membrane forms a phagocytic vacuole, the phagosome. Lysosomes present in the cytosol fuse with the phagosome, discharging the contents of their granules into the vacuole. The fusion product of the phagosome and lysosome is called a phagolysosome. Lysosomal granules contain many enzymes that are bacteriostatic and bactericidal. Bactericidal products are also produced following activation of the NADPH oxidase complex. See also Figure 11.6.

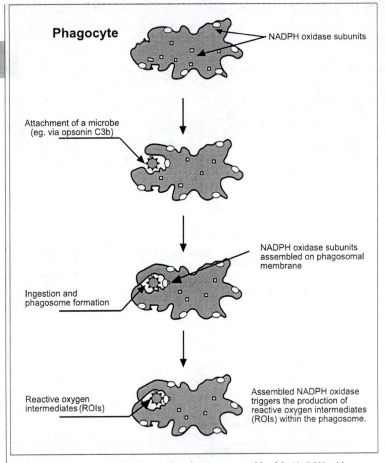

Fig. 2.6. Binding pathogens directly, or indirectly, triggers assembly of the NADPH oxidase complex, which becomes a component of the phagocytic vacuole.

Production of nitric oxide and other reactive nitrogen intermediates

Nitric oxide (NO) is a lipid and water soluble gas that is cytotoxic/cytostatic to invading microorganisms. Many parasites and other intracellular organisms including viruses, intracellular bacteria, parasites, and fungi are susceptible to NO. While the nitric oxide is harmful to microorganisms, even more potent bactericidal agents are produced when nitric oxide reacts with reactive oxygen intermediates and generates **reactive nitrogen intermediates** (RNIs). In host defense, NO (and other RNIs) are particularly important for the elimination of intracellular organisms that are resistant to reactive oxygen intermediates (ROIs) and lysosomal enzymes in the phagolysosomes, such as *Mycobacteria* species, intracellular bacteria and *Leishmania* species. These organisms not only resist degradation in phagolysosomes, but actually seem to thrive within that microenvironment. NO has a number of molecular targets including iron sulfur proteins in the electron transport chain. This would inhibit the respiratory cycle. In addition, key enzymes required for the synthesis of DNA are inhibited.

In phagocytes, synthesis of NO requires the induction of **nitric oxide synthase (iNos)**, a cytosolic enzyme that catalyzes the conversion of L-arginine to L-citrulline and NO in the presence of oxygen (Fig. 2.7).

$$\text{L-Arginine} + \text{Oxygen} \xrightarrow{\text{iNOS}} \text{L-Citrulline} + \text{Nitric oxide (NO)}$$

High levels of NO are not only toxic to microbes but may even be toxic to the phagocytes producing it, and to surrounding cells, because NO is both lipid and water-soluble. The short half-life of NO (seconds) confers some protection. However, host tissues may be damaged in a nonspecific manner.

Regulation of nitric oxide synthase
Induction of nitric oxide synthase (NOS) occurs in response to inflammatory products, microbial products, and/or cytokines. In vitro studies show that the induction of NOS occurs in response to phagocytosis of *Mycobacteria*, *Leishmania*, gram negative organisms, or the cytokine IFNγ. Other studies have reported

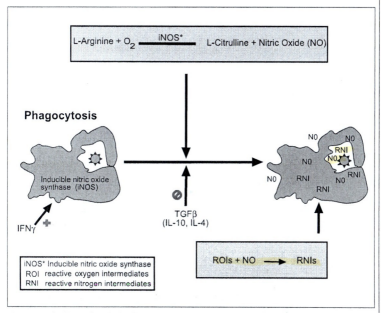

Fig. 2.7. Induction of iNOS leads to the production of nitric oxide (NO) and other reactive nitrogen intermediates (RNIs). In the presence of IFNγ, phagocytosis induces the cytosolic enzyme nitric oxide synthase (iNOS), which in the presence of oxygen, catalyzes the conversion of L-arginine to L-citrulline and nitric oxide. Nitric oxide reacts with ROIs to form RNIs.

that the induction of NOS requires two signals, a priming signal delivered by bacterial products or the cytokine, tumor necrosis factor, and a second signal reportedly delivered by INFγ. Down regulation of NO synthesis occurs in response to the cytokines interleukin-10 (IL-10), IL-4, and transforming growth factor beta (TGFβ). Of these, TGFβ is the most effective inhibitor of NO synthesis. Mice deficient in TGFβ spontaneously over express inducible nitric oxide synthase.

GENETIC DEFECTS IN NADPH OXIDASE: CHRONIC GRANULOMATOUS DISEASE

Chronic granulomatous disease (CGD) is an inherited immunodeficiency disorder in which individuals are susceptible to normally nonpathogenic, as well as pathogenic organisms. Clinically CGD manifests as severe recurrent bacterial and fungal infections. CGD is characterized biochemically by the absence of a respiratory burst and associated production of reactive oxygen intermediates (ROIs) (Fig. 2.8). Genetic defects in any of the NADPH oxidase components can decrease the activity of this enzyme complex. A diagnosis of CGD is made by demonstrating the absence of, or severely decreased, NADPH oxidase activity in neutrophils. One assay, the nitroblue tetrazolium (NBT) test, is used to demonstrate this defect in neutrophils. A droplet of the patient's blood is placed onto a slide along with a neutrophil activator and NBT. NBT is a yellow dye that becomes insoluble and turns purple in the presence of NADPH oxidase activity. This genetic disorder emphasizes the role of ROIs in host defense to microbes.

NATURAL KILLER CELLS

Phagocytosis and activated complement are effective mechanisms for eliminating bacterial infections. Viral infections, however, require a different approach because viruses are sequestered within the host's cells until they bud and infect other cells. For a brief period of time following budding from the cell, the virus is susceptible to the action of phagocytes. The released viral particles rapidly infect other cells, where they escape immune surveillance. The primary immune mechanism to eliminate viral infections is destruction of host cells that harbor the virus before significant viral replication occurs (Fig. 2.9). This depends upon an ability of host defense mechanisms to recognize that a cell has been infected by virus (producing alterations at the cell surface) before the virus has finished its intracellular replication cycle. In innate immunity, recognition and destruction of virally infected cells is mediated by **natural killer** (**NK**) **cells**. Natural killer cells express receptors that recognize cell surface proteins an infected cell and thereafter *kill* the infected cell. The receptors used by NK cells to recognize proteins on the surface of virally infected cells are still being characterized.

Viruses have developed an *escape* mechanism to avoid killing by NK cells, which operates as follows. NK cells also express **killer inhibitory receptors** (KIRs), whose ligand is class I MHC molecules. When NK cells interact with class I MHC positive cells, the NK cell receives a signal that inhibits killing of the cell expressing the

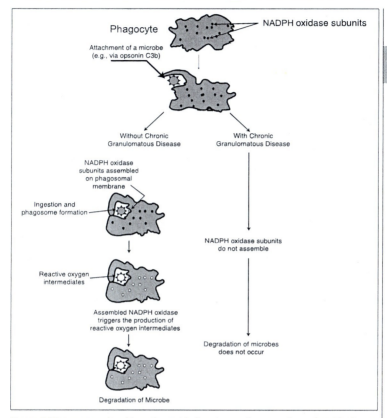

Fig. 2.8. ROIs are not produced in patients with chronic granulomatous disease (CGD). Chronic granulomatous disease, an inherited immunodeficiency disorder, is characterized by the absence of a respiratory burst and reactive oxygen intermediate (ROI) production following phagocytosis.

class I MHC. Therefore, if a virus triggers mechanisms causing up-regulation of MHC molecules on the cell surface it inhibits the ability of the NK cell to destroy the cells it has infected. Under these conditions, however, killing of virally infected cells by CTL (cells of adaptive immunity) is enhanced! Thus the "battle" between viral infection and host defense represents one of "attack and counter-attack". Some tumors also decrease expression of MHC on their cell surface. Again, while this makes the tumor cells more susceptible to the lytic action of NK cells, it provides an escape from detection by adaptive immune processes (CTL).

Recognition of virally infected cells by NK cells occurs directly, using NK receptors as described above. **NK cells also recognize targets indirectly via the FcγR when IgG molecules have bound to the viral proteins** (Fig. 2.9). Direct recognition via the NK cell receptor, leading to lysis, is referred to as **receptor-mediated cytotoxicity**. Indirect interaction via the

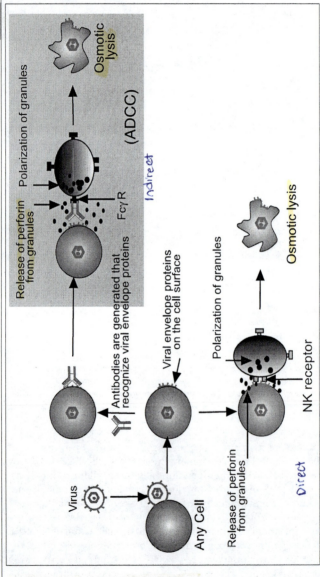

Fig. 2.9. Interaction of virally infected cells with NK cells leads to osmotic cell lysis. Recognition of virally infected cells occurs in one of two ways. NK cells interact directly with residual viral proteins on the infected cell membrane via the NK receptor, or indirectly via the FcγR after IgG molecules have bound to viral proteins. Regardless of the mode of interaction with the infected target cell, conjugate formation with NK cells leads to the release of lytic granules containing a protein, perforin. Perforin inserts into the cell membrane and induces osmotic cell lysis.

FcγR, leading to lysis, is referred to as **antibody-dependent cellular cytotoxicity** (ADCC). Regardless of the mode of interaction with the infected target cell, conjugate formation with NK cells leads to the release of lytic granules that contain a protein, termed **perforin**. Perforin inserts into the cell membrane and induces osmotic cell lysis. The ability of NK cells to kill is enhanced by exposure to cytokines (interleukin-2, interleukin 12, or interferon gamma (IFNγ)). NK cells arise from bone marrow precursors and are found predominantly in the blood, spleen, and peritoneal exudate.

Eosinophils

Eosinophils are bone marrow derived cells that exist both in the circulation and in tissues. Only a small percentage of eosinophils released from the bone marrow remain in circulation. The half-life of eosinophils is 8-10 hours. Eosinophils play a major role in immunity to parasites, particularly helminths, which are relatively resistant to destruction by neutrophils and macrophages. While eosinophils are categorized as cells of the innate immune system, their role in host defense against parasites requires antibodies (IgE) generated in adaptive immunity. Recognition of helminths by eosinophils is indirect (Fig.2.10). Eosinophils have FcεR that bind to IgE antibodies themselves bound to epitopes on helminths. This interaction triggers degranulation of eosinophils leading to the release of several molecules, including **major basic protein** (MBP), and **eosinophil cationic protein** (ECP). MBP and ECP are very toxic to helminths and some other parasites.

Summary

The innate immune system is mobilized once natural physical and chemical barriers, that typically prevent microbes from entering our bodies, have been penetrated. Complement activation, phagocytosis, and cell-mediated cytotoxicity are the principal means of innate host defense. Inflammatory cell products, chemokines, and cytokines all contribute to the enhancement of innate immunity. One of the earliest responses to infection is the activation of a system of serum proteins, the alternative pathway of the complement. Phagocytosis is another early response.

In phagocytosis organisms are engulfed and destroyed by phagocytes. This ingestion of microorganisms occurs when a portion of the plasma membrane extends outward and surrounds the microbe, thus forming a phagocytic vacuole that becomes a component of the cytoplasm. The phagocytic vacuoles become sites of microorganism destruction by lysosomal enzymes, nitric oxide, and other reactive nitrogen intermediates. Phagocytosis and complement are very effective at eliminating bacteria that live outside cells. Viral infections, however, require a different approach because the viruses are sequestered within the host's cells until they bud and infect other cells. Natural killer (NK) cells have the capacity to lyse virally infected autologous cells and provide the first line of antiviral defense, before the activation of adaptive immunity. Parasites, particularly helminths, are handled by an entirely different cell type in the immune system, the eosinophil.

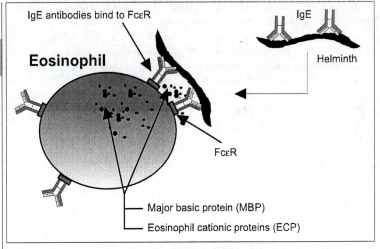

Fig. 2.10. MCP and MBP secreted by activated eosinophils kill helminths. FcεR on eosinophils binds to IgE antibodies bound to epitopes on helminths. This interaction triggers degranulation of eosinophils, leading to the release of several molecules, including major basic protein (MBP), and eosinophil cationic protein (ECP). MBP and ECP are toxic to helminths and some other parasites.

These organisms are relatively resistant to destruction by neutrophils and macrophages. However, proteins released from activated eosinophils readily destroy helminths.

CLINICAL CASES AND DISCUSSION

Clinical Case #3
RD is an 8-year old boy who has had a surprisingly high number (8) of severe recurrent bacterial and fungal infections. Each has responded to the appropriate medication, but you want to find the underlying cause of his problem. Routine analyses of serum Igs, B and T-cell counts (and function) show no clear abnormality. How might you proceed?

Discussion Case #3
Background
This defect looks suspiciously as though it is associated with problems in innate immunity, and/or one of those associated with cell trafficking (adhesion molecule defects). Microorganisms are handled by the innate immune system (macrophages/neutrophils, etc.) after ingestion and activation of a variety of intracellular killing pathways. Amongst these are intracellular killing pathways associated with: (i) reactive oxygen species generated following activation of NADPH oxidase; (ii) reactive nitrogen species generated following the activation of nitric

oxide synthase; and (iii) lysosomal enzymes released when lysosomes fuse with phagosomes.

A defective NADPH oxidase leaves individuals susceptible to bacterial infection. Some bacterial destruction can still occur in the phagocytic vacuoles of those individuals lacking NADPH oxidase if they are infected with bacteria which are hydrogen peroxide producing but catalase negative. Here the hydrogen peroxide produced in the phagocytic vacuole by the bacteria acts as a substrate for myeloperoxidase (a lysosomal enzyme) to generate bactericidal hypochlorite when chloride ion is present.

Chronic granulomatous disease (CGD), one of the more common of the immunodeficiencies of the innate immune defense system, is an immunodeficiency disorder which is characterized by the absence of a respiratory burst and associated reactive oxygen intermediates (ROIs). Genetic defects in any of the NADPH oxidase components produce similar disease manifestations, and a diagnosis of CGD is made by demonstrating decreased NADPH oxidase activity (in neutrophils), using the nitroblue tetrazolium (NBT) test. NBT is a yellow dye that turns purple in the presence of NADPH oxidase activity.

Tests
The NBT test would be the first step in the "work up" of this child. Assuming that the dye remains yellow, what treatment is available for this child?

Treatment Options
Prophylactic administration of antibiotics to combat bacterial infections and itraconazole for fungal infections represent the mainstay for treatment. Recently, prophylactic administration of the cytokine, IFNγ, has gained popularity. In one study, seventy percent of CGD patients treated with IFNγ had a reduction in the number of severe infections. In normal individuals IFNγ has been shown to enhance production of ROIs. However, in the absence of a functional NADPH oxidase, this is unlikely to represent the mechanism by which IFNγ mediates its effects. Increased protection afforded to CGD patients treated with IFNγ may result from enhanced production of nitric oxide. There are several reports indicating that IFNγ enhances nitric oxide production in macrophages. In more severe cases, bone marrow transplantation to replace hematopoietic cells has been performed when a suitable donor has been available. However, bone marrow transplantation carries a high mortality risk (Chapter 17).

In the future, treatment may rely on gene therapy. One preliminary report described successful treatment of five adult patients with CGD using a gene therapy approach. These patients were first treated with the cytokine granulocyte monocyte colony stimulating factor (GM-CSF), a growth factor for CD34+ stem cells (precursors of hematopoietic cells), in order to expand this population. CD34+ peripheral blood stem cells were isolated from the patients and transduced ex vivo with a retroviral vector containing an insert of the normal gene known to be defective in these patients. The transduced cells were then infused back into the patients. In all five patients, the functionally corrected neutrophils were detected in circulation and activity peaked at about one month. In some of the patients, the transduced cells were still detectable six months later. No toxicity of treatment was observed. A more extensive gene therapy trial is underway.

Clinical Case #4
You see a young child with a persistent herpes virus infection (x 8 weeks). Subsequent blood work reveals increased liver enzymes, which becomes understandable when you find evidence for a chronic infection with cytomegalovirus (CMV). Further questioning reveals a strong family history of an inability to clear viral infections, and early death of close family members. How would you proceed?

Discussion Case #4
Background
In all cases of immunodeficiency disorders, one starts with simple concepts about how the body deals with infection. In general, adaptive immune responses to bacteria (extracellular) are a function of B cells/immunoglobulin, with/without auxiliary roles for cells of the macrophage species. Viral infections, intracellular organisms and fungi are generally handled by T-cell mediated immunity. Thus, in an individual suffering from chronic viremias we should think of defects in cell-mediated rather than B-cell (antibody-mediated) immunity. T cells recognize antigen presented in association with class I MHC ($CD8^+$ T cells) or class II MHC ($CD4^+$ T cells). The former develop into lytic cells (CTL) which kill virally infected cells directly.

There are multiple innate viral defense mechanisms. First, viral infection of cells leads to production of interferons (α/β), which activate a number of genes encoding for antiviral activity. In addition there exists a particular defense mechanism active against influenza virus infection, encoded by the so-called Mx gene. Finally, so-called Natural Killer (NK) cells are known to be crucial for the early stages of antiviral immunity, particularly for Herpes viruses (including CMV). NK activity is stimulated by IFNγ, and thus defects in IFNγ production/function can lead to defective viral immunity.

Tests
In this case, there is no evidence for diseases of macrophages associated with abnormalities in reactive oxygen/nitrogen species production. Therefore tests for phagocytic function are unnecessary. Tests for immunoglobulin levels, T-cell and B-cell numbers and functions, would be ordered in the "work up" of this patient. Assuming these are normal, how would you proceed?

With no obvious defect in T-cell numbers and/or function, we have to consider other forms of antiviral immunity besides acquired immunity (dependent upon lymphocyte function). The most likely defect, in this case, is in NK cell number and/or function. A familial genetic disorder of this type is known (Chediak-Higashi syndrome), which often presents in the manner described for this person. A mouse model of this disease, the *beige* mouse, also lacks NK function and is

Innate Immune Responses to Pathogens

highly susceptible to CMV infection. In man, NK cells express the CD16 surface antigen, and measurement of this antigen (by fluorescence activated cell sorting) becomes a simple test to quantify NK cells.

Treatment

Assuming that this patient has low numbers of CD16+ cells, how would you treat?

The only definitive strategy is a bone marrow transplant to regenerate the missing cell population. However, given the risk/problems inherent in this therapy, one should ask, "How severe is the problem?" and "Can it be treated in less toxic ways?" In this patient, passive Ig (which should contain enough antiviral Ig for day-to-day problems) is an alternative, coupled with immune Ig (e.g. zoster immune globulin; hepatitis immune globulin) whenever there is evidence of severe infection.

TEST YOURSELF

Multiple Choice Questions
1. All of the following may serve as opsonins for phagocytosis EXCEPT
   a. C5a
   b. C3b
   c. CRP
   d. IgG
2. Which one of the following lysosomal enzymes destroys muramic acid in bacterial cell walls?
   a. lactoferrin
   b. lysozyme
   c. defensins
   d. myeloperoxidase
3. Which one of the following is NOT classified as a reactive oxygen intermediate?
   a. nitric oxide
   b. superoxide
   c. hydrogen peroxide
   d. hydroxyl radical
4. Helminths are destroyed by the action of enzymes released by which one of the following cell types?
   a. eosinophils
   b. natural killer cells
   c. macrophages
   d. neutrophils

5. Activation of complement generates proteolytic fragments and activated proteins that facilitate
   a. opsonin mediated phagocytosis
   b. mast cell degranulation
   c. osmotic lysis of cells
   d. all of the above

Answers: 1a; 2b; 3a; 4a; 5d

Short Answer Questions
1. In general terms explain " opsonin-mediated" as it relates to recognition and binding of microbes by phagocytes.
2. List the reactive oxygen intermediates formed in the cascade of reactions initiated by NADPH oxidase activation. Define the term " respiratory burst".
3. Individuals with a defective component in the NADPH oxidase enzyme complex have a disorder known as "Chronic Granulomatous Disease" (CGD). Explain why these individuals have recurrent bacterial and fungal infections.
4. Explain how hypochlorite may be produced in the phagocytic vacuoles of CGD individuals following phagocytosis of catalase negative, hydrogen peroxide producing bacteria.
5. Which cytokine has been shown to be effective as prophylactic treatment for CGD? Explain the rationale for gene therapy for individuals with CGD.

Antigen Presenting Cells

Objectives 51
Antigen Presenting Cells 51
Antigen Presenting Molecule: General Features 53
Antigen Presenting Molecule: Class I MHC Molecules 56
Antigen Presenting Molecules: Class II MHC Molecules 61
Antigen Presenting Molecules: CD1 Molecules 64
Summary 64
Clinical Cases and Discussion 65
Test Yourself 67

OBJECTIVES

This chapter documents the essential differences in antigen presentation to CD4+ T cells vs CD8+ T cells and the role played by major histocompatibility complex (MHC) molecules in the delivery of antigenic peptides to those different cells. The reader will find that CD4+ T cells are *restricted* to seeing antigen in association with class II MHC, while CD8+ T cells are *restricted* to seeing antigen in association with class I MHC. This restriction in itself is a function of the nature of the processing steps involved in antigen presentation to T cells, and the essential differences between *professional* antigen presenting cells (needed for presentation to CD4+ T cells) vs conventional cells which present antigen to CD8+ T cells.

ANTIGEN PRESENTING CELLS

General features
Micro-organisms, many of which are pathogens, are present throughout our microenvironment. For the most part, we are protected from this microbial onslaught by inherent physical and chemical barriers. When these barriers are penetrated, nonspecific innate mechanisms are activated in an attempt to destroy these invaders. Activation of various innate mechanisms is accompanied by cytokine release. These cytokines, in conjunction with the presentation of foreign antigen by antigen presenting cells, serve as a link between innate and adaptive immunity. While antigen presenting cells actually deliver antigen to T lymphocytes, the cytokines that are present in the local microenvironment have a profound influence on the subsequent course of T lymphocyte differentiation following interaction with antigen presenting cells.

Professional **antigen presenting cells** deliver antigen to CD4+ T cells, a process termed **antigen presentation**. For effective presentation, an antigen fragment is displayed within the groove of special antigen presenting molecules. These *antigen* *presenting molecules* are proteins encoded by the **major histocompatibility complex (MHC)**, a gene complex originally identified because of its role in graft rejection. Professional antigen presenting cells include **dendritic cells, macrophages and B cells**. Of these, the dendritic cell is the most efficient presenter of antigen during a **primary immune response** to antigen. All antigen presenting cells express, and require for their T-cell stimulatory function, cell surface class II MHC molecules and other molecules, the so-called costimulatory molecules, (including B7 and CD40). Although all antigen presenting cells express these molecules constitutively in varying degrees, antigen capture and/or cytokines further regulates their expression. Cells that present antigen to CD8+ T cells are not generally termed "antigen presenting cells". Rather, they are called **target cells** because the antigen displayed on their cells surface (with class I MHC) *targets* them for CD8+ T-cell-mediated death. Any nucleated cell is a potential target cell because, in general, all nucleated cells express class I MHC.

Dendritic cells

Immature dendritic cells are present in virtually all lymphoid and non lymphoid tissues (except the brain) including the mucosal epithelium of the oral cavity, anus, and vagina. In the skin epidermis these cells are referred to as Langerhans cells. For the most part, immature dendritic cells function as sentinel cells (or gatekeepers) in peripheral tissues where they capture antigens and carry them to secondary lymphoid tissues. Some immature dendritic cells are also resident in secondary lymphoid tissues where they capture antigens that have invaded that site (Fig. 3.1). Phenotypically immature dendritic cells express high concentrations of **FcγR**, and low concentrations of both class II MHC and **costimulatory molecules** (e.g., **B7**). Unlike their immature counterpart, mature dendritic cells cannot endocytose antigen. Rather their role is to display antigen for T-cell scrutiny and to secrete cytokines (e.g., interleukin-12 (IL-12)) which are important in further T-cell development.

Interestingly dendritic cells also express CD4, a molecule that, on T cells, determines T-cell lineage and function. **CD4** is one receptor for the human immunodeficiency virus, type 1 (HIV-1). Infection with HIV-1 is initiated by interaction of viral envelope proteins with (at least) two receptors, the CD4 molecule and a **chemokine receptor**, CCR5 and/or CXCR4. Immature dendritic cells express both CD4 and the chemokine receptors. The important role of chemokine receptors in the process of HIV infection became evident when individuals with defective CCR5 receptors were shown to be relatively resistant to infection with HIV-1.

Macrophages

For primary immune responses the macrophage is not as effective in antigen presentation as is the dendritic cell. The role of macrophages in antigen presentation during secondary immune responses can be explained, in part, by their tissue distribution. Secondary immune responses generally occur at the site of infection. In contrast, primary immune responses occur in secondary lymphoid tissues and not at the site of infection. This explains why dendritic cells are probably more

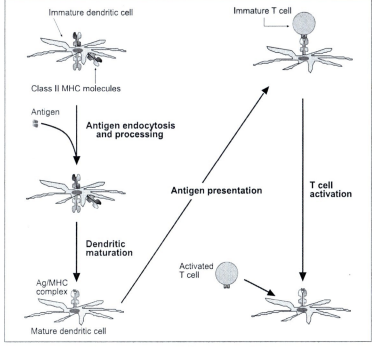

Fig. 3.1. Dendritic cells present antigen to T cells. Immature dendritic cells capture antigen, process it, and display the complex on the cell surface for presentation to CD4+ T cells.

important in primary immune responses than macrophages since, unlike macrophages, dendritic cells can capture antigen in the periphery and transport it to the appropriate lymphoid tissue. Like dendritic cells, macrophages also express CD4 and the chemokine receptors CCR5 and/or CXCR4. Consequently, macrophages can readily be infected with HIV-1.

B cells

B cells recognize antigen via antigen specific receptors (membrane antibody). Because antigen recognition by B cells is so specific, B cells can bind antigen even when it is present in low concentration. As a result, B cells serve as the predominant antigen presenting cells when antigen is limiting. Binding of antigen by B cells is followed by internalization of both the receptor and the antigen into an endosomal vesicle. Thereafter, processing is the same as that observed for other antigen presenting cells.

ANTIGEN PRESENTING MOLECULE: GENERAL FEATURES

Antigen presenting molecules encoded by the MHC locus fall into two major classes, **class I MHC molecules**, and **class II MHC molecules** (Fig. 3.2). All

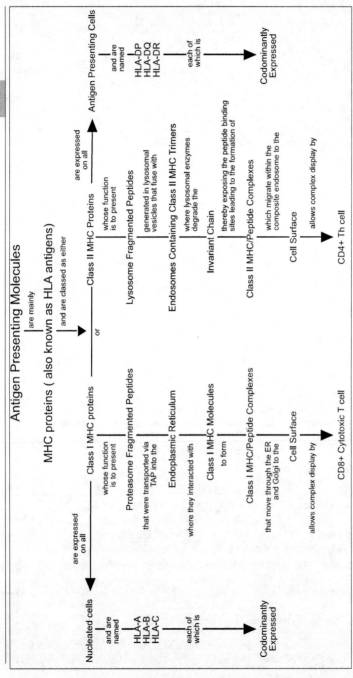

Fig. 3.2. Concept map for class I and class II MHC molecules. Class I MHC molecules are expressed on all nucleated cells, whereas class II MHC molecules are expressed only on professional antigen presenting cells.

nucleated cells express class I MHC molecules, while only professional antigen presenting cells express class II MHC molecules. Thus, antigen presenting cells express both class I and class II MHC molecules. In humans the MHC, located on chromosome 6, is referred to as the "**HLA**" in recognition of the fact that the proteins are human leukocyte antigens. In this text, the terms MHC and HLA are used interchangeably. In humans, the class I MHC molecules are encoded by three loci (A, B, and C), whereas the class II MHC molecules are encoded by a "D" locus that is further subdivided into three loci, DP, DQ, and DR (Fig. 3.3).

Polymorphism is the distinguishing characteristic of class I and class II MHC molecules. Genes encoding each MHC locus are present in multiple forms (alleles) within the population. From an evolutionary perspective, this is advantageous for population survival because antigen fragments must associate with MHC molecules to be delivered to T cells, cells that are absolutely required for adaptive immunity. The likelihood that one of the MHC alleles present in individuals within a population will bind to, and present, an antigen fragment of any particular microorganism to T cells, is increased by the existence of numerous alleles. In the absence of such polymorphism one could envisage the evolution of a lethal organism that failed to associate with (a restricted set of) MHC determinants and was thus unable to induce T-cell immunity, with disastrous consequences for the species. This importance of MHC presentation and adaptive T-cell immunity is exemplified by consideration of immunity to HIV, the etiological agent responsible for AIDS. Differences in susceptibility to infection are believed to be a reflection of unique presentation of antigen to T cells by the MHC of susceptible versus resistant individuals.

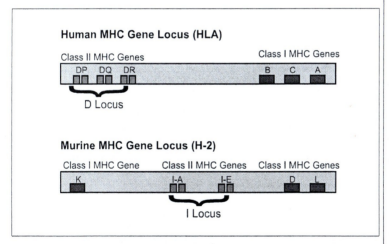

Fig. 3.3. Schematic of class I and class II MHC loci. In humans, the class I MHC molecules are encoded by three loci (A, B, and C), whereas the class II MHC molecules are encoded by a "D" locus that is further subdivided into three loci, DP, DQ, and DR.

Antigen Presenting Molecule: Class I MHC Molecules

Role of class I MHC molecules and class I MHC restriction

Infected cells are identified for destruction by CD8+ T cells following expression of a complex on the target cell surface, composed of an antigen fragment displayed in association with class I MHC molecule. CD8+ T cells, ONLY recognize cells infected with virus, or other cytosolic pathogens, if these cells display the antigenic peptide in association with class I MHC molecules on their cell surface. In other words, they are RESTRICTED to "seeing" antigen in association with class I MHC, a phenomenon referred to as **class I MHC restriction**. In the absence of an antigenic peptide/class I MHC complex, CD8+ T-cell recognition does not occur.

Structure of class I MHC

Each class I MHC molecule is composed of a transmembrane polymorphic polypeptide "heavy" chain (~45 kD) noncovalently associated with a smaller polypeptide (~12 kD), termed β2–**microglobulin**. β2-microglobulin is a nonpolymorphic molecule (Fig. 3.4). It does not have a transmembrane domain, and unlike class I MHC molecules, it is encoded on chromosome 15. β2-microglobulin does not bind antigenic fragments, but its significance is indicated by evidence that the class I MHC 45 kD chain does not fold properly in its absence. There are human diseases characterized by increased susceptibility to intracellular (viral) pathogens that result from a deficiency in β2-microglobulin. The class I MHC 45 kD polypeptide chain binds antigenic fragments that are approximately 10 amino acids in length. The tertiary structure of class I MHC molecules provides a "platform" or "groove" into which the peptide fits.

Nomenclature and codominant expression of class I MHC molecules

In humans, the class I MHC molecules are HLA-A, HLA-B, and HLA-C, each of which is codominantly expressed on all nucleated cells. **Codominant expression** of HLA molecules means that one copy of each HLA (A, B, and C) that is inherited from each parent will be transcribed and translated into protein. Therefore, each cell has the potential to express six different class I HLA (MHC) molecules (Fig. 3.5). The HLA molecules are polymorphic, with numerous allelic forms of each gene present in the population. These allelic forms are given numbers to designate different alleles, e.g., HLA-A11, HLA-B21. For newly identified HLA molecules, the letter "w" (for workshop) is included in the designation, e.g., HLA-Aw19. Each human cell expresses hundreds of thousands of copies of each of the six HLA (A, B and C) proteins, but only a fraction of these are "loaded" with foreign antigenic fragments during an infection.

Antigen processing

Microorganisms that are present in the cytoplasm, but are not enclosed within a vacuole, are susceptible to the proteolytic action of an enzyme complex termed a **proteosome** (Fig. 3.6). Cytosolic proteins are targeted for degradation following the attachment of ubiquitin, a small peptide found in the cytosol of all cells. Peptide

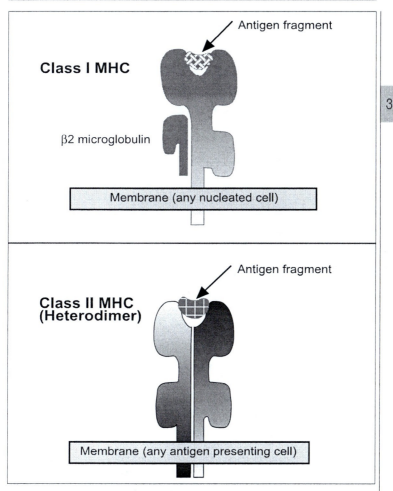

Fig. 3.4. Schematic illustration of class I MHC and class II MHC molecules. Each class I MHC molecule is composed of a transmembrane polymorphic polypeptide chain noncovalently associated with a small polypeptide, termed β2-microglobulin. Each class II MHC molecule is a heterodimer consisting of two transmembrane polypeptide chains in noncovalent association.

fragments generated by the proteosome, in turn, bind to the **transporter of antigen processing (TAP) proteins,** and are transported into the endoplasmic reticulum where they contact coassembled class I MHC molecules i.e., the 45 kD and β2 microglobulin. Complexes are released from the Golgi into vesicles that fuse with the cell membrane, thus displaying the antigen peptide/class I MHC complex on the cell surface. This expression of foreign antigen, in association with class I MHC, in turn signals the immune system that this particular cell is infected.

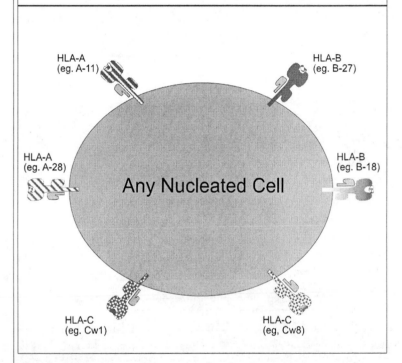

Fig. 3.5. Class I MHC is codominantly expressed on all nucleated cells. Codominant expression of HLA molecules means that one copy of each HLA (A, B, and C) inherited from each parent is expressed.

Class I MHC molecules and viral evasion of immune defenses

Sabotaging the expression of the peptide/class I MHC complexes on the cell surface effectively protects the virus and the infected cells can serve as veritable "factories and reservoirs" for viruses (Fig. 3.7). An understanding of these evasion mechanisms would stimulate the development of strategies for antiviral therapies.

Herpes simplex virus (HSV), a DNA virus, is sequestered inside neurons where it maintains a life-long infection, marked by bouts of recurrent overt infection.

Antigen Presenting Cells

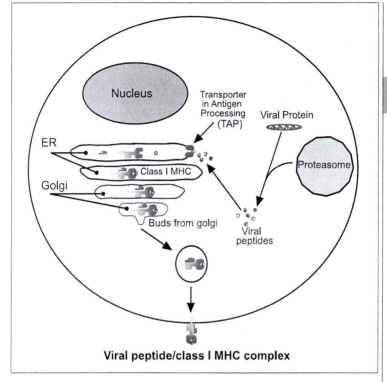

Fig. 3.6. Fate of viral proteins in an infected cell. Microorganisms present in the cytoplasm, but not enclosed within a vacuole, are susceptible to the proteolytic action of an enzyme complex termed a proteosome. Peptides are transported to the endoplasmic reticulum (ER) where they encounter class I MHC. Subsequently the complex is displayed on the cell surface for presentation to CD8+ T cells.

Neurons express little cell surface class I MHC molecules, and so they provide a relatively safe haven for viruses. Recurrent infections of non-neuronal tissues occur because HSV also produces an immediate early protein that binds to the cytosolic portion of the TAP transporter. This effectively inhibits TAP-mediated translocation of peptides from the cytosol into the endoplasmic reticulum. In the absence of peptide transport to the endoplasmic reticulum, antigenic peptide/ class I MHC complexes do not form, and the infection (by virus) in the cell remains undetected.

Epstein Barr virus (EBV), the causative agent of mononucleosis, is another virus that has evolved mechanisms by which it can establish permanent (latent) infection of cells, in this case, of B cells. One of the mechanisms by which EBV thwarts the immune system is by inhibiting the activity of proteasomes. In so doing the virus prevents hydrolysis of viral proteins into peptide size fragments.

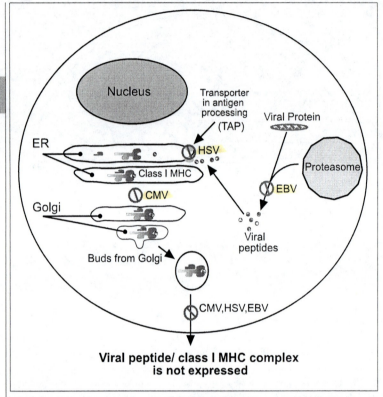

Fig. 3.7. Some viruses thwart the expression of viral peptide/class I MHC on the cell surface. Herpes simplex virus (HSV), Epstein Barr virus (EBV), and cytomegaloviruses (CMV) have evolved mechanisms that thwart the display of viral peptide/class I MHC on the cell surface.

Only peptides (antigenic fragments) of a suitable size can bind in the "groove" of class I MHC molecules. Whole virus, or even whole viral protein, is too large to bind in this groove. In the absence of a peptide/MHC complex on the cell surface, EBV remains safely sequestered in the B cell.

Cytomegalovirus (CMV), a member of the herpes family, infects immunocompetent individuals without causing symptoms. In immunocompromised individuals, infection with CMV may cause numerous disorders including encephalitis, pneumonia, hepatitis, retinitis or blindness. CMV has evolved several mechanisms that hinder the expression of antigen peptide/class I MHC complexes on the cell surface. As one example, CMV encodes proteins that redirect newly synthesized class I MHC molecules from the endoplasmic reticulum back into the cytoplasm where they themselves are degraded by the proteasome.

ANTIGEN PRESENTING MOLECULES: CLASS II MHC MOLECULES

Role of class II MHC molecules and class II MHC restriction
Class II MHC molecules present antigen to CD4+ T cells (Fig. 3.2). CD4+ T cells ONLY recognize antigenic peptides if they are displayed with class II MHC molecules present on the surface of so-called "professional" antigen presenting cells. Thus CD4+ T cells are RESTRICTED to "see" antigen in association with class II MHC, a phenomenon referred to as **class II MHC restriction**. In the presence of appropriate costimulatory signals, T cells are then further activated to secrete cytokines.

Structure of class II MHC molecules
Each class II MHC molecule is a **heterodimer consisting of two transmembrane polymorphic polypeptide chains** (~29 kD each) in noncovalent association (Fig. 3.4). The three heterodimers, DP, DQ, and DR, are structurally similar and each binds antigenic fragments that vary between 15-30 amino acids in length. A third molecule, the **invariant chain, (Ii)**, transiently associates with class II MHC molecules in the endoplasmic reticulum, forming a trimeric complex (class II MHC heterodimer and Ii). This invariant chain blocks the binding of superfluous peptides that the MHC heterodimer might encounter in the endoplasmic reticulum. In addition, the invariant chain serves to direct the transport of class II MHC molecules through the Golgi, from where they are released within endosomes.

Nomenclature and codominant expression of class II MHC molecules
In humans, the class II MHC molecules are HLA-DP, HLA-DQ, and HLA-DR, each of which is codominantly expressed on all antigen presenting cells. Codominant expression of HLA molecules means that one copy of each HLA (DP, DQ, and DR) inherited from each parent will be expressed (Fig. 3.8). Therefore a minimum of six different class II molecules will be expressed on the cell surface providing the parents are genetically unrelated. Antigen presenting cells will also express a complete set of class I MHC molecules. Class II MHC molecules are polymorphic (numerous alleles). These allelic forms are given numbers to designate different alleles, e.g., HLA-DPw1, HLA-DQ3, HLA-DR 4. The letter "w" represents a newly identified molecule (assigned a "workshop" number).

Processing of microorganisms and association with class II MHC molecules
When microbes that thrive extracellularly penetrate the host's physical defenses some of the microbes are endocytosed by antigen presenting cells. This uptake of antigen by antigen presenting cells is the first step in the sequence of events that leads to the display of a microbial peptide with class II MHC on the cell surface (Fig. 3.9). Subsequent steps include the fusion of the endocytotic vesicle with lysosomes that release their contents into the endosome. In a second fusion process, this newly formed vesicle fuses with an endosome that contains the class II MHC, creating a chimeric endosome. In so doing, the class II MHC/Ii complex is exposed to lysosomal enzymes, the Ii chain is degraded, and an antigenic peptide

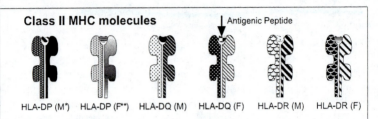

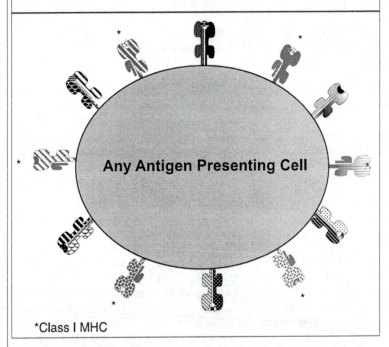

Fig. 3.8. Codominant expression of class I and class II MHC molecules on APC. Codominant expression of HLA molecules means that one copy of each HLA class I (A, B, and C) and class II (DP, DQ, and DR) gene product inherited from each parent is expressed.

binds in the newly exposed groove of the class II MHC. Another MHC encoded molecule (DM) facilitates this process in an, as yet, ill understood fashion. The chimeric endosome migrates to, and fuses with, the cell membrane such that the antigen peptide/class II MHC complex is displayed on the surface of the antigen presenting cell. When these complexes are recognized by T-cell receptors present on CD4+ T cells, in the presence of appropriate costimulatory signals, the T cell is activated to secrete cytokines.

Disease association with class I and class II MHC expression

Population studies have shown that particular diseases and disorders are associated with specific HLA alleles. These associations do not imply causality, though they do reflect the existence of susceptibility genes. Thus, in the Caucasian population of the USA 90% of the individuals with ankylosing spondylitis are males who have inherited the HLA-B27 allele (though the majority of HLA-B27 individuals are disease-free). Ninety percent of individuals with Type 1 diabetes, an autoimmune disorder associated with destruction of the insulin producing beta cells of the pancreatic islets of Langerhans, express either HLA-DR3 or HLA-DR4. If both HLA-DR3 and HLA-DR4 are present, the risk of developing Type 1 diabetes is greatest. Again, however, Type 1 diabetes occurs in only a small percent of individuals that express the HLA-DR3 and HLA-DR4 phenotype, indicating that other factors are operative, perhaps protective genes in unaffected individuals. These genes may be encoded by DQ alleles.

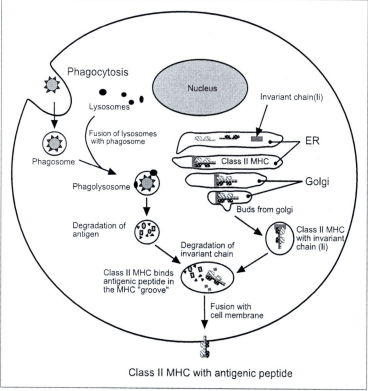

Fig. 3.9. Processing and presentation of exogenous proteins with class II MHC molecules. Extracellular organisms are endocytosed and processed in a series of steps leading to the display of antigenic peptide/class II MHC on the antigen cell surface.

Antigen Presenting Molecules: CD1 Molecules

Nomenclature and structure

"CD1" molecules are specialized antigen presenting proteins encoded by genes on chromosome 1. In humans, five genes have been identified that encode for proteins CD1 a, b, c, d, and e. Structurally, the CD1 molecules resemble class I MHC molecules in that they associate with β2-microglobulin. However, unlike class I MHC molecules, there is no evidence for allelic polymorphism, which implies that their function may be different from that of classical class I MHC molecules (below).

Tissue distribution and function

With the exception of CD1d and CD1e, CD1 molecules have a tissue distribution similar to that of class II MHC molecules, being constitutively expressed on cortical thymocytes, peripheral B cells, and dendritic cells. Only CD1-c is constitutively expressed on peripheral B cells, though during hepatitis B infections, for instance, both CD1-a and CD1-b molecules are also expressed. CD1 proteins (a-c) are also induced on macrophages during the chronic inflammation associated with mycobacterial infections. CD1 molecules present nonpolymorphic lipid and/or glycolipid microbial antigens to discrete classes of both CD4+ $\alpha\beta$ and $\gamma\delta$ T cells, particularly following mycobacterial infection. This specialized form of antigen presentation has heightened interest in this novel class of molecules.

Summary

Antigen presenting cells are required to deliver antigen to T cells. Professional antigen presenting cells including dendritic cells, macrophages and B cells are needed for stimulation of CD4+ T cells. Of these, the dendritic cell is the most efficient antigen presenting cell during primary immune responses to antigen. Cells that present antigen to CD8+ T cells are not "professional" antigen presenting cells, but are often called target cells because once identified, they are targeted for destruction (by CD8+ CTL).

Antigen presenting molecules are cell surface proteins that bind and present peptides, or antigen fragments, to T lymphocytes. Generally antigen presenting molecules are proteins encoded by the MHC locus, which fall into two major classes, class I and class II MHC molecules. In humans the MHC is referred to as the "HLA" in recognition of the fact that the proteins are human leukocyte antigens. Both class I and class II MHC molecules are polymorphic and codominantly expressed. However, the distribution of these proteins differs. Whereas class I MHC is constitutively expressed on all nucleated cells, class II MHC molecules are constitutively expressed only on antigen presenting cells. CD8+ T cells can only recognize antigen peptides when presented by class I MHC molecules and so CD8+ T cells are said to be *class I MHC restricted*. Likewise, CD4 + T cells can only recognize antigen peptides when presented by class II MHC molecules, and so CD4+ T cells are said to be *class II MHC restricted*.

CLINICAL CASES AND DISCUSSION

Clinical Case #5
A young 20-year old male complains of increasing stiffness in the hips and low back, and general malaise for several months. The family history reveals that the patient's father and uncle have suffered from similar disorders for many years, and the uncle is now essentially an invalid. Blood work is essentially normal, but an ESR (erythrocyte sedimentation rate) is high (100; normal range 5-15), and X-rays of the hips and low back indicate widespread significant joint space loss, with signs of fusion of at least two vertebrae. HLA-typing of this patient is positive for HLA-B27, as is that of the affected relatives. What is the likely diagnosis? How does this explain the observations above? What is one popular model for the etiology of this disorder?

Discussion Case #5
Background
The picture of general malaise, along with a personal and family predisposition to arthritic symptoms strongly suggests an inflammatory arthritic disorder of some kind. The joint space narrowing is common with arthritic disorders, but in the hip and low back one should think of ankylosing spondylitis. The association with HLA-B27 is of interest, because of the insight it is thought to give on the etiology of this disorder. While not a common HLA-haplotype, greater than 90% of individuals with ankylosing spondylitis are found to be HLA-B27 (the relative risk is of the order of 100). Current thought is that individuals with this HLA-haplotype inherit a predisposition to produce an autoimmune-mediated destruction of self bony tissue following infection with *Klebsiella* organisms. One of the prominent immunological determinants of an antigen in *Klebsiella* is a protein sequence that corresponds to a region in HLA-B27. This represents an example of molecular mimicry. Inheritance of both HLA-B27 and exposure to the inciting environmental trigger (Klebsiella) thus induces disease in the population at risk.

Tests
It is important that other potential causes of joint inflammation be eliminated. Thus, blood tests to lessen the likelihood of rheumatoid arthritis (looking for rheumatoid factor, Ig complexes etc) and/or systemic lupus erythematosus (blood tests to look for antinuclear antibody, other defined lupus-associated blood or cell markers) or other so-called connective tissue diseases (e.g., scleroderma) should be done.

Treatment
Nonsteroidal anti-inflammatory agents are used first, before a slow move to more potent agents (with greater risk of side effects), such as steroids, and even (nonspecific) antimetabolic reagents that prevent proliferation of all cells (methotrexate etc).

Clinical Case #6

A fair-haired blue-eyed boy is brought to see you by his mother who is concerned over his failure to gain weight. He is currently 30 months of age, and was developing normally until age 12 months. He also has rather severe intermittent stomach cramps, especially when he eats bread and other cereal-type foods. A cousin allegedly had the same problem which the mother tells you resolved after his diet was changed. She is concerned that her son might suffer from a similar "food allergy". What would your approach be to such a problem? What is a common disorder like this? What is the cause?

Discussion Case # 6

Background

Complaints of food allergies are quite common, but often are more imagined than real. However, in association with the failure to thrive, and the family history, you should be more concerned. In this case there is strong evidence that something in cereal is causing the problem. Allergies to gliadin (wheat-germ), present in cereal, are not uncommon, and this is the likely culprit. For individuals with allergy to gliadin, exposure to foods containing gliadin leads, as in this child's case, to intestinal hypersensitivity reactions, with release of histamine (causing smooth muscle contractions and stomach cramps), and general symptoms of diarrhea, and unwellness.

An interesting MHC association has been found for this disorder. Individuals expressing the HLA-B8 and HLA-D23 molecules are found some ten times more commonly in populations suffering from this disorder than in the general population (that is, the relative risk for this disorder in HLA-B8, HLA-D23 positive individuals is approximately 10 times that in non-HLA-B8 (D23) persons). Most likely this is because these MHC molecules can bind to the offending gliadin epitopes (antigen determinants responsible for the problem), and display the complex on the cell surface, while other MHC haplotypes do not. The disease is often referred to as coeliac disease; individuals with this MHC haplotype also often have blue eyes/fair-hair, probably due to a gene linkage phenomenon.

Tests

Classically one attempts to identify the allergic reaction (if it exists) by moving first to a minimal, elemental diet (proven, over time, to be acceptable even to those with intolerance to multiple foods) which the patient can tolerate. You then gradually add in those choices you think are likely most responsible for the initiating problem and observe symptoms.

Treatment

Use a modified diet. Starches (complex carbohydrates) are important dietary foods, but there are number of nongliadin natural starchy foods (rice and other legumes).

Test Yourself

Multiple Choice Questions
1. Which one of the following associates with class II MHC molecules to prevent the peptide binding in the "groove" formed by the two polypeptide chains?
   a. β2-microglobulin
   b. adapter protein
   c. invariant chain (Ii)
   d. clathrin
2. The multipeptide unit that degrades cytosolic viral proteins is called
   a. calnexin
   b. TAP
   c. proteasome
   d. NADPH oxidase
3. Class I MHC presents antigen to which one of the following?
   a. CD4+ Th1 cells
   b. CD4+ Th2 cells
   c. Natural killer cells
   d. CD8+ T cells
4. Which one of the following cells is not an antigen presenting cell?
   a. Neutrophil
   b. B cell
   c. Macrophage
   d. Dendritic cell
5. A 12-year-old boy has a one month history of increased urination, appetite and thirst. Tests reveal a very high (8-fold elevation) blood sugar, with high levels of sugar in the urine. Which of the following HLA molecules would you anticipate on his father's and/or mother's white blood cells?
   a. HLA-DR3
   b. HLA-B27
   c. HLA-A2
   d. HLA-DQ5
   e. HLA-C4

Answers: 1c; 2c; 3d; 4a; 5a

Short Answer Questions
1. What is meant by polymorphism? Of what advantage is MHC polymorphism to a species?
2. What is meant by codominant expression? Why is it advantageous to the individual?
3. Describe how some viruses prevent the display of antigenic peptide/class I MHC on the infected cell surface.

4. Compare and contrast antigen processing and presentation when the antigen is: (a) within a cytosolic endosome; (b) in the cytosol, but not limited by a vesicle.
5. Which antigen presenting cells are: (a) most effective under limiting antigen concentrations? (b) optimum for primary immune responses?

Soluble Mediators of Immunity I: Antibodies

Objectives	69
Antibodies	69
General Features of Antibodies	69
Structure Function Relationship of Antibodies	71
Properties of Immunoglobulin Isotypes	72
Monoclonal Antibodies	77
Monoclonal Antibodies as Therapeutic Agents	78
Clinical Trials	79
Summary	80
Clinical Cases and Discussion	81
Test Yourself	84

Objectives

At the end of this chapter the reader will understand the essential common features of the molecular structure of **antibody** molecules, as well as the manner by which we discriminate between molecules of different **classes**, **sub-classes**, **allotypes** and **idiotypes**. The biological functions associated with these differences will be explored.

The reader will be introduced to the concept of monoclonal antibodies, and their production. The interest in the use of such antibodies in a wide variety of clinical scenarios will be explored, including tumor immunotherapy, diagnostic decision making, and the regulation of inflammatory cascades.

ANTIBODIES

GENERAL FEATURES OF ANTIBODIES

Structure

Antibodies, also known as **immunoglobulins**, are heterogenous bifunctional glycoproteins secreted by differentiated B cells termed plasma cells. Monomeric antibody units consist of two identical **light chains** covalently linked to two identical **heavy chains** (Fig. 4.1). Each light chain and each heavy chain has a **variable region** (N-terminal) and a **constant region** (C-terminal). Dimeric, trimeric and pentameric forms of immunoglobulin are composed of two, three and five monomeric units.

Clinical Immunology, by Reginald Gorczynski and Jacqueline Stanley. 2001 Landes Bioscience

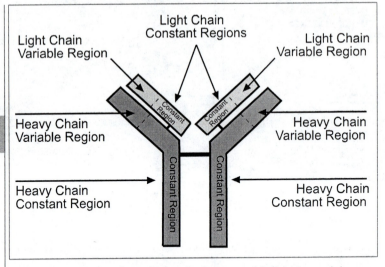

Fig. 4.1. General structure of an antibody molecule (immunoglobulin). Monomeric immunoglobulin molecules consist of two identical light chains covalently linked to two identical heavy chains.

Antibodies possess both antigen binding capacity and biological activity. The antigen binding capacity resides in a structure(s) conferred by amino acid sequences in the so-called variable regions. Amino acid differences in this region also confer exquisite specificity, with respect to antigen recognition and binding. The biological activities of different antibody molecules are the result of amino acid differences in the constant region, although the basic molecular structure of the antibodies is the same. The different constant regions define the **isotype** (family) of immunoglobulins, **IgA, IgD, IgE, IgG** and **IgM**, where **Ig** refers to the term immunoglobulin.

Light chains
Light chains are composed of variable and constant regions. The constant region, **kappa** or **lambda**, distinguishes the two classes of light chains. A single antibody molecule will have either two kappa or two lambda light chains, but never a mixture of the two. In humans, the predominant light chain is kappa. Although lambda chains are invariant in the population, kappa chains demonstrate allotypy. Allotypy refers to the presence of allelic forms of the same protein in the population. Kappa chain **allotypes** are referred to as Km.

Heavy chains
Heavy chains are composed of a variable and a constant region. Five major classes of heavy chains can be distinguished with different constant regions, designated by the Greek letters alpha (α), delta (δ), epsilon (ε), gamma (γ) or mu (μ).

These constant regions give rise to the antibody isotypes IgA, IgD, IgE, IgG and IgM respectively. Allotypic forms of the IgA and IgG heavy chains gives rise to allotypes designated Am and Gm, respectively.

STRUCTURE FUNCTION RELATIONSHIP OF ANTIBODIES

Discovery by proteolysis
Antibodies possess both an antigen binding capacity and a biological activity. This bifunctional nature of antibodies was initially demonstrated following proteolytic cleavage of antibody (Fig. 4.2). Digestion with papain yields three molecules, two copies of a single antigen binding region, **F(ab)**, and one readily crystallizable fragment (**Fc**) that cannot bind antigen. Digestion of antibodies with pepsin generates one molecule possessing two antigen binding sites, **Fab2**. In pepsin digests, the Fc portion is proteolytically degraded.

Antigen binding region
The combined variable regions of the light and heavy chains define the antigen binding site. There are two identical binding sites on each monomeric antibody molecule. The interaction between the antigen and the antibody binding site involves both hydrophobic and ionic components. The strength of the interaction between one antigen binding site and its monovalent antigen determines the **affinity** of the interaction. Antibody *avidity* describes the overall binding energy of all of the antigen binding sites with antigen.

Although each variable region is unique, a comparison of the variable regions from both light and heavy chains shows that some positional sequences are

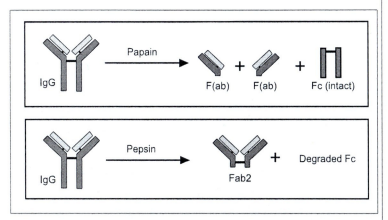

Fig. 4.2. Products of proteolytic digestion. Immunoglobulins are heterogenous bifunctional glycoproteins that possess both antigen binding capacity and biological activity. Proteolysis with papain yields two antigen binding fragments, F(ab) and one readily crystallizable fragment (Fc) which cannot bind antigen. In contrast, pepsin generates one fragment that can bind two antigen molecules (Fab2). The Fc portion is degraded.

relatively invariant, while others differ considerably. Regions that differ extensively are termed hypervariable and represent amino acid sequences that are unique to a particular antibody and complementary to a particular antigenic epitope. Hence hypervariable regions are also termed **complementary determining regions, CDRs**.

Hypervariable regions can also serve as antigenic determinants (idiotopes). The collection of **idiotopes** in a given antibody defines the **idiotype**. Consequently, antibodies generated to the collection of idiotopes on a single antibody molecule are termed **anti-idiotypic antibodies**.

Biological effector region

The Fc region is determined by the constant region of the antibody and mediates the antibody effector function. Because the constant region of the antibody also defines the antibody isotype, the antibody isotype thus correlates with the antibody's biological role in an immune response. The properties of the antibody isotypes IgA, IgD, IgE, IgG, and IgM are discussed below.

PROPERTIES OF IMMUNOGLOBULIN ISOTYPES

Immunoglobulin A

Immunoglobulin A (IgA) exists as a monomer, dimer or a trimer (Fig. 4.3, Table 4.1). IgA has a half-life of approximately one week. In humans, IgA is further subtyped as IgA1 and IgA2. Dimeric and trimeric forms of IgA are associated with an additional component termed a **J chain**. Most of the IgA is found in mucosa-associated lymphoid tissue, although traces of IgA are also found in the circulation. IgA is found predominantly in the gastrointestinal tract and in secretions such as tears, sweat, and saliva. IgA is present at all external surfaces (except skin), impeding microbial binding to epithelia. IgA is also the major antibody of milk and colostrum. Consequently, infants who are breastfed are endowed with the mother's immunity to gastrointestinal pathogens.

Mucosa-associated IgA is secreted as dimeric IgA by plasma cells present in the lamina propria (Fig. 4.4). Transport from the lamina propria to the lumen is initiated when dimeric IgA binds to a protein, the **secretory component**, present on the basolateral face of the epithelial cells. The attached dimeric IgA, along with the secretory component, is endocytosed and transported through the epithelial cell in this vesicle. When the vesicle containing the complex reaches the lumenal side of the epithelial cell, the secretory component is cleaved with the IgA retaining a fragment of the secretory component, while the remainder of the protein remains attached to the epithelial cell (Fig. 4.4). The IgA released into the intestinal lumen is referred to as secretory IgA in recognition of the fact that it retained a piece of the secretory component. Secretory IgA functions in immunosurveillance binding to organisms before they bind to M cells, their port of entry into the lamina propria. In addition to its pathogen neutralizing function, aggregated IgA activates the alternative pathway of complement.

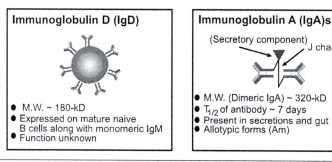

Immunoglobulin G (IgG)
- M.W. ~ 150-kD
- Percentage of total Ig: ~75-80
- $T_{1/2}$ ~three weeks for IgG 1,2,4
- $T_{1/2}$ ~one week for IgG 3
- Crosses placenta
- Fc/FcγR: Opsonization and ADCC
- Activates complement (IgG 1,2,3)
- Neutralization (viruses, toxins)
- Allotypic forms (Gm)
- Subclasses IgG 1, 2, 3, 4

Immunoglobulin E (IgE)
- M.W. ~ 195-kD
- $T_{1/2}$ of non-bound antibody ~ 2 days
- Reaginic antibody (allergies)
- Mainly bound to FcεR on mast cells and basophils

Pentameric IgM (Secreted form)
- M.W. ~ 900-kD
- $T_{1/2}$ of antibody ~ 7 days
- Predominates in primary responses
- Monomeric form on immature + naive B cells
- Isohemagglutinins are of the IgM isotype
- Activates complement (classic pathway)

Immunoglobulin D (IgD)
- M.W. ~ 180-kD
- Expressed on mature naive B cells along with monomeric IgM
- Function unknown

Immunoglobulin A (IgA)s
- M.W. (Dimeric IgA) ~ 320-kD
- $T_{1/2}$ of antibody ~ 7 days
- Present in secretions and gut
- Allotypic forms (Am)

Fig. 4.3. Immunoglobulin isotypes. Properties of immunoglobulins and their biological roles are determined by the immunoglobulin isotype.

Immunoglobulin D

In contrast to other isotypes, **immunoglobulin D** (IgD) exists only as a membrane bound form. It is expressed on naive B cells, along with IgM (Fig. 4.3). Low detectable serum levels of IgD likely reflect products of B-cell death. The function(s) of IgD remain under investigation.

Table 4.1 Structural and biological properties of immunoglobulin isotypes

	IgG	IgA	IgM	IgD	IgE
[Serum] (mg/dl)	~1200	~100	~150	Negligible	Negligible
Percent of Total Ig	~80	~14	~7	Negligible	Negligible
Form in Serum (typical)	Monomer	Monomer, Dimer	Pentamer	Monomer	Monomer
Molecular Weight (kD)	~150	~160 (Monomer)	~900	~180	~200
% Carbohydrate	~3	~7	~10	~10	~12
Covalent Attachments	–	J chain, Secretory Component	J Chain	–	–
Distribution	Vascular (intra and extra)	Vascular (intra) + Mucosa	Vascular (intra)	Membrane (naive B cells)	FcεR on Mast cells, Basophils
Subclasses	4	2	–	–	–
Allotypes	20 (Gm)	2 (Am)	–	–	–
# Fabs (Valence)	2	2 or 4	10	2	2
Milk and Colostrum	+	+++	–	–	–
Placental Transfer	++	–	–	–	–
Agglutinating Capability	+	+ (Monomer)	+++	–	–
Complement Activation (Classical Pathway)	+ (not IgG4)	–	+++	–	–
Complement Activation (Alternative Pathway)	–	Aggregated Form	–	–	–
Reaginic Antibody (Allergic Activity)	–	–	–	–	+++
Half Life	IgG 1,2,4 ~21 days IgG3 ~ 7 days	~ 5 days	~ 5 days	~ 3 days	~ 2 days (unbound)

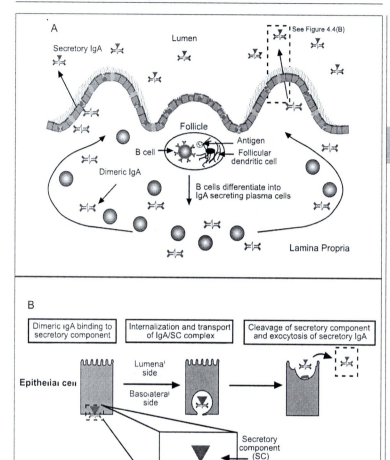

Fig. 4.4. Immunoglobulin A (IgA): A. Production of dimeric IgA B. Transport of IgA from the lamina propria to the lumen. A. Plasma cells in the lamina propria secrete dimeric IgA into the lamina propria region. Dimeric IgA binds to the basolateral surface of epithelial cells via a molecule termed secretory component, (SC). B. Upon binding to SC, dimeric IgA is internalized, and transported across the epithelial cell via intracellular vesicles. At the lumenal side, bound SC-IgA complex is cleaved and exocytosed into the lumen. A portion of the secretory component remains bound to the IgA, which is referred to as secretory IgA; the other remains bound to the epithelial cell.

Immunoglobulin E

Immunoglobulin E (IgE) is a monomeric antibody, normally barely detectable in serum because most IgE is bound to FcεR on mast cells and basophils (Fig. 4.3, Table 4.1). Multivalent antigen binding to IgE (bound to mast cells and basophils via the FcεR) results in a crosslinking of FcεRs leading to release of inflammatory and vasoactive mediators from preformed granules present in mast cells and basophils.

Immunoglobulin G

Immunoglobulin G (IgG) is a 150 kD monomer (Fig. 4.3, Table 4.1) that constitutes approximately seventy five percent of the total circulating immunoglobulin. IgG circulates between blood and interstitial fluid [~ 12 mg/ml], and has a half-life of about three weeks. IgG antibodies can be transported across the placenta and enter the fetal circulation so that the mother's immunity is transferred to the fetus.

Immunologically, IgG plays a major role in elimination of microbes by facilitating: (i) opsonization by phagocytes; (ii) antibody-dependent cell mediated cytotoxicity (ADCC) by natural killer cells; (iii) complement activation; and (iv) neutralization of viruses and toxins.

i	Opsonization	Opsonization refers to phagocytosis that is triggered following binding of the Fc region of antibodies, bound by the pathogen, to FcγR on phagocytes.
ii	ADCC	ADCC refers to the process by which natural killer cells interact with, and destroy, target cells coated with antigen specific IgG. Natural killer cells express a low affinity FcγR whose interaction with target cell-bound IgG triggers the release of molecules cytotoxic to target cell.
iii	Complement	Complement activation by IgG requires that IgG is a component of an immune complex. A complement protein binds the complex and triggers the activation of the complement cascade.
iv	Neutralization	Neutralization of viruses or toxins results when IgG antibody binds antigen to inhibit the antigen's ability to bind to a cell surface receptor.

In humans, IgG is further subclassified as IgG1, IgG2, IgG3, and IgG4, subtypes differing from one another in their constant regions. Because biological potential is mediated via the Fc portion of IgG, it is not surprising that minor differences in function are observed among subtypes, including differences in serum concentration, half life, and relative biological potency. IgG1 is present in the highest concentration (9 mg/ml) and IgG4 the lowest (0.5mg/ml); IgG3 has a half life of only one week, but is the most effective (classic pathway) activator of complement of all IgG subtypes. IgG4 does not activate complement at all, nor does it bind to FcγR. All IgG subtypes cross the placenta.

Immunoglobulin M

Immunoglobulin M (IgM) exists as a monomer when membrane associated, but is secreted from plasma cells in a pentameric form (Fig. 4.3, Table 4.1). Pentameric IgM consists of five covalently attached monomeric units, and a single short J chain, thought to facilitate polymerization of the monomers. Pentameric IgM constitutes about 7% of total immunoglobulin; is largely intravascular [2 mg/ml]; is the only isotype expressed on immature B cells; and is expressed on naive mature B cells along with IgD. IgM has a half-life of approximately 5-7 days.

The pentameric form of IgM has ten antigen binding sites, but steric hindrance impedes the simultaneous occupation of all sites by antigen. Although IgM antibodies have a low intrinsic affinity for antigen, the number of antigen binding sites confers a relatively high avidity for antigen. The importance of IgM to an immune response lies in its unparalleled ability to activate the classical pathway of complement, requiring only one IgM antigen/antigen complex. Because complement activation leads to enhanced phagocytosis and osmotic lysis of bacteria, the role of IgM in an immune response is significant.

MONOCLONAL ANTIBODIES

Generation of monoclonal antibodies

Monoclonal antibodies are a collection of antibody molecules arising from a single clone of antibody secreting plasma cells, all of which recognize the same, and only one, epitope on the immunizing antigen. Immunization of B cells with protein antigens leads to their activation and differentiation to memory B cells or antibody secreting plasma cells. Most protein antigens have several different epitopes. Therefore, several plasma cell clones, each secreting antibodies of a unique specificity will be generated in response to one antigen. The total antibody collection from all the different clones is **polyclonal**, but antibodies secreted by each clone of cells are **monoclonal**. By isolating single B-cell clones, and immortalizing the plasma cells, the commercial production of large quantities of monoclonal antibodies that can be used for therapeutic purposes has become commonplace.

Monoclonal antibodies are generated from immunized animals (e.g., mice). Single cell suspensions from the spleen of immunized animals are fused with myeloma cells, a malignant plasma cell tumor (Fig. 4.5). This generates hybrid cells termed **hybridomas**, which are both immortal and secrete the antibodies of interest (from the immunized animal). Hybridomas are now screened to detect the relevant antibodies. For this, the hybridoma cells are separated into single cell cultures by plating in microtiter plates, generally screening some 2000 wells for each hybridoma suspension. An aliquot of the supernatant is removed from each well and added to other microtiter plates precoated with the antigen of interest. Reactivity is determined in **enzyme-linked immunosorbent assays** (ELISAs), looking for plate-bound antibody. Once the hybridoma cells of interest have been identified, they are subcultured to serve as *antibody factories* that secrete the appropriate monoclonal antibody.

A. Immunization and production of splenic single cell suspensions

Repeated immunization of a mouse with the antigen of interest
Sacrifice the mouse and remove the spleen
Make a single cell suspension of the spleen

B. Fusion with a malignant plasma cell and selection of fused cells

Fuse the spleen cells with maliganant plasma cells
Incubate in special media to remove malignant cells that did not fuse
Spleen cells that did not fuse die in a few days

C. Identifying the fused cell that is secreting the antibody of interest

Remove supernatant samples from each of the wells
Incubate in a microtiter plate in limiting dilution (one cell per well)
Test for the presence of antibody using ELISA techniques
Identify the microtiter well(s) containing the plasma cell of interest

D. Purification of monoclonal antibody

Culture in sequentially larger volumes
Remove supernatant, purify by column chromatography
Identify the fraction of interest using spectrophotometry

Store monoclonal antibody at 4°C

Fig. 4.5. Monoclonal antibody production. Monoclonal antibodies are generated in animals (e.g., mouse). In accordance with the stepwise procedures described in this figure, large quantities of monoclonal antibodies can be generated.

MONOCLONAL ANTIBODIES AS THERAPEUTIC AGENTS

General Features

In theory, the intravenous injection of monoclonal antibodies should provide the long sought *magic bullet* for cancer or autoimmune therapy. The term *magic bullet* refers to the use of a treatment that *magically* localizes only to the desired target, in contrast to conventional treatment (e.g., drugs, irradiation or surgery) where no such specific target localization can be achieved. The use of monoclonal antibodies (which can co-opt complement and/or ADCC/phagocytosis in vivo) has not been as effective as one would have predicted. Consequently, toxic agents are covalently linked to antibodies that target cells, or tissues, for destruction. The efficacy of monoclonal antibody therapy is limited by many factors.

Limitations

(i) Mice are often used for immunization to produce the monoclonal antibodies, and the human recipient of those antibodies often mounts an immune response that destroys these foreign antibodies. This is termed a HAMA (human anti-mouse antibody) response. Often the beneficial effect of the antibody used for treatment is transient, and a second treatment with antibody from the same species is ineffective. One approach to eliminate the HAMA response is to use genetic engineering technology to generate chimeric antibodies that retain the mouse variable regions (antigen-specificity domains) but have human constant regions. These are known as humanized chimeric antibodies.

(ii) The use of humanized antibodies has eliminated the problems associated with the HAMA response to the constant region of the antibody, but generation of anti-idiotypic antibodies (directed against the mouse variable region domains) continues to be a problem.

(iii) The size of the antibody molecule is a limiting factor for therapies requiring that antibodies leave the circulation and enter tissue sites, if there is no coexisting inflammation (inflammation makes blood vessels leaky). The use of Fab2 fragments facilitates access to tissue sites because these fragments are considerably smaller than the intact antibody. Unfortunately, the fragments now enter many tissues nonspecifically, and if a toxic molecule or radioactive label has been attached to the Fab2 fragments (to improve killing potency for the specific target), the incidence of bystander damage is also increased.

(iv) The formation of immunoconjugates (antibody plus drug or radioactive molecule) requires a stable linkage to prevent the deposition of free drug or radioisotope into healthy tissues. Formation of stable linkages has been a challenge.

(v) Treatment of cancers with immunoconjugates is limited by the general lack of tissue specific antigens on most cancer cells. Ensuring selectivity of treatment to the malignant tissue (but not the normal tissue) is a problem (Chapter 16).

CLINICAL TRIALS

Hodgkins's Disease
Clinical trials using Yttrium-90 labeled anti-ferritin polyclonal Fab2 has met with some success (62% response rate) in patients with end stage Hodgkin's for whom no other curative treatment is available. These patients also receive autologous bone marrow transplants following treatment (Chapter 17).

Immunodiagnosis

Even if a proposed monoclonal antibody does not reach the high titer/selective toxicity needed for immunotherapy, these molecules can have other value. Monitoring carcinoembryonic antigen (CEA) levels using monoclonal antibodies to CEA, following colon tumor resection, has proven to be a useful means of assessing recurrence, as has following βHCG levels following treatment for choriocarcinoma. Other studies are investigating the use of radiolabeled monoclonal anti-tumor antibodies (along with a Gamma camera) to detect (by radiography) the localization of tumor deposits in those patients.

Septic shock

There has been interest in the use of anti-tumor necrosis factor (anti-TNF) monoclonal antibodies in the treatment of septic shock. The *shock* response, with concomitant low blood pressure, increased vascular permeability, pyrexia etc. is believed to be initiated by massive release of TNF by activated macrophages. The "shock" response is a particular problem in instances of gram negative sepsis, where lipopolysaccharide (LPS) released by such organisms has profound TNF inducing capacity, leading to a high morbidity/mortality. Numerous clinical trials of infusion of anti-TNF monoclonal antibodies have been reported in the last several years, though to date none has shown the profound effect hoped for.

Xenotransplantation

Xenotransplantation (transplantation of organs across species) is initially limited by hyperacute rejection responses, attributed to xenoantibodies. These xenoantibodies are naturally occurring antibodies directed to tissue antigens of the donor species. When these antibodies bind to the donor antigens, complement activation occurs which leads to early (minutes/hours) graft thrombosis and graft loss. Strategies to overcome this problem include the use of anti-complement component antibodies, or even artificial antigen-columns for removal of the natural antibodies in recipient serum.

Drug abuse

The interaction of antibody with a drug should neutralize the drug by preventing binding to its receptor. Animal studies using anti-drug Fab2 fragments, instead of intact antibodies, to counteract the effects of an overdose of PCP (angel dust) have reported that behaviors associated with the drug were eliminated in a matter of minutes.

SUMMARY

Antibodies, or immunoglobulins, are heterogenous bifunctional glycoproteins that possess both antigen binding capacity and biological activity. Monomeric immunoglobulin molecules consist of two identical light chains covalently linked to two identical heavy chains, with each chain composed of a variable region and a constant region. The variable regions are so termed because they differ between immunoglobulins, whereas the constant regions may be shared by many immunoglobulins.

Specific amino acid sequences in the variable regions of both light and heavy chains confer specificity to the antibody and serve as the antigen-binding site, regardless of the constant region. These unique amino acid sequences, also known as idiotopes, can themselves serve as antigenic determinants. In addition to recognition and binding of antigen, immunoglobulins have biological functions, delineated by the constant region of each heavy chain, the antibody isotype. The five major antibody isotypes, IgA, IgD, IgE, IgG and IgM, are so designated according to their heavy chain constant regions, $\alpha, \delta, \epsilon, \gamma$ and μ respectively. The effectiveness of antibodies as tools to eliminate infection relies on the bifunctional nature of antibodies. That is, the variable regions binds antigen; the constant region (isotype) determines the biological role of the antibody in the immune response.

Differentiated B cells, termed plasma cells, secrete antibodies. Each plasma cell clone secretes antibodies that recognize one epitope of the immunizing antigen. Antibodies secreted by a plasma cell clone are termed monoclonal. The development of protocols to isolate single B-cell clones, as well as techniques for the immortalization of plasma cells, has enabled the commercial production of monoclonal antibodies that can be used for therapeutic purposes. In theory, the intravenous injection of monoclonal antibodies should provide the long sought *magic bullet* for cancer or autoimmune therapy. In practice, the antigenicity, and the size of antibodies, limits the efficacy of monoclonal antibody therapy. The efficacy of monoclonal antibodies as therapeutic agents has been enhanced by the conjugation of radioactive isotopes or drugs to the antibody molecule. In these situations, the specificity of the antibody targets the tissue and the drug or radioactive isotope destroys the tissue. Several clinical trials using antibodies as therapeutic agents are in progress.

CLINICAL CASES AND DISCUSSION

Clinical Case # 7
Joan is a 17-year old girl who comes to your Emergency Department in the terminal stages of delivery. You determine this to be an uneventful pregnancy (she is now 39 weeks of gestation). She has had essentially no antenatal care. She delivers a healthy baby boy, and the delivery itself is uncomplicated. You order the nurse to give an injection of RhoGam to Joan. What is the basis of this treatment?

Discussion Case #7
Background
The mother:fetus relationship is an interesting one immunologically, as it represents essentially a *natural* allograft. There are a number of examples indicating that the mother is quite capable of recognizing foreign antigens on this allograft. Prominent amongst these are the so-called blood group polysaccharide antigens (A, B, O and Rh) present on red blood cells. Individuals have natural antibodies to the blood group polysaccharide antigens A, and/or B, following immunization with crossreactive antigens present on bacteria that comprise the natural gut flora.

Individuals do not have antibodies to the antigens present on their own tissues. As example,
  i   "A" blood group individuals have " A" antigens on their red blood cells, and circulating natural anti-B antibodies.
  ii "B" blood group individuals have "B" antigens on their red blood cells, and circulating natural anti-A antibodies.
  iii "AB" blood group individuals have both the "A" and the "B" antigens on their red blood cells. They have no circulating natural anti-A antibodies or anti-B antibodies.
  iv "O" blood group individuals have neither the "A" nor the "B" antigens on their red blood cells. They have both circulating anti-A antibodies and anti-B antibodies.

When individuals are confronted with red blood cells that express antigens to which they have natural antibodies, complement is activated and the red blood cells are lysed. Interestingly, anti-Rh antibody is only made (in Rh negative individuals) after exposure to Rh antigen. However, anti-Rh IgG antibodies cross the placenta easily. It is this issue that we are addressing in this case.

Tests
In this scenario we do not have time to determine the Rhesus status of the mother and father. However, we should assume the worst. We must assume that it is possible that Joan is Rh negative, and the father is Rh positive.

Treatment
Treatment is an injection of anti-Rh antibodies, *RhoGam*, to the mother just before/after the birth of the baby. The rationale for this treatment is based on the assumption that the baby is Rh positive. In the event of bleeding during birth, some of the baby's red blood cells could immunize the mother, whom we assume to be Rh negative, against the Rh antigen. This risk of immunization occurs during any bleeding episodes during pregnancy, and during bleeding at birth.

The problems associated with such immunization come not with the first pregnancy, but with the second (and subsequent) pregnancies involving a Rh positive child. IgG anti-Rh antibodies generated after the first pregnancy (in the absence of RhoGam treatment) could cross the placenta, cause lysis of the fetal red cells, and lead to hemolytic disease (of pregnancy). It is crucial that we inhibit such sensitization.

Passive delivery of anti-Rh antibody has been shown to be effective at inhibiting sensitization to Rh antigen in this scenario. How it does so still remains obscure. One notion suggests that the anti-Rh antibodies merely *mask* the antigen so that the mother cannot be sensitized. Estimates of the density of antigen (compared with the amount of IgG given) suggest this is not the explanation. Current thought is that some complex immunoregulatory network is set up following treatment with Rhogam. This in turn causes active suppression of the production of anti-Rh antibodies by the mother.

Clinical Case #8

Sam is a 9-year-old boy who has had repeated bacterial sinus infections. As his family doctor you wonder if there may be an underlying immunological defect which is contributing to this problem, or whether he is merely "unlucky". Further investigations show normal numbers/function of B and T cells, granulocytes and macrophages. Immunoglobulin levels are grossly normal. Electrophoresis reveals only IgM and IgG antibodies in the immunoglobulin pool. Does this help in understanding Sam's problem?

Discussion Case #8

Background

Provision of resistance to microbial pathogens represents a key role for the immune system. In general, antibodies (with complement and macrophages/other accessory cells) provide prominent resistance to bacterial infection. T cells (and their products) provide resistance against viral, fungal and intracellular pathogens, either by direct lysis of the infected cells, or by activating (by released cytokines) endogenous *killer pathways* within the infected cell. In this particular case we are told that this young boy is prone to bacterial sinus infections.

Defects important to rule out, in the face of recurrent bacterial infections include, for instance, genetic defects in the NADPH oxidase system (chronic granulomatous disease) and in the complement system. In the absence of defects in the phagocytic or complement systems, we are drawn to consider the B-cell system and deficiencies therein as a prime suspect in the problem. However, B- and T-cell numbers and function are normal, as are the levels of IgG and IgM. Therefore, the defect in this patient does not appear to be associated with defects in B-cell development/differentiation, as would occur in Bruton's X-linked hypogammaglobulinemia.

Tests

The normal numbers for IgG and IgM do not necessarily mean that this individual has normal numbers of other antibody isotypes, and plasma IgA levels should be determined. No IgA is detected.

Treatment

IgA is an antibody prominent at mucosal surfaces, where it is believed to play an essential "first line" of defense against mucosal pathogens. Indeed, there is a specialized system selected during evolution that enables this IgA to be delivered and secreted at these surfaces (so-called "secretory piece" for IgA). In the absence of secreted IgA it is not surprising to find that the body's resistance to pathogens at mucosal surfaces is impaired, leading to an increased susceptibility to bacterial infections at this site.

Note that there are other natural resistance mechanisms operating at mucosal surfaces, so in general this defect is not life threatening. The usual treatment is, in fact, antibiotics (given as needed). Some thought has been given to trying to develop a nasal insufflation of passive IgA.

TEST YOURSELF

Multiple Choice Questions
For questions 1-10, choose a, b, c, or d. Use each choice once, more than once, or not at all.
- a. IgG
- b. IgE
- c. IgM
- d. IgA
- e. IgD

1. crosses the placenta
2. has the longest half life
3. is present in the highest concentration in circulation
4. isotype of isohemagglutinins
5. expressed on immature B cells
6. in aggregated form activates the alternative pathway of complement
7. "stored" bound to FcεR on mast cells and basophils
8. most efficient (when bound to antigen) at activating the classical pathway of complement
9. is known as the reaginic antibody
10. transferred to the infant during breast feeding

1. (a) 2.(a) 3. (a) 4. (c) 5. (c) 6. (d) 7. (b) 8. (c) 9. (b) 10 (d) and to a lesser degree (a).

Short Answer Questions
1. Describe the action of papain and pepsin on the IgG molecule. Explain how studies with these enzymes led to the discovery that immunoglobulins are bifunctional molecules.
2. Where does the antigen binding site reside in the immunoglobulin molecule?
3. What are complementary determining regions? What is meant by the term hypervariable regions within a variable region? What are framework regions?
4. What is the relationship between IgE and allergies? Explain.
5. Why is breastfeeding important in developing countries?

Soluble Mediators of Immunity II: Complement

Objectives	85
Complement	86
Complement Pathways: General Features	86
Complement Biological Activities	93
Complement Regulation	95
Complement and Coagulation Pathways Are Linked via Kallikrein	99
Complement Genetic Deficiencies	99
Role of Complement in Medicine	103
Xenotransplantation: Complement Is Deleterious	103
Summary	104
Clinical Cases and Discussion	105
Test Yourself	108

Objectives

This chapter introduces the reader to the complement system, a family of proteins whose proteolytically derived fragments facilitate elimination of microorganisms, particularly extracellular bacteria. Activation of complement takes place in a cascade, following two pathways (the classical and the alternative pathways), with characteristic initial triggering events and some unique early steps in each pathway. Each pathway produces key convertase molecules, C3 convertase and C5 convertase for the classical/alternative pathways, respectively, and thereafter the pathways are identical. Natural regulatory molecules also exist that are important physiologically for homeostasis of the complement cascades.

A primary function of the activated complement cascade is the elimination of extracellular organisms. Common triggering events for complement activation are molecules expressed by these microorganisms themselves (or the adaptive immune responses to them). Other endogenous molecules have the ability to trigger the complement cascade. Understanding these other triggering mechanisms takes on added importance as we understand that during complement activation a number of the other biologically active molecules produced are important in inflammation and in altering vascular permeability.

The importance of complement activation to host defense will become evident as the reader appreciates the pathology attributable to genetic deficiencies of several complement components.

Clinical Immunology, by Reginald Gorczynski and Jacqueline Stanley. 2001 Landes Bioscience

COMPLEMENT

COMPLEMENT PATHWAYS: GENERAL FEATURES

The complement system is a family of numerous (~30) activation and regulatory proteins found either bound to the cell membrane or in circulation (Fig. 5.1). Complement proteins are synthesized mainly by the liver. However, some of these proteins are also synthesized by macrophages and fibroblasts. Many circulating complement proteins are proenzymes whose activation requires their proteolytic hydrolysis. These proteolytic fragments can function as effector molecules for the immune system (Fig. 5.2). These effector molecules: (i) facilitate the interaction of phagocytes to induce opsonin-mediated phagocytosis; (ii) induce osmotic lysis of microbes; (iii) enhance vascular permeability by inducing degranulation of mast cells/ basophils; (iv) induce chemotaxis of neutrophils; and (v) facilitate immune complex elimination.

The complement system is one of the earliest defense mechanisms activated in response to microbial infections. Complement proteins that function as enzymes are sequentially activated in a cascade, often referred to as a complement *pathway*. There are two pathways for activation of the complement cascade, the alternative and the classical pathways, but each pathway generates the fragment "C3b", a pivotal molecule in host defense. Thereafter, both pathways converge in a final common pathway.

Many cells have receptors for the proteolytically derived complement fragments and this dictates which cells respond to complement activation (Table 5.1). Osmotic lysis of cells or microbes, however, requires the terminal pathway of the complement cascade (Fig. 5.2). The product of terminal pathway activation is the formation, and insertion into the target cell membrane, of a protein complex, the membrane attack complex (MAC), which induces osmotic lysis of the target cells/ microbes.

Complement activity and the deleterious complement effects on autologous cells are minimized by a number of soluble, or membrane bound, regulatory proteins (Fig. 5.1). The role of the complement system in host defense is underscored when one considers the clinical consequences of microbial evasion strategies and complement genetic deficiencies.

Alternative complement pathway: Activation

The **alternative pathway of complement** activation (Fig. 5.3), so named because it was identified secondary to the classical complement pathway, is considered, in evolutionary terms, the older of the two activation pathways. When microbes penetrate the body's intrinsic physical and chemical barriers, they are confronted by numerous innate host defenses, including the alternative complement pathway. The prompt mobilization of the alternative pathway following invasion by an infectious agent is contingent on the availability of small amounts of a spontaneously generated complement fragment, C3b. The C3b is derived from circulating C3 in a process which can be referred to as complement pathway

Soluble Mediators of Immunity II: Complement

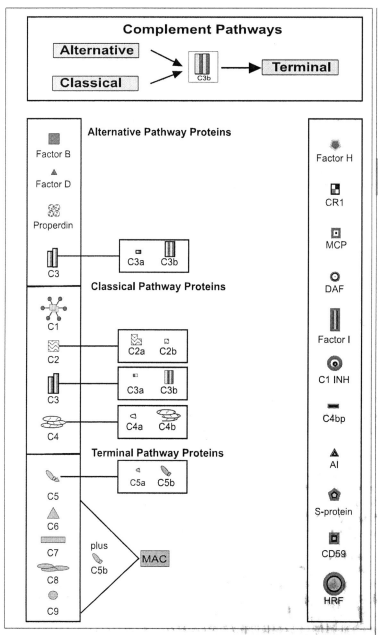

Fig. 5.1. Complement proteins: A, Effector molecules. B, Regulatory proteins. Complement proteins form a family of numerous (~30) activation and regulatory molecules found membrane bound, or in circulation.

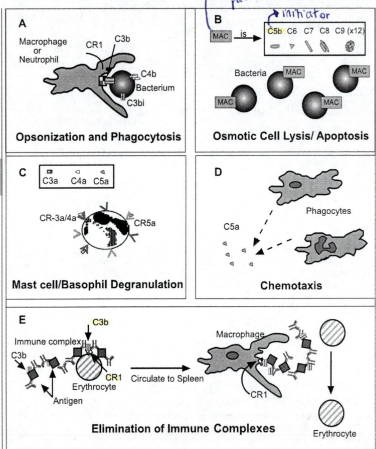

Fig. 5.2. **Biological activities of complement**. Opsonization and Phagocytosis: A. Macrophages and neutrophils express the **complement receptor CR1** whose **ligands include** complement fragments **C3b**, C3bi, and C4b. When deposited onto microbial surfaces these complement fragments serve as opsonins to facilitate phagocytosis by cells expressing CR1 receptors. B. Osmotic Cell Lysis: **Activation of the terminal pathway** involves the **formation of a membrane attack complex** (MAC) on a microbial cell surface, which induces osmotic lysis and microbial destruction. C. Mast Cell or Basophil Degranulation: Mast cells and basophils express the complement receptors CR-3a/4a and CR-5a. Binding of the anaphylatoxins to their cognate receptors on mast cells and basophils induces degranulation and release of inflammatory mediators. D. Chemotaxis: The anaphylatoxin C5a is chemotactic for phagocytes. E. Elimination of Immune Complexes: Complement activation generates C3b that may be deposited on immune complexes. **Interaction of CR1 present on red blood cells with its ligand, C3b, present on the immune complexes, facilitates delivery of complexes to the spleen where phagocytes, again bearing CR1 receptors, interact with free C3b molecules on the immune complexes inducing phagocytosis of the complexes.**

Soluble Mediators of Immunity II: Complement

Table 5.1 Complement receptors

Complement Receptor	Ligand	Cells on Which the Receptor Is Expressed
CR1	C3b, C3bi, C4b	Phagocytes, B cells, RBC
CR2	C3bi	B cells
CR3a/4a	C3a, C4a,	Mast cells, Basophils
CR5a	C5a	Mast cells, Basophils

"tickover" (Fig. 5.4). In the absence of microbial infection, the spontaneously generated C3b is rapidly inactivated either by interaction with water or complement regulatory proteins.

In the presence of microorganisms, particularly bacteria, the spontaneously generated C3b binds to the microbial surfaces, providing an initiating step for complement activation (Fig. 5.3). This is rapidly followed by the deposition, adjacent to C3b, of another complement protein, **Factor B**, and its hydrolysis to Ba and Bb by **Factor D**. The C3bBb complex generated on the microbial surface is known as the **alternative pathway C3 convertase**. This C3 convertase is stabilized by a tetrameric protein, **properdin**, that extends its half-life 6- to 10-fold.

The formation of the C3 convertase is the hallmark of the alternative complement pathway activation because the products generated (C3a and C3b) play a key role in host defense, and further progression (C3b) of the complement cascade. C3b is required for the formation of the **alternative pathway C5 convertase** (C3bBbC3b), which cleaves C5 to generate C5a and C5b (Fig. 5.3). The formation of C5b is the initiating step for the formation of the **membrane attack complex**, which characterizes the terminal (common) pathway of complement activation. The biological roles of the proteolytically derived complement proteins are described below.

Classical complement pathway: Activation

Activation of the **classical pathway of complement** occurs only after adaptive host defenses have been recruited (Fig. 5.5). Specifically, IgM, or IgG (subclasses 1, 2, or 3) antibodies specific for an antigen (e.g., infectious agent) must be generated and bind to that antigen. In this antigen/antibody complex, or **immune complex**, antigen is bound via the Fab region of antibody leaving the Fc regions available to bind the complement protein, C1. C1 is composed of three components, C1q, C1r, and C1s. C1s possesses an esterase activity, which is activated when C1 binds to two adjoining Fc regions of antigen bound IgM or IgG.

Immune complexes containing IgM are more efficient at complement activation than those containing IgG because IgM is a pentamer. Thus even one IgM molecule provides two adjacent Fc regions, the minimum number required for C1 activation. In contrast to IgM, about 600 IgG molecules are required to generate two IgG molecules that are sufficiently close for simultaneous binding by C1.

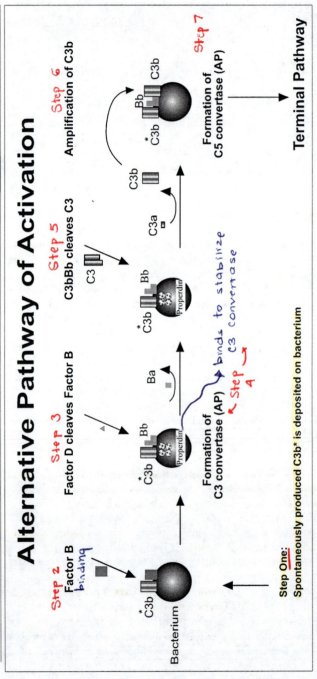

Fig. 5.3. Complement activation: alternative pathway. Activation of complement by the alternative pathway begins when spontaneously generated C3b* is deposited on a microbial surface. Factor B binds to membrane bound C3b*. Factor D proteolytically cleaves Factor B to generate Bb and Ba. Ba is released. Bb remains bound to C3b* forming a C3 convertase complex covalently attached to the microbial surface. This complex is stabilized by properdin. The C3 convertase binds to C3, cleaving it into two fragments, C3a and C3b. C3a, an anaphylatoxin, is released. Newly generated C3b remains bound to the C3b*Bb complex forming a C5 convertase (C3b*BbC3b) which cleaves C5 to generate fragments initiating activation of the terminal pathway.

Soluble Mediators of Immunity II: Complement

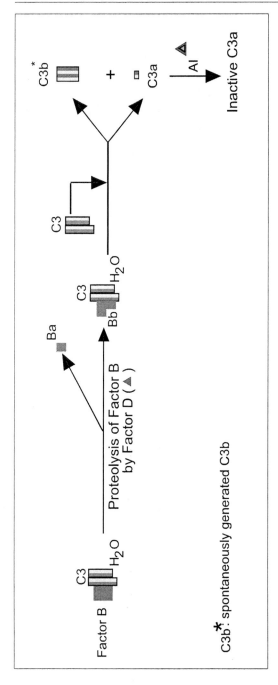

Fig. 5.4. Spontaneous generation of C3b ("tickover"). C3 interacts with water to form the C3 (H$_2$O) molecule that binds Factor B. In this form Factor B can be cleaved by Factor D to generate C3 (H$_2$O)-Bb. This fluid phase complex hydrolyzes C3 and generates C3a and C3b. In the absence of an appropriate activating surface, C3b is inactivated by Factor I using Factor H as cofactor. The anaphylatoxin inhibitor, AI, inactivates C3a.

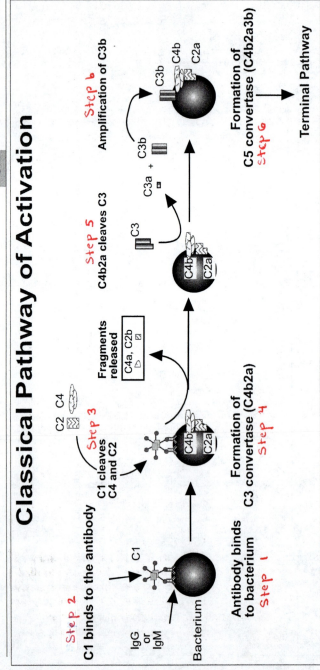

Fig. 5.5. Complement activation: classical pathway. Classical pathway activation occurs following binding of an antigen/antibody complex (IgG or IgM) by C1. C1 cleaves C4 and C2. Fragments C4a, an anaphylatoxin, and C2b, a kinin, are released into the fluid phase. Fragments C4b and C2a form a C3 convertase complex covalently linked to the microbial cell surface. The C3 convertase binds to C3, cleaving it into two fragments, C3a and C3b. C3a, an anaphylatoxin, is released. C3b remains bound to the C4bC2a complex forming a C5 convertase (C4bC2aC3b), cleaving C5 to generate fragments that activate the terminal pathway.

C1 cleaves C4 into two fragments, C4a and C4b. Deposition of C4b onto a microbial (or other antigen) surface is rapidly followed by C2 binding adjacent to the C4b. C2 is also cleaved proteolytically by C1. The C4b2a complex so generated is the **classical complement pathway C3 convertase**. This C3 convertase is an enzymatic complex that cleaves C3 to C3a and C3b. The formation of this C3 convertase is the hallmark of classical complement pathway activation, with the products generated (C3a and C3b) playing a major role in host defense, and further progression (C3b) of the complement cascade. C3b is required for the formation of the **classical complement pathway C5 convertase** (C4b2a3b), which cleaves C5 proteolytically to generate C5a and C5b. Subsequent events are the same as for the alternate complement pathway. The biological roles of the proteolytically derived complement proteins are described below.

Terminal complement pathway: Activation
Activation of either the alternate or the classical complement pathways generates C5b, the initiator molecule for the formation of the **membrane attack complex (MAC)** in the **terminal complement pathway** (Fig. 5.6). Insertion of the MAC into the target membrane induces osmotic lysis and death of the microbe (or cell).

COMPLEMENT BIOLOGICAL ACTIVITIES

Although the alternative and classical pathways differ with respect to their components and their mode of activation, many of the proteolytically derived fragments are the same for both pathways (Fig. 5.2). The role of these products is the same regardless of how they were generated.

C3a and C5a
C3a and C5a are **anaphylatoxins** generated by the action of the C3 and C5 convertases on the complement proteins C3 and C5, respectively. These molecules bind to cognate receptors on mast cells and basophils inducing degranulation, resulting in the release of histamine and other inflammatory mediators. Histamine increases vascular permeability, a requirement for recruiting cells from the blood into tissues. C5a is also chemotactic for phagocytes, recruiting these cells to the site of infection. Both the induction of histamine release and **chemotaxis** of neutrophils contribute to the initiation of the inflammatory response. The anaphylatoxin **C4a** is generated only following activation of the classical pathway.

C3b
C3b has numerous biological roles. When deposited on microbial surfaces it serves as an opsonin; when deposited on immune complexes it facilitates the elimination of immune complexes; when utilized by the alternative pathway, it amplifies complement activity because C3b is a component of the alternative pathway C3 convertase. In addition, C3b is required for the formation of the C5 convertases of both the alternative (C3bBbC3b) and the classical (C4b2a3b) complement pathways.

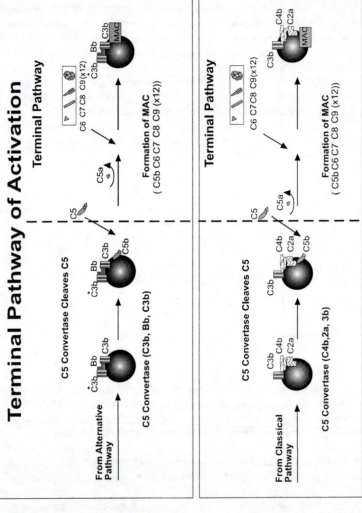

Fig. 5.6. Complement activation: terminal pathway. C5 convertases, derived from the classical or alternate pathways, generate C5a and C5b from C5. C5a, an anaphylatoxin, is released. C5b is deposited on the microbial cell membrane. Formation of MAC is initiated when C5b is deposited on the microbial surface. Components C6, C7, C8, and C9 (x12) are sequentially deposited on the microbial surface.

C5b

C5b is generated by the action of C5 convertases on the complement protein, C5. The formation and deposition of the proteolytically derived C5b proteolytic fragment onto cell surfaces serves as the stimulus for the formation of the membrane attack complex (C5b, C6, C7, C8, C9). The membrane attack complex induces osmotic lysis of the cells (or microbes) on which it forms.

C2b

C2b is produced by C1 acting on C2 in the classical pathway. C2b is a weak kinin that increases vascular permeability, and in doing so contributes to the genesis of inflammation.

COMPLEMENT REGULATION

Complement activity and deleterious complement effects on autologous cells are minimized by a variety of membrane-associated and soluble proteins (Figs. 5.7-5.9). Some are associated exclusively with one complement activation pathway or another, while others have a more general action. These proteins function in a species-specific manner, a fact that takes on great significance in the field of xenotransplantation (transplantation of organs/tissues across different species).

- **Factor I**   In the presence of any one of the cofactors, complement receptor 1 (CR1), Factor H, or membrane cofactor protein (MCP), C3b (soluble or membrane bound) is cleaved by Factor I to yield the inactive form, C3bi. Factor I also cleaves C4b to its inactive form, C4bi, in the presence of cofactors CR1, MCP, or C4 binding protein (C4bp).

- **Factor H**   As well as being a cofactor for Factor I, Factor H binds to C3b in the fluid phase thus preventing C3b from binding to the cell surface. When the alternative pathway C3 convertase has formed, Factor H competitively binds with C3b, inducing the dissociation of this convertase.

- **DAF**   Decay accelerating factor (DAF) binds to membrane bound C4b and C3b, blocking the formation of the alternative and classical pathway C3 convertases. When the C3 convertases have already formed, DAF competitively binds with C3b, or C4b, promoting their dissociation.

- **C4bp**   In addition to its role as a cofactor for Factor I, C4 binding protein (C4bp) binds to fluid phase C4b, preventing its attachment to cells. When the classical C3 convertase has already formed, C4bp competitively binds with C4b, promoting its dissociation.

- **CR1**   As well as being a cofactor for Factor I, complement receptor 1 (CR1) binds to membrane bound C4b and C3b, blocking the formation of the alternative and classical pathway C3 convertases. When the C3 convertases have already formed, CR1 competitively binds with C3b, or C4b, promoting their dissociation. In addition,

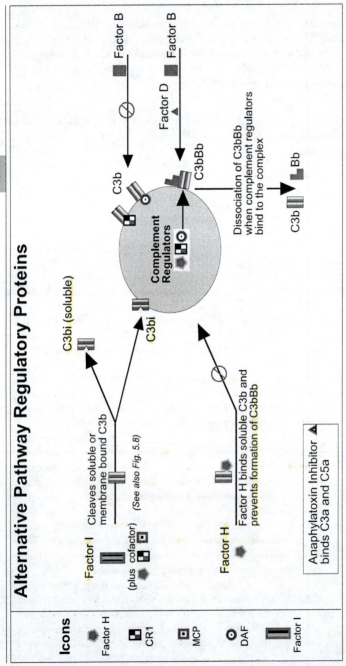

Fig. 5.7. Regulatory proteins: alternative complement pathway. Regulatory complement proteins protect autologous cells from alternative pathway complement mediated damage—see text for details.

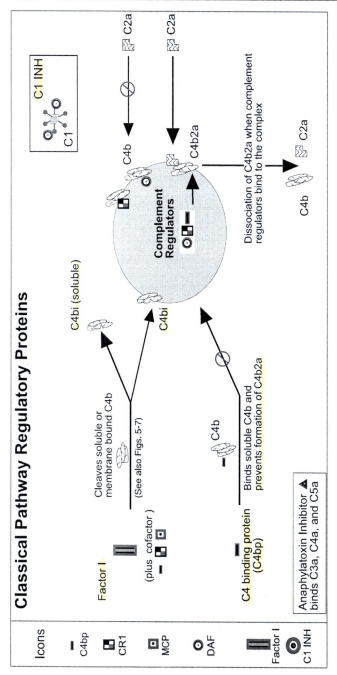

Fig. 5.8. Regulatory proteins: classical complement pathway. Regulatory complement proteins protect autologous cells from classical pathway complement mediated damage—see text for details.

Terminal Pathway

MAC is → C5b C6 C7 C8 C9 (x12)

HRF → MAC (Autologous Cell)
MAC ← S-protein
CD59 → MAC

Anaphylatoxin Inhibitor ▲ binds C5a

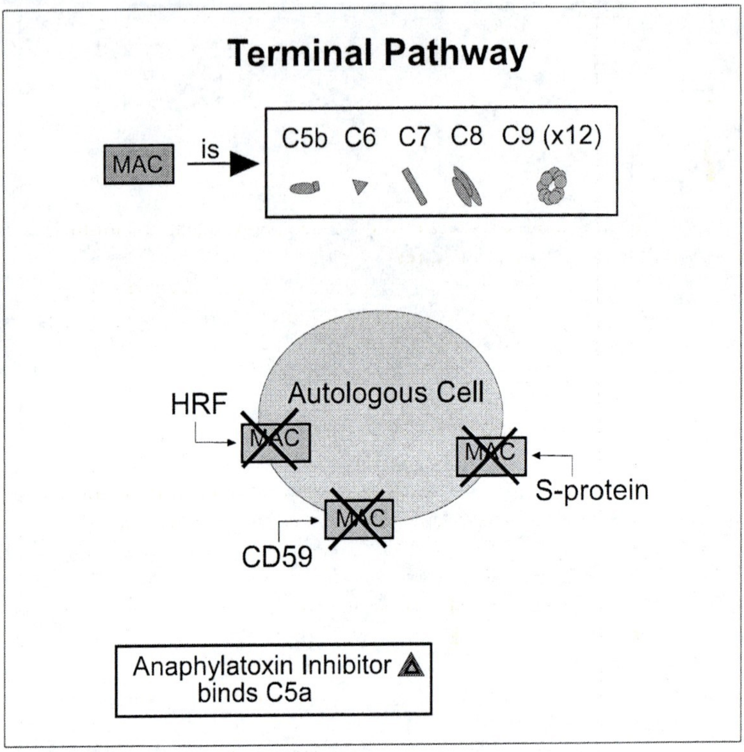

Fig. 5.9. Regulatory proteins: terminal complement pathway. S protein, HRF (homologous restriction factor) and CD59 all inhibit the formation of the membrane attack complex (MAC). S-protein, or vitronectin, binds to soluble C5bC6C7 complex preventing insertion into autologous membranes. CD59 and HRF bind to C8 preventing the binding and polymerization of C9 and concomitant formation of MAC.

	CR1 binds to membrane bound C3bi and C4bi, preventing their degradation to biologically active molecules
MCP	Membrane cofactor protein (MCP) is a cofactor for Factor I.
AI	The anaphylatoxin inhibitor (AI) binds to C3a, C4a, and C5a, inhibiting their binding to receptors on mast cells and basophils.
C1 INH	The C1 esterase inhibitor (C1 INH) forms a complex with C1, preventing the spontaneous activation of the classical complement pathway. In addition to inhibiting C1, the C1 INH inactivates kallikrein. Kallikrein links the complement and intrinsic coagulation pathways (see below).
MAC INH	MAC inhibitors (MAC INH) include homologous restriction factor (HRF), S-protein, and CD59. These inhibit formation of MAC on autologous cells. S-protein, or vitronectin, binds to soluble [C5b,

C6, C7] complexes preventing their insertion into autologous membranes. CD59 and HRF bind to C8, preventing the binding and polymerization of C9 and formation of MAC.

COMPLEMENT AND COAGULATION PATHWAYS ARE LINKED VIA KALLIKREIN

Intrinsic coagulation pathway generates kallikrein
The complement and the contact intrinsic coagulation systems are intimately linked via the plasma protein **kallikrein**, the enzymatic form of the zymogen, prekallikrein (Fig. 5.10). The conversion of prekallikrein to its enzymatic form follows activation of the intrinsic coagulation system. This coagulation system is activated in response to tissue damage. More specifically, tissue damage triggers the activation of Factor XII, one of the components of this coagulation pathway. The mechanism by which contact with damaged tissue activates Factor XII remains an enigma. The activated form of Factor XII is designated Factor XII(a). Factor XII(a), in the presence of kininogen, cleaves prekallikrein to form the active protease kallikrein. Interestingly, kallikrein serves to enhance the intrinsic coagulation pathway by proteolytically converting Factor XII to Factor XII(a) in the presence of a cofactor, kininogen. In doing so, the amount of available Factor XII(a) is amplified and so is the coagulation process. The two proteins, Factor XII (a) and kallikrein reciprocally activate one another.

The interactive roles of Factor XII and prekallikrein in the intrinsic coagulation pathway have been well studied. More recent reports have shown that the complement protein, C5, serves as a kallikrein substrate, in vitro, with C5a and C5b as products of the reaction (Figs. 5.10, 5.11). Another kallikrein substrate is **kininogen**. Proteolytic hydrolysis of kininogen generates kininogen(a) and **bradykinin**, a potent vasodilator that increases vascular permeability. Bradykinin is important in the establishment of an inflammatory response. Activated kallikrein is inhibited when it forms a complex with the complement C1 esterase inhibitor (C1 INH).

COMPLEMENT GENETIC DEFICIENCIES

General features
Genetic deficiencies have been reported for virtually every component of complement. Only a few are considered here. Clinical manifestations in those patients with complement deficiencies depend on the role of the defective complement component. Deficiencies in proteins required for initiation, or further progression, of the complement cascade result in an increased susceptibility to microbial infections. In contrast, deficiencies in the regulatory components lead to uncontrolled complement activation and damage to host tissues, generally reflected by the secondary effects of increased vascular permeability (edema) and of mediator release (histamine-induced smooth muscle contraction, with bronchoconstriction/abdominal cramps etc.).

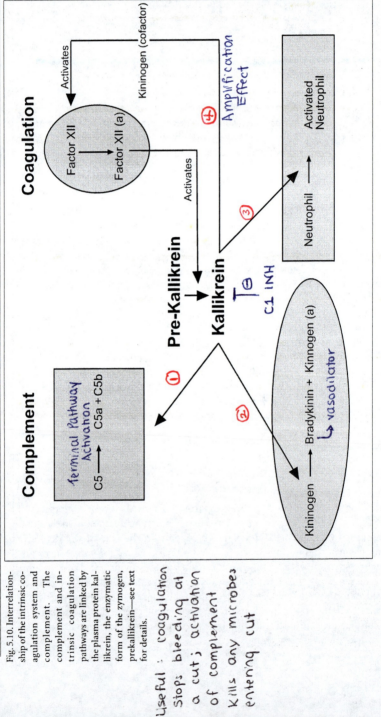

Fig. 5.10. Interrelationship of the intrinsic coagulation system and complement. The complement and intrinsic coagulation pathways are linked by the plasma protein kallikrein, the enzymatic form of the zymogen, prekallikrein—see text for details.

4 Effects of Kallikrein

Useful: coagulation stops bleeding at a cut; activation of complement kills any microbes entering cut

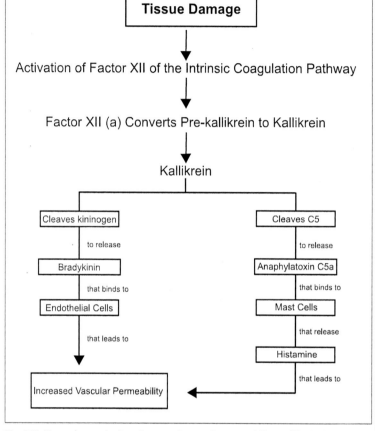

Fig. 5.11. Tissue damage leads to increases in vascular permeability. Kallikrein is a protease acting on kininogen and C5 of the complement system. Hydrolysis of kininogen produces bradykinin, while one of the products of C5 proteolysis is C5a, an anaphylatoxin. C5a binds to receptors on basophils and mast cells inducing degranulation and histamine release. Histamine alters vascular permeability, while bradykinin mediates vasodilatation and increased vascular permeability.

C1 esterase inhibitor deficiency: Disrupted regulation

C1 esterase inhibitor (C1 INH) deficiency is an inherited autosomal and recessive complement disorder associated with the disease **hereditary angioedema** (HAE). HAE may result from the synthesis of a mutated C1 INH protein or insufficient production of a normal protein. Clinical manifestations are recurrent episodes of facial/tongue and laryngeal edema that may cause obstruction of the upper airways. C1 INH deficiency may lead to edema of the gastrointestinal tract which presents as colic or diarrhea. These clinical manifestations occur following dysregulation of the normal inflammatory mechanisms that induce increases in vascular permeability.

C1 INH normally inhibits spontaneous activation of the classical complement protein, C1, and inactivates kallikrein, a protease that functions in the intrinsic blood coagulation cascade. Without adequate C1 INH inhibition, C1 spontaneously triggers the classical complement cascade, with cleavage of C4 and C2, along with formation of the C3 convertase (C4b2a). Various regulatory proteins ensure that the C3 convertase is readily dissociated, should it form on the host cell surface. However, the other products generated, C4a and C2b, are molecules which increase vascular permeability. C4a is a weak anaphylatoxin that binds to receptors on mast cells and basophils to induce degranulation and histamine release. The C2b fragment is a kinin that causes vasodilatation of the postcapillary venules and subcutaneous edema.

Complement activation often causes local tissue damage, reflecting the innocent bystander effect of proximity to nonspecific inflammatory agents. Tissue damage triggers the activation of Factor XII of the intrinsic coagulation pathway enzyme, which initiates a series of activation events leading to the generation of kallikrein, whose enzymatic activity generates the potent vasodilators C5a and bradykinin. Under normal circumstances, C1 INH inactivates kallikrein, and the associated production of C5a and bradykinin.

In the absence of C1 INH protein, normal inflammatory mechanisms that increase vascular permeability are unregulated. These mechanisms include the uncontrolled production of anaphylatoxins (C3a, C4a, and C5a) and kinins (C2b and bradykinin), again resulting in edema. The unregulated production of anaphylatoxins overwhelms the capability of the anaphylatoxin inhibitors.

Deficiencies in glycosylphosphatidylinositol anchors: Disrupted regulation

The regulatory proteins, decay accelerating protein (DAF), CD59, and homologous restriction factor (HRF) are anchored to cell membranes via glycosylphosphatidylinositol (GPI). DAF accelerates the decay of the C3 convertases, blocking amplification of both the alternative and classical pathways. CD59 and HRF block the formation of the membrane attack complex.

A rare defect in the ability of cells to synthesize the glycosylphosphatidylinositol anchoring molecules results in a deficiency in these proteins, leaving these cells susceptible to lysis by complement. This disorder is known as **paroxysmal nocturnal haemoglobulinuria** (PNH). PNH is an inherited disorder that can manifest as hemolytic anemia. Because DAF is expressed as a GPI linkage in red blood cells but can be expressed as a normal transmembrane protein in other cells, the defect affects only the red cell lineage.

C3 protein deficiency: Disrupted activation

C3 is the major component of both the classical and the alternative pathways. Its serum concentration is the highest of all complement proteins. C3 deficiency is inherited as an autosomal recessive trait, predisposing individuals to severe recurrent pyogenic infections, further underscoring the significance of opsonin mediated phagocytosis in the elimination of infectious agents. During the normal course of complement activation, C3 is cleaved into two fragments, one of which is C3b. The deposition of C3b, an opsonin, on the microbial cell surface facilitates the interaction of phagocytes with the infectious agent.

In addition to opsonin mediated phagocytosis, C3 impacts on virtually all effector functions of complement, including opsonization, immune complex elimination, and "downstream" complement activation through formation of the C5 convertases of both the alternative and classical complement pathways. A secondary, or acquired, C3 deficiency occurs in individuals who have a primary deficiency in any of the complement regulatory components that would normally inactivate the C3 convertases. In the absence of regulatory mechanisms, C3 is consumed in an uncontrolled manner.

Terminal pathway protein deficiencies: Disrupted activation

Although activation of the alternative and classical complement pathways leads to the formation of MAC on target cells, most microbial destruction is mediated by opsonin mediated phagocytosis. Bacteria that belong to the *Neisseria sp* are not readily phagocytosed in this manner. Complement mediated destruction of these bacteria requires the insertion of MAC complexes in their cell (membranes). Therefore, individuals who have genetic deficiencies in any of the complement proteins that comprise MAC will be predisposed to recurrent meningococcal and gonococcal *Neisserial* infections.

ROLE OF COMPLEMENT IN MEDICINE

Complement activation represents one of the earliest and most powerful mechanisms of host defense, particularly in response to infections with bacteria that thrive outside cells. While the activation of complement may be protective in some situations, in other situations it is deleterious to the host.

XENOTRANSPLANTATION: COMPLEMENT IS DELETERIOUS

Xenotransplantation refers to the transplantation of a graft across species. For humans, porcine grafts may represent a solution to the shortage of human organs. A major barrier to **xenotransplantation** is the hyperacute rejection that manifests minutes to hours after the graft has been transplanted. This hyperacute rejection occurs because humans have natural (IgM) antibodies that react with the α1,3 galactosyl linkage of porcine carbohydrate antigens present on the endothelial lining of graft blood vessels. When these circulating natural human antibodies bind these porcine antigens they form immune complexes on the blood vessel wall. Because human complement proteins are always in circulation, the classic complement pathway is activated as C1 binds to the Fc regions of the bound antibodies. Complement activation leads to destruction of the endothelial cells lining the graft blood vessels and to graft thrombosis.

Damage to the endothelial cells occurs as phagocytes recruited to this site secrete inflammatory mediators that cause local tissue damage and thrombosis. The events are summarized as follows:

i	Anaphylatoxins (C3a, C4a, and C5a) are generated.
ii	Anaphylatoxins bind to receptors on mast cells and basophils.
iii	Mast cells and basophils degranulate and release histamine.
iv	Histamine enhances vascular permeability.
v	C5a is chemotactic for phagocytes. It also activates phagocytes.
vi	Phagocytes try to ingest the immune complexes and in doing so secrete inflammatory mediators that damage the endothelial cells.
vii	Damage to cells activates the intrinsic coagulation pathway, thrombosis, and the activation of kallikrein that, in turn, generates bradykinin.
viii	Bradykinin is a potent vasodilator and activator of neutrophils.
ix	Complement activation leads to the formation of membrane attack complexes on the porcine endothelial cells because these cells lack human regulatory proteins.
x	Osmotic lysis and death of the cell (porcine graft) occurs. In addition activation of macrophages leads to release of a novel procoagulant activity (fibroleukin or fgl-2) distinct from tissue factor or other known Factor X11 activators. This triggers extensive fibrin deposition (from fibrinogen) and thrombosis.

Xenografts are more susceptible to complement mediated damage than allografts because complement regulatory proteins are species specific. Therefore, even though the porcine tissue may express complement regulatory proteins, they fail to protect the graft against the effects of human complement. Theoretically, the introduction of appropriate human regulatory proteins into the xenograft should protect the graft from complement mediated damage initiated by hyperacute rejection.

Human CD59 or DAF genes have been expressed in transgenic pigs. The presence of these human proteins in the porcine tissue provided some protection from complement mediated damage when the tissue was exposed ex vivo to human complement activating proteins.

SUMMARY

Complement describes a family of proteins whose proteolytically derived fragments facilitate elimination of microorganisms, particularly extracellular bacteria. These proteolytically derived fragments: (i) facilitate the interaction of phagocytes to induce opsonin-mediated phagocytosis; (ii) induce osmotic lysis of microbes; (iii) enhance vascular permeability by inducing degranulation of mast cells/basophils; (iv) induce chemotaxis of neutrophils; and (v) facilitate immune complex elimination. The facilitated interaction of phagocytes with microbes, particularly bacteria, in a manner that leads to phagocytosis of the microbe, is most significant.

The complement system is comprised of numerous (~30) activation and regulatory proteins synthesized mainly by the liver. Many circulate as dormant enzymes whose activation requires their proteolytic hydrolysis. Complement activation gives rise to a cascade of reactions in which complement proteins serve as substrates in a sequential manner. Consequently, complement activation and the ensuing cascade of biochemical reactions is best described as *the complement pathway*.

There are two pathways of complement activation, the *alternative* and the *classical*, each converging into a common/terminal pathway, that generates a membrane attack complex on the surface of susceptible cells to induce their osmotic lysis. Before this terminal pathway, complement activation by either the alternative or classical pathway leads to the formation of two enzymatic complexes, the C3 and C5 convertases, on the target cell. While not identical, the predominant differences in the convertases of the two pathways reflect more the different biologically active proteolytic fragments produced during their generation than major differences in their activity.

The initiating stimulus for activation of the alternative pathway of complement is the deposition of spontaneously generated C3b fragment onto a microbial cell surface. The initiating stimulus for activation of the classical pathway of complement is the binding of C1 to immune complexes in which either IgM or IgG is bound to antigen. Although the activation of either pathway leads to the formation of a C3 and a C5 convertase, the components of the convertases differ (*vide supra*).

The role of complement in host immunity is underscored by the pathogenicity of microbes that have evolved mechanisms to evade complement mediated destruction. As well, deficiencies of virtually all components of complement, regulatory proteins, or complement receptors have been documented. Clinical manifestations of complement deficiencies depend on the role of a given component.

Complement activity and deleterious complement effects on autologous cells are minimized by a variety of soluble, or membrane bound proteins. Some of these proteins are associated exclusively with one complement activation pathway or another, while others are protective in a more general way.

CLINICAL CASES AND DISCUSSION

Clinical Case #9
Peter is a 16-year-old boy whom you see in consultation for repeated episodes of spontaneous swelling of the lips over the last three to five years. None has been of particular medical consequence until this morning, when he came to your Hospital's Emergency Department. In addition to the swelling of lips, Peter was also experiencing some difficulty swallowing and taking a deep breath. What is a potential problem here? How would it be investigated? How would it be treated?

Discussion Case #9
Background
The complaints of difficulty swallowing and breathing sound like the complaints of a hyperallergic individual and/or asthmatic. This occurs when there is β-antagonist activation of smooth muscles and airway spasm. Further questioning and lung function tests are used to determine if this is an allergic reaction. Lung

function is determined by measuring conventional parameters. It turns out that Peter does not have asthma or a known allergy to environmental allergens. Indeed, while these might help explain these latest symptoms, they would not address the issue of the intermittent lip swelling.

This edema in the lips is caused by intermittent changes in the permeability of blood vessels, with fluid leaking from the blood into the extracellular space. This is seen in a variety of conditions where release of inflammatory mediators (including cytokines such as tumor necrosis factor (TNF), interleukin-1 (IL-1)) cause an increase in blood vessel permeability. Another physiological mechanism that regulates membrane permeability is the complement system. Factors released, or recruited, by the complement cascade have profound inflammatory effects, including alterations in vascular permeability. Spontaneous activation of the complement cascade is held in check by a number of inhibitory molecules, amongst which is the C1 esterase inhibitor (C1 INH). C1 INH binds to C1 and in so doing prevents activation of the classical complement cascade.

Tissue damage leads to the activation of the intrinsic coagulation pathway with subsequent activation of kallikrein, and generation of bradykinin, a potent vasodilator (see xenotransplantation). C1 INH also binds to and inhibits kallikrein. In the absence of C1 INH, intermittent, though generally transient, episodes of complement activation occur, with release of vasoactive byproducts leading to the lip and laryngeal edema described above.

Tests

Further investigation of this individual involves determining whether he has a congenital defect in C1 INH. The presence of C1 INH is identified by enzyme linked immunosorbent assay (ELISA) replacing the (older) functional tests for independent complement components.

Treatment

Therapy for this disorder is artificial replacement of C1 INH (intramuscular injection). The half-life of the molecule is long, so replacement therapy is intermittent.

Clinical Case #10

A patient of yours returns to the Intensive Care Unit from the Operating Room after her third renal transplant in the last ten years. The two previous grafts failed as a result of chronic rejection. Thirty minutes later she complains of severe abdominal crampy pain, has a fever, and becomes hypotensive (low blood pressure). She is returned immediately to the OR. She is not bleeding, but her graft shows extensive thrombosis. She did not receive transfusion during the surgery. What has happened and why?

Discussion of Case #10

Background

Organ graft rejection (Chapter 17) generally falls into one of two categories, acute and chronic rejection. **Acute rejection** develops over days to weeks and results from the activation of host T cells by alloantigens on the graft. This rejection is generally treated with increased immunosuppressive therapy to inhibit T-cell activation.

In contrast to acute rejection, the etiology of **chronic rejection** remains an enigma. It develops over a prolonged period of time (months to years postgrafting), and seems to follow repeated episodes of acute rejection. Although it is believed to have an immunological basis it is nevertheless relatively refractory to immunosuppressive treatment.

There are two, not uncommon, scenarios where humoral (antibody mediated) immunity plays an important role in graft rejection. Both scenarios involve **hyperacute rejection**. This reaction occurs within minutes to hours of grafting and is due to preformed antibodies that recognize antigens on the graft tissue. In a **xenotransplant** scenario (across species), the antibodies involved are preformed anti-carbohydrate antibodies that recognize species-unique sugar residues on grafted cells. In an **allotransplant** scenario (between individuals of the same species), hyperacute rejection is seen in patients who have been previously exposed (immunized) to alloantigens. **Alloantigens** are molecules present on cells of other members of the same species. Individuals most at risk for hyperacute rejection include (i) women with multiple previous pregnancies; (ii) individuals who have had multiple transfusions; and (iii) those who have had previous organ/tissue grafts. Hyperacute rejection is unresponsive to treatment, and graft removal is the only option.

Pretransplantation tests are performed to match the donor and the recipient. The laboratory *types* for antibody incompatibility between the graft and recipient (using peripheral blood cells). Sometimes, the relevant antigens are weak, and are not detected in this fashion. Alternatively, the relevant antigens are not present on the blood cells used for typing, but are tissue-specific. In this case, the relevant antigens would be unique to the kidney and not present on the peripheral blood cells used for testing.

The pathophysiology of hyperacute rejection is thus one of rapid deposition of antibody on the graft, with formation of immune complexes. C1 proteins subsequently bind to the Fc regions of antibodies present in the immune complexes. This initiates activation of the classical complement pathway, leading to the generation of anaphylatoxins and C3b deposition on the immune complexes. The anaphylatoxins bind to cognate receptors on mast cells and basophils, inducing degranulation and histamine release. The anaphylatoxin, C5a, is chemotactic for neutrophils. The presence of C3b on the immune complexes, as well as the Fc region of bound IgG antibodies, targets the immune complexes for ingestion by the neutrophils, a process termed opsonin mediated phagocytosis. This process activates neutrophils to secrete inflammatory molecules that damage the endothelium. As the endothelium is exposed, it serves to activate Factor XII, a component of the intrinsic coagulation pathway, and activation of this coagulation pathway leads to fibrin deposition and the formation of blood clots (**thrombi**) in the graft. The neutrophil mediated damage, along with the formation of thrombi, constitutes hyperacute graft failure.

For xenotransplants, a number of manipulations are under consideration to overcome the problem of hyperacute rejection. Included in these manipulations are: (i) preabsorption of host blood onto an artificial support containing xenogeneic tissue to remove anti-xenoantibodies; (ii) use of transgenic organs in which the transgene is a human complement regulatory protein (e.g., DAF); and (iii) infusion of anticomplement proteins (e.g., cobra venom factor). These molecules, found in a number of venomous species, are proteases that in some cases inactivate key complement protein molecules.

Tests
Simple inspection of the graft provides all the clinical information needed to indicate whether hyperacute rejection (and attendant thrombosis) has occurred. There are other more subtle tests for fibrin deposition, etc., but generally these are NOT be required, given the urgency of treatment.

Treatment
Remove the graft immediately and return the patient, as far as possible, to his/her initial pretransplant state. In the event of renal transplantation, hemodialysis (artificial blood filtering) could be reinstituted. Temporizing measures for patients receiving cardiac or hepatic grafts are less well-worked out.

TEST YOURSELF

Multiple Choice Questions
1. The classical pathway C5 convertase is composed of all the following EXCEPT
    a. C4b
    b. C5b
    c. C2a
    d. C3b
2. All the following are anaphylatoxins and induce degranulation of mast cells and basophils EXCEPT
    a. C2a
    b. C3a
    c. C4a
    d. C5a
3. All the following directly inhibit the formation of MAC EXCEPT
    a. S-protein
    b. CD59
    c. HRF
    d. CR1
4. When C3b is deposited onto a bacterial surface, the alternative pathway of complement is activated and a C3 convertase is assembled on the micro-

bial surface. Complement components directly/indirectly required for formation/stabilization of this C3 convertase include all the following EXCEPT
   a. Properdin
   b. Factor B
   c. Factor D
   d. Factor H
   e. C3b
5. A young girl has documented Neisseria meningitis. No family history is available (the girl was adopted) but review of her medical record from a forwarding hospital reveals an otherwise previously well child with three episodes of Neisseria over 2 years. Which is not an explanation of these findings?
   a. Low C3
   b. Low C6-C8
   c. Absent factor D
   d. Absent properdin
   e. C1 INH deficiency

Answers: 1b ; 2a ; 3d ; 4d ; 5e

Short Answer Questions
1. Complement serves primarily as a first line of defense against which class of organisms?
2. Which tissue synthesizes most of the complement proteins?
3. List the five biological activities of complement. Which components mediate each function?
4. Explain why IgM is more effective at activating complement than IgG.
5. List the steps that lead to the destruction of a porcine graft in hyperacute rejection.

Soluble Mediators of Immunity III: Cytokines

Objectives	110
Cytokines	111
General Features	111
Cytokine Receptors That Engage the JAK/STAT Pathway	111
Cytokine Receptors That Engage SMADs	117
Biological Activities of Cytokines That Signal via the JAK/STAT Pathway	117
Clinical Relevance of Cytokines	120
Chemokines	124
Summary	125
Clinical Cases and Discussion	126
Test Yourself	128

Objectives

Cytokines are produced by cells of both the acquired immune system (lymphocytes) as well as the cells of the innate system (macrophages, mast cells etc.). Other cells (e.g., fibroblasts) not considered classically to belong to the immune system, per se, can also produce such molecules. The importance of cytokines lies in their ability to influence a number of functions in different cells/cell systems. In addition to contributing to the regulation of cell:cell communication and differentiation in the immune system, inflammatory cytokines are themselves activators of the inflammatory cascade.

Despite the multiplicity of cytokines described, order to the complexity in their numbers comes from the manner in which the different cytokines deliver signals to cells. These signaling cascades are complex, involving activation of kinases through a series of phosphorylation/dephosphorylation steps, and ultimately the delivery of transcriptional regulators to the cell nucleus for differential gene activation. Many cytokines use similar receptors to deliver their signals, which helps us understand some of the redundancy in the cytokine, and cytokine receptor, families. This redundancy exists at the functional level, implying they play a critical role in normal homeostasis.

We conclude with a brief discussion of a newly discovered family of molecules, the chemokines. These molecules are involved in multiple facets of immunity, beyond their role in cell chemotaxis (the role for which they were first recognized). Current clinical interest has focused on the role chemokine antagonists might play in regulating inflammation.

Clinical Immunology, by Reginald Gorczynski and Jacqueline Stanley. 2001 Landes Bioscience

CYTOKINES

GENERAL FEATURES

Cytokines are small peptides secreted mainly by activated leukocytes. Different **cytokines** may trigger the same biological responses, a characteristic termed "functional redundancy". Additionally, cytokines are pleiotropic, with each cytokine mediating numerous seemingly unrelated biological effects. The cells targeted by cytokines constitutively express low affinity receptors, whose conversion to a high affinity state requires association with one or more transmembrane signaling molecules to form a receptor complex. For some cytokine receptors, the signaling molecule(s) is/are unique to that receptor, while for others, the signaling molecule(s) is/are component(s) of several cytokine receptor complexes. This may help explain the functional redundancy referred to earlier (Fig. 6.1).

The pleiotropic nature and functional redundancy of cytokines presents a challenge for simplified and concise presentation. Our approach is to consider that cytokine binding to cognate receptors triggers signal transduction events that determine the biological response of the cell expressing the cytokine receptor. The organization of this chapter, therefore, describes families of cytokines whose receptors share common signaling molecules, as well as individual cytokines which signal via receptors that function independently, without sharing signaling molecules (Table 6.1). Clinical scenarios in which genetic deficiencies in one signaling molecule inhibit the activities of numerous cytokines, using the same molecule, underscores the significance of shared signaling molecules.

Cytokine receptors can be classed as: (i) molecules not possessing any catalytic activity but recruiting, or associating with, catalytic proteins, usually tyrosine kinases; (ii) molecules that are intrinsic serine/threonine kinases; and (iii) molecules associated with several, poorly defined, pathways (Fig. 6.2).

CYTOKINE RECEPTORS THAT ENGAGE THE JAK/STAT PATHWAY

Janus tyrosine kinases

Cytokine receptors that engage the JAK/STAT pathway possess no intrinsic activity. These receptors associate with one or more members of the family of tyrosine kinases, named the **Janus tyrosine kinases (JAKs)**. Four JAK kinases have been identified that participate in cytokine signaling, **JAK 1, JAK 2, JAK 3**, and **TYK2**. JAK association with the cytokine receptor complex has some element of specificity because JAKs preferentially associate with distinct receptor molecules (Table 6.2). JAK 1 and JAK 2 association with the interferon gamma receptor (IFNγR) is illustrated in Figure 6.3.

JAK substrates

In resting cells, JAK kinases are inactive. **JAK kinases** are activated by transphosphorylation when they are brought into close proximity to one another following cytokine binding to one or more cytokine receptor components. The cytokine

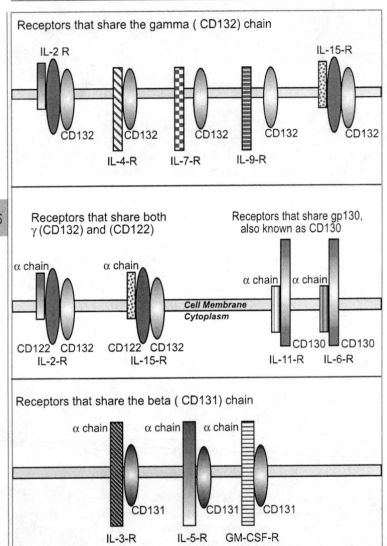

Fig. 6.1. Cytokine receptor families defined by shared signaling molecules. Many cytokine receptors share components, which is useful in their classification.

receptors themselves serve as JAK substrates. Cytokine receptors that signal via the JAK/STAT pathway exhibit common structural properties such as the characteristic *src* homology 2 (SH2) domain, within which is located the tyrosine residue(s) that serve as JAK target(s). When phosphorylated, the SH2 binding motifs become docking sites for binding proteins that structurally link the recep-

Table 6.1. Receptor families, signaling pathways, and cytokines

Receptor	Pathway	Cytokines
Independent	JAK/STAT	IFNγ, IL-10, IL-12, and IFNα/β
Utilize CD130	JAK/STAT	IL-6, and IL-11
Utilize CDw131	JAK/STAT	IL-3, IL-5, and GM-CSF
Utilize CD132	JAK/STAT	IL-2, IL-4, IL-7, IL-9, and IL-15
Utilize CD122	JAK/STAT	IL-2, and IL-15
Independent	Poorly Resolved	TNF, IL-1
Ser./Thr. Kinase	SMAD	TGFβ

tor complex to signaling pathways. Proteins that are recruited to the docking site include the **STAT proteins**. STAT protein family members, named STAT 1 through to STAT 6, are latent transcription factors for genes that are expressed in response to cytokines.

Signaling via the JAK/STAT pathway

One of the most extensively studied cytokine receptors is the IFNγR. This receptor is unique because it recruits only one STAT protein. However, the overall concept associated with IFNγR signaling is generalizeable to other cytokine receptors that use the JAK/STAT pathway. IFNγ binds to the monomeric alpha chain and induces its noncovalent homodimerization (Fig. 6.3). The homodimeric nature of IFNγ facilitates this association. Alpha chain homodimerization is followed by the interaction of two IFNγR beta subunits with this intermediary complex, forming a functional IFNγ/IFNγR complex (IFNγ, two IFNγR alpha subunits, and two IFNγR beta subunits).

The ligand-induced association of alpha and beta subunits brings into juxtaposition the JAK 1 and JAK 2 tyrosine kinases that transphosphorylate one another and then phosphorylate the alpha subunit of the IFNγ receptor. The phosphorylation of tyrosine residues on the IFNγR alpha subunit creates binding sites recognized by proteins with SH2 domains. The latent transcription factor, STAT 1α, expresses an SH2 domain, and is recruited to the alpha subunit where it is activated when phosphorylated by JAKs. Phosphorylated STAT 1α molecules dissociate from the alpha subunit, homodimerize, and translocate to the nucleus. STAT dimers bind to related GAS (interferon **g**amma **a**ssociated **s**equences) and activate transcription. For cytokine receptors where more than one STAT protein becomes recruited to the receptor, these STAT proteins also heterodimerize.

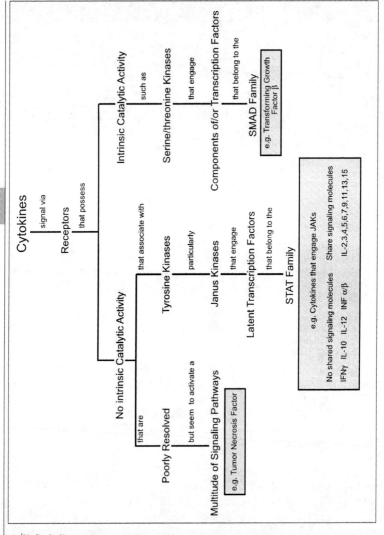

Fig. 6.2. Concept map depicting signaling properties of cytokine receptors. Cytokine receptors are classified according to their intrinsic enzymatic properties.

Soluble Mediators of Immunity III: Cytokines 115

Table 6.2. Cytokine receptors that share receptor components and use the JAK/STAT pathway of signaling

Receptor	Receptor Components	CD Designation	CD122 IL-2Rβ	CDw130 Gp130	CD131 βc	CD132 γc	JAK	STAT
IL-6	alpha subunit gp130	CD126 CD130	—	+	—	—	1,2, T2	1, 3
IL-11	alpha subunit gp130	——— CD130	—	+	—	—	1,2, T2	1, 3
IL-3	alpha subunit β common chain	CD123 CDw131	—	—	+	—	2	5
IL-5	alpha subunit β common chain	CDw125 CDw131	—	—	+	—	2	5
GM-CSF	alpha subunit β common chain	——— CDw131	—	—	+	—	2	5
IL-4	alpha subunit γ common chain	CD124 CD132	—	—	—	+	1 3	6 5
IL-7	alpha subunit γ common chain	CD127 CD132	—	—	—	+	1 3	3 5
IL-9	alpha subunit γ common chain	——— CD132	—	—	—	+	1 3	3 5
IL-2	alpha subunit IL-2-R β γ common chain	CD25 CD122 CD132	+	—	—	+	1 3	3 5
IL-15	alpha subunit IL-2-R β γ common chain	——— CD122 CD132	+	—	—	+	1 3	3 5

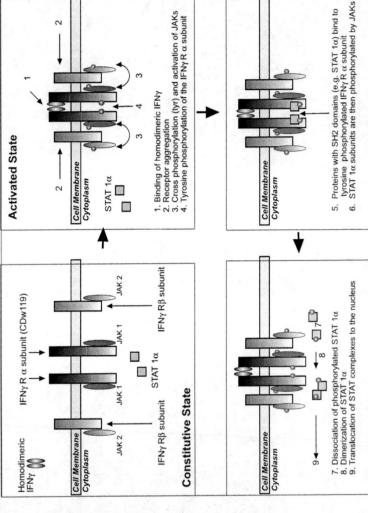

Fig. 6.3. Signaling via the IFNγ receptor complex. Interferon gamma binds to the monomeric alpha chain and induces its noncovalent homodimerization. Interaction of two beta subunits with this intermediary complex forms a functional IFNγR complex. The ligand-induced association of alpha and beta subunits brings into juxtaposition the JAK tyrosine kinases that transphosphorylate one another, and then phosphorylate the receptor alpha subunits. The latent transcription factor, STAT 1α, expresses an SH2 domain and is recruited to the alpha subunit where it is activated following phosphorylation by JAKs. STAT 1α molecules dissociate from the alpha subunit, homodimerize, and translocate to the nucleus.

Cytokine Receptors that Engage SMADs

Intrinsic serine/threonine receptor kinases
In contrast to cytokine receptors that associate with JAK tyrosine kinases, the transforming growth factor beta (TGFβ) cytokine receptor is an intrinsic serine/threonine kinase. TGFβ signals through a receptor complex formed by two types of serine/threonine kinase polypeptides, termed type I and type II. Type II polypeptides are the ligand binding moiety, while the type I polypeptide mediates signaling (Fig. 6.4). The emerging model of signaling via the TGFβ receptor complex suggests that it is a tetramer containing two copies of each type I and type II polypeptides.

The intrinsic serine/threonine kinases of the receptor are activated by cross phosphorylation following ligand binding. The activated receptor complex is a scaffold for proteins, many of which are substrates for the receptor kinase. Members of a family of proteins, termed SMADs, are activated by receptor mediated phosphorylation (Fig. 6.4). Phosphorylated SMADs dissociate from the receptor, forming either hetero-oligomeric or dimeric complexes with a cytosolic SMAD that is not recruited to the receptor complex. These SMAD complexes translocate to the nucleus where they complex with multiple DNA binding proteins to initiate transcription in response to TGFβ. SMAD complexes may also regulate transcription by binding directly to DNA.

Biological Activities of Cytokines That Signal via the JAK/STAT Pathway

The biological activities of cytokines are determined by two major factors, the physiological function of the cell expressing the cytokine receptor (the cytokine target) and the signaling molecules that link the receptor to signal transduction cascades and gene transcription (Table 6.3). Many cytokines mediate their effects through receptors that signal via the JAK/STAT pathway, and these cytokines can be classified according to the signaling molecules that they share. When cytokines, signal via receptors that have a single signaling molecule shared with other cytokine receptors, there is a great overlap with respect to biological function (e.g., interleukin-6 (IL-6) and IL-11) (Table 6.4). For some cytokines the overlap in biological function is not as great as one would predict, which may reflect undetermined signaling via other components of the receptor complex (e.g., IL-3, IL-5, and granulocyte monocyte colony stimulating factor (GM-CSF) (Table 6.5). The degree of functional redundancy, observed for the IL-2 and the IL-15 cytokines, reflects the fact that their receptors share two signaling molecules (Table 6.6). Other cytokines (IL-4, IL-7 and IL-9) that share only one of these signaling molecules with IL-2 and IL-15, exhibit less functional redundancy with them (Table 6.6). Some cytokines signal via the JAK/STAT pathway, but exhibit no overlap in biological function (IFNγ, IFNα/β, IL-10 and IL-12 (Table 6.7). The signal transduction cascades recruited following binding of tumor necrosis factor (TNF) to its

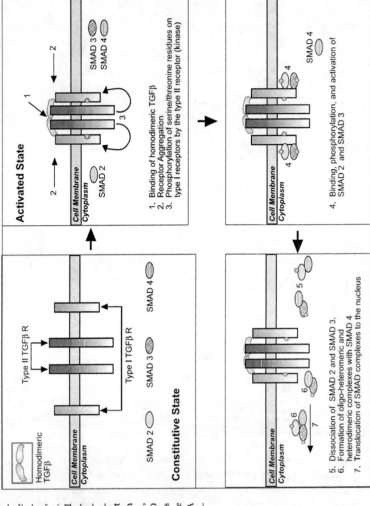

Fig. 6.4. Signaling via the TGFβ receptor complex. TGFβ binds to type II TGFβ receptors, triggering receptor aggregation with type I receptors, as well as their phosphorylation. SMAD2 and SMAD3 bind to type I receptors where they are phosphorylated and released from the receptor complex. Released SMADs associate with SMAD 4 (which does not bind to the TGFβ receptor) to form either hetero-oliogmeric (SMAD 2, 3, 4) or dimeric (SMAD 2, 4; SMAD 3, 4) complexes. These complexes translocate to the nucleus where they complex with multiple DNA binding proteins to initiate transcription.

Soluble Mediators of Immunity III: Cytokines

Table 6.3. The major cell sources and cell targets of cytokines

Cytokine	Major Cell Source	Major Immunological Cell Target
Cytokines that use CD130		
IL-6	Monocytes, macrophages, fibroblasts, keratinocytes	B cells, hepatocytes, pluripotent stem cells
IL-11	Bone marrow stromal fibroblasts	B cells, hepatocytes, pluripotent stem cells
Cytokines that use CD122 and CD132		
IL-2	CD4+ T cells	CD8+ T cells, NK cells, preactivated CD4+ T cells and B cells
IL-15	Fibroblasts, epithelial cells, adherent PBM cells*	CD8+ T cells, NK cells, preactivated CD4+ T cells and B cells
Cytokines that use CD132 (not CD122)		
IL-4	CD4+ Th2 cells, mast cells	T cells, B cells, neutrophils, fibroblasts, monocytes/macrophages
IL-7	Bone marrow stromal cells	Thymocytes, Pre-B cells, NK cells, T cells, macrophages
IL-9	CD4+ Th2 cells	Activated T cells, activated B cells
Cytokines that use CDw131		
IL-3	T cells, mast cells	Hematopoietic cells, myeloid progenitors,
IL-5	T cells, mast cells	Hematopoietic cells, eosinophils, myeloid progenitors
GM-CSF	T cells, macrophages, bone marrow stromal fibroblasts	Hematopoietic cells, myeloid progenitors
Cytokines that do not share signaling chains		
IFNγ	CD4+ Th1 cells, NK cells	Monocytes, macrophages, NK cells, T cells, B cells
IL-10	CD4+ Th2 cells	Monocytes, macrophages, NK cells, T cells, B cells
IL-12	Dendritic cells, macrophages	NK cells, CD4+ T cells
IFN α/β	Virally infected cells	Most cells
Cytokines whose receptors are not resolved		
TNF	Macrophages, CD4+ Th1 cells	Most cells
IL-1	Macrophages	T cells, B cells monocytes, macrophages, neutrophils
Cytokines whose receptors are intrinsic kinase		
TGFβ	T cells, macrophages	T cells, B cells, NK cells

* peripheral blood mononuclear cells

Table 6.4. Biological activities of cytokines that utilize CD130 and signal via JAK/STATs

	IL-6	IL-11
1. Differentiation of activated B cells to Ig secreting plasma cells	+	+
2. Induction of acute phase proteins by hepatocytes	+	+
3. Stimulate pluripotent stem cells to respond to IL-3, IL-5, GM-CSF	+	+
4. Maturation of megakaryocytes	+	+
5. Osteoclastogenesis and thus osteoporosis	+	?

Table 6.5. Biological activities of cytokines that share CDw131 and signal via JAK/STATs

	IL-3	IL-5	GM-CSF
Hematopoietic growth factor	+	+	+
Induces growth and differentiation of myeloid progenitors	+		
Growth and differentiation factor for eosinophils		+	
Growth and differentiation of myeloid progenitor to monocytes and neutrophils			+

receptor are poorly understood, although the biological activities of TNF are well documented (Table 6.8).

CLINICAL RELEVANCE OF CYTOKINES

Interferon gamma (IFNγ)

Immunosuppressed individuals, particularly those with deficiencies in CD4+ T cells (e.g., HIV patients) are unable to produce significant quantities of IFNγ. These individuals are at significant risk for uncontrolled proliferation of *Mycobacterium sp.*, a problem further exacerbated by the evolution of drug resistance in several strains of *Mycobacterium tuberculosis*.

Children with mutations in one chain of the IFNγ receptor have a predisposition to infection with weakly pathogenic strains of mycobacteria, but not to viral infections, or to most strains of bacteria. In these individuals infection with *Mycobacterium tuberculosis* generally causes disseminated infection (not one localized to the respiratory tract as in most healthy individuals) with high mortality. In many third world countries, immunization with **Bacillus Calmette-Guerin (BCG)**, an attenuated strain of *Mycobacterium bovis*, provides some protection against tuberculosis. In healthy individuals, BCG vaccination is typically innocuous. In immunocompromised individuals or in individuals with inactivating mutations in the IFNγ receptor, this immunization can be fatal.

Soluble Mediators of Immunity III: Cytokines

Table 6.6. Biological activities of cytokines that signal via CD122 and/or CD132

	IL-2	IL-15	IL-4	IL-7	IL-9
Differentiation of pre-B cells to B cells				+	
Differentiation of pre-T cells to T cells	+		+		
Differentiation of pre-T cells to NK cells		+			
Differentiation of naive CD4+ T cells to Th2			+		
Differentiation of naive CD8+ T cells to CTL	+				
Isotype switching to IgE			+		
Stabilize mRNA for IL-3 and GM-CSF					+
Stimulates production of nitric oxide		+			
Regulation of erythropoiesis					+
Proliferation of pre-B cells				+	
Proliferation of pre-T cells	+		+		
Proliferation of preactivated B cells	+		+		+
Proliferation of preactivated T cell subsets	+	+	+	+	+
Proliferation of preactivated NK cells	+	+	+		

Table 6.7. Biological activities of independent receptors that engage the JAK/STAT pathway

	IFNγ	IL-10	IL-12	IFNα/β
Differentiation of Monocytes to Macrophages	+			
Differentiation of Th0 to Th1	+		+	
Isotype Switching of B cells (IgG2a and IgG3)	+			
Enhances Macrophage Cytotoxicity	+			
Inhibits Cytokine Secretion by Macrophages		+		
Inhibits Cytokine Secretion by NK and Th1 Cells		+		
Enhances NK Cell Cytotoxicity			+	
Antiviral Effects				+

Interleukin-12

IL-12 is a potential therapeutic agent for individuals infected systemically by protozoa of the species *Leishmania*. *Leishmania sp.* are intracellular parasites that infect and thrive within macrophages. Macrophages productively infected with these parasites express decreased levels of class II MHC and produce less IL-12. Since IL-12 activates natural killer (NK) cells to secrete IFNγ, which is required for

Table 6.8. Biological activities of tumor necrosis factor

1. TNF induces endothelial cells to secrete chemoattractants for leukocytes.
2. TNF induces endothelial cells to express adhesion molecules that facilitate leukocyte emigration.
3. TNF activates neutrophils and monocytes.
4. TNF enhances the cytotoxicity of macrophages by enhancing production of ROIs and RNIs.
5. TNF induces macrophages to secrete cytokines, IL-1 and IL-6.
6. TNF enhances its own secretion by macrophages.
7. TNF acts on the hypothalamus to induce fever (need systemic concentrations).
8. TNF upregulates acute phase protein synthesis indirectly by inducing IL-6 secretion by macrophages.
9. TNF produced chronically leads to cachexia.
10. TNF produced acutely, in very high concentration, leads to septic shock.

the differentiation of naive CD4+ T cells to a Th1 phenotype, secreting IFNγ and IL-2 (Type 1 cytokines), the defect in IL-12 production has far reaching consequences. Administration of IL-12 would, in theory, stimulate NK cells to secrete IFNγ and shift the differentiation of naive T cells to a Th1 phenotype secreting IFNγ. In experimental animal models (using mice susceptible to *L. tropica*), concomitant treatment with IL-12 leads to resolution of infection and increased IFNγ production.

The ability of IL-12 to enhance immunity to viral infections is under investigation in a phase I, randomized, double blind, placebo controlled study with human immunodeficiency virus (HIV) patients on stable antiretroviral therapy. Previous studies showed that in the later stages of HIV infection a polarization to Type 2 cytokine production (Th2 cells) was seen. In the presence of IL-12 the differentiation of naive CD4+ T cells should become biased toward a Th1 subset instead of a Th2 subset, and since cytokines secreted by Th1 cells are required for the immunity to viruses, IL-12 is expected to enhance immunity to HIV.

Interferon α/β

Type I interferons (IFN α/β) have been administered as therapeutic agents for a number of years. In 1986, type I interferon received FDA approval as a therapeutic agent for hairy cell leukemia. In 1998 the FDA approved type I interferon as a therapeutic agent for sexually transmitted genital warts and for Kaposi's sarcoma. More recently, type I interferon has been approved as adjunctive therapy in patients with metastatic melanoma, as well as for patients with renal cell carcinoma. Preliminary results of these trials suggest that adjunctive therapy with interferon type 1 may prolong survival and delay disease progression. Some types of tumors are, however, refractory to the effects of type I interferon. Although the mechanism of action of type I interferon on tumor growth remains unresolved, a regulatory effect on the cell cycle is probably important.

Type I interferon has also received FDA approval as a therapeutic agent for the treatment of relapsing-remitting multiple sclerosis because this cytokine seems to slow the progressive disability associated with this disease. Investigations into the mechanism of action of interferon on disease progression indicate that treatment with type 1 interferon leads to: (i) a decrease in one subclass of B cells; (ii) an increase in soluble adhesion molecules suggesting that the effect of this cytokine is to interfere with the recruitment of leukocytes to the site of inflammation; and (iii) inhibition of T-cell proliferation.

Type I interferon is one current therapy for chronic infection caused by hepatitis B and hepatitis C virus. Based on liver biopsies of patients with hepatitis C, the efficacy of interferon therapy correlates with the number of type I interferon receptors present on hepatocytes. However, whether the effects of interferon represent a modulation of the immune system, or direct antiviral effects remains to be determined. The antiviral effects are lost rapidly following cessation of treatment, implying no active immune process develops during therapy that induces sterile immunity.

Cytokines that signal via CD132

Human X-linked severe combined immunodeficiency (XSCID) is characterized by a deficiency in T cells, natural killer cells, and, less profoundly, B cells. These individuals present with severe and persistent infections early in life. Most patients with XSCID carry a genetic mutation in CD132 (common γ chain), with mutations ranging from nonsense mutations to deletion of entire exons. One diagnostic procedure for identifying individuals with XSCID is genomic sequencing of CD132. The only *cure* for XSCID at present is a successful bone marrow transplant. Genetic dysfunction in CD132 has far reaching effects because CD132 is the common signal transducing chain for IL-2, IL-4, IL-7, IL-9, and IL-15. Consequently, multiple cytokine systems are simultaneously affected resulting in profound impairment of immune function.

The impairment in immune functioning associated with mutations in CD132 may result from the inability of CD132 to bind JAK kinases, given that in normal cells, JAK 3 associates constitutively with CD132. Stable cell lines derived from XSCID patients are unable to activate JAK kinases in response to IL-2. However, insertion of a retroviral vector expressing a normal CD132 restores the ability of these cell lines to phosphorylate, and activate, JAK 3 in response to IL-2.

JAK 3 deficient patients have a clinical phenotype virtually identical to that of XSCID individuals, with recurrent infections leading to death in infancy. Stable cell lines established from JAK 3 deficient patients do not proliferate in response to IL-2. Again, insertion of a retroviral vector containing JAK 3 restores JAK 3 expression and the response to IL-2. In those cells expressing this retroviral vector, JAK 3 phosphorylation and activation is followed by normal proliferation. The success of in vitro reconstitution studies for CD132 and JAK 3 kinases provides the basis for trials of gene therapy, rather than bone marrow transplantation, as treatment for these two genetic disorders.

Tumor necrosis factor
Considering the role of TNF in sepsis, it is not surprising that clinical trials using anti-TNF antibodies to block TNF have received FDA approval. In one trial in patients with bacterial sepsis, early (three day) mortality was reduced, although mortality rates after one month were not affected.

One of the problems associated with the use of mouse antibodies for therapy is the development of human anti-mouse antibodies (i.e., the HAMA response). To overcome this problem, human/mouse chimeric antibodies have been engineered. These humanized/chimeric antibodies are human IgG antibodies constructed with murine complementary determining regions/idiotopes (those amino acids in the variable region that interact with the TNF). Therefore, human anti-mouse antibodies are NOT generated against the antibody framework regions. However, some antibodies that interact with the idiotopes (anti-idiotypic) do arise. As an alternative approach, fusion proteins, entirely of human origin, were engineered, where the recognition moiety (e.g., for TNF) was not of antibody origin, but rather was a component of the TNF receptor. These fusion proteins are comprised of the IgG heavy chain constant region fused to two copies of the extracellular domain of the TNF receptor (the recognition moiety). These fusion proteins are soluble and should "mop up" the TNF. Additionally, since the entire fusion protein is of human origin, no anti-mouse antibodies are generated. Unfortunately, results of clinical trials using this fusion protein were not as positive as those results from trials that used anti-TNF chimeric/humanized antibodies.

TNF expression is increased in chronic inflammatory diseases including cerebral malaria, rheumatoid arthritis, and Crohn's disease. Blocking TNF using anti-TNF antibodies or the fusion protein as treatment for both rheumatoid arthritis and Crohn's disease seems a promising approach, based on multicenter phase III clinical trials, using only a single injection of anti-TNF. Clinical improvement was seen that lasted some 4-6 weeks.

Chemokines

Chemokines have been grouped into four families, the CXC, CC, C, and CX3C families, depending upon the existence of one or more cysteines and the number of amino acids separating the first two cysteine residues. Prominent members of the CXC family are IL-8 and IP-10. CXC chemokines are chemotactic for neutrophils, but not for monocytes. CC chemokines (MCP-1,2 or 3), RANTES etc. are chemotactic for monocytes and lymphocytes, but not for neutrophils. Lymphotaxin, the only member of the C family, is chemotactic for CD8+ T cells; CX3C chemokine is chemotactic for monocytes and neutrophils.

Production of the CC chemokines MIP-1α and MCP-1 in the CNS has been implicated in experimental allergic encephalomyelitis (EAE) in animals, a model of the human disease multiple sclerosis. It has been speculated that chemokine production acts as a local attractant for leukocyte recruitment. More recently it has been shown that chemokines can also act as cofactors to regulate cytokine production from stimulated lymphocytes, and that chemokines can induce intracellular signaling in T cells. Thus, recent data in the mouse analyzing oral tolerance induction to soluble peptides suggested that early local (within the Peyer's patch) production of the chemokine MCP-1 is implicated in down regulation of IL-12 production. This leads to a subsequent polarization towards Type 2 cytokine production and inhibition of disease.

SUMMARY

Cytokines are small peptides secreted mainly by activated leukocytes. Different cytokines may trigger the same biological responses, a characteristic termed functional redundancy. Additionally, cytokines are pleiotropic in that each cytokine can mediate numerous seemingly unrelated biological effects. In the main, cell targets constitutively express low affinity cytokine receptors whose conversion to a high affinity state requires association with another molecule to form a cytokine receptor complex. For some cytokine receptors, the signaling molecule(s) is/are unique to that receptor. For other cytokines receptors, the signaling molecule(s) is/are component(s) of several cytokine receptor complexes, and may serve as the basis for the overlap in biological function (functional redundancy). The common signaling molecules CD130, CDw131, CD132, and CD122 may be used to categorize families of cytokines or cytokine receptors.

In general cytokine receptors associate with members of a family of tyrosine kinases, Janus tyrosine kinases (JAKs). Four JAK kinases have been identified that participate in cytokine signaling, JAK 1, JAK 2, JAK 3, and TYK2. JAK association with cytokine receptor complexes has some element of specificity because JAKs preferentially associate with distinct receptor molecules.

In resting cells, JAK kinases are constitutively inactive. JAK kinases are activated by transphosphorylation when they are brought into close proximity to one another, which occurs when receptor molecules associate to form receptor complexes. Activated JAKs phosphorylate tyrosine residues within the unique binding sites of receptor complexes. Cytoplasmic proteins are recruited to receptor complexes and bind to the unique site via SH2 domains. Some of the recruited proteins are adapter proteins that structurally link the receptor complex to signaling pathways. Others are latent transcription factors such as the STAT proteins, named STAT 1 through to STAT 6.

Some cytokine receptors are intrinsic serine/threonine kinases that are activated following ligand binding (e.g., TGFβ). These activated receptor complexes also serve as scaffolds for proteins that link the receptor complex to various signaling pathways. By analogy with the JAK/STAT pathway of activation, these receptors recruit members of a family of proteins termed "SMAD". These proteins are molecules whose activation by phosphorylation is required for their function as components of transcription factors.

The signaling mechanisms of some cytokine receptors is poorly defined, although they do not seem to be associated with the JAKs, STATS, or SMADs. Receptors that fall into this category are IL-1R and TNFR.

CLINICAL CASES AND DISCUSSION

Clinical Case #11
A patient suffers from severe environmental and food allergies. His mother, after browsing through some immunology literature at the local library, comes to you to inquire about the possibility of trying an "oral tolerance inducing regime" to help overcome his problem. Will this be helpful, and if not, why not?

Discussion Case #11
Background
Data in patients with food allergies, and from severe asthmatics, indicates that exposure to allergen induces rapid production of histamine, a consequence of crosslinking IgE on the surface of basophils/mast cells (in the skin, lining of GI tract). Production of IgE is predominantly under the control of the Th2 cytokines, IL-4 and IL-5. Individuals prone to hyperallergic states are found to be *overproducers* of IL-4 and IL-5, inducing a *class-switch to* IgE production in activated B cells. Novel therapies thus center on decreasing IgE production (by decreasing production of IL-4 and IL-5).

Oral exposure to antigen induces *unresponsiveness to* a number of foreign agents and thus promotes *tolerance*. Often this tolerance represents more an *immune deviation* from one type of immune response (e.g., a cell-mediated response) to another (e.g., a humoral response). These responses are sustained by Th1 (IL-2, IFNγ, and TNF) and Th2 cytokines, respectively. In some autoimmune disorders where pathology is related to production of Th1 cytokines, "tuning down" Th1 stimulation by oral feeding of crude antigen has proven to be of some benefit.

The mechanism by which oral feeding "works" is probably quite multifactorial. Recent data implicates a role for altered chemokine production, as well as altered production of the cytokines IL-12 and TGFβ in the local (mucosal) milieu, in regulating the altered cytokine networks. Blockade of MCP-1 in fact abolished the switch to type 2 cytokine production, and increased IL-12 production (with decreased TGFβ), after oral feeding in laboratory animals.

Tests
First you should check if this individual is predisposed to allergies (environmental and/or food related). Beware that some of these reactions can be fatal and a judicious use of tests is appropriate! Allergies can be familial, so more history would be useful. Skin testing can often pick up a number of environmental allergens (pollen; animal dander etc.), while food allergies are documented by placing the patient on a minimalist (hypoallergenic) diet and slowly adding in foods, observing the subsequent response.

Treatment

Generally the best treatment is avoidance of the allergen. In some instances desensitization therapy is undertaken for medical reasons (the allergic reaction itself is particularly severe and thus potentially life-threatening), or even personal ones (the patient does not like the chronic, albeit nonlethal, symptoms). Desensitization involves immunization with the allergen, but by another route (e.g., intramuscular), which has been associated with production of cell-mediated immunity and Th1 cytokines, with a decline in Th2 cytokines, a decline in IgE production, and promotion of IgG production. All of these effects might induce improvement in this patient's condition.

Clinical Case #12

Ms. P. is a 55-year-old lady who has had erosive deforming rheumatoid arthritis for 20 years. She has failed all conventional treatments (including anti-inflammatory medications, gold, methotrexate, etc.) You are considering her for inclusion in a clinical trial in which anti-TNF monoclonal antibody is injected as a therapeutic agent. Why might this work?

Discussion Case #12

Background

Rheumatoid arthritis is an autoimmune disorder of unknown etiology, associated with inflammatory changes in joints. Excessive oligoclonal or even polyclonal activation of B cells leads to hypergammaglobulinemia and often the production of rheumatoid factor (antibodies recognizing the Fc region of autologous IgG). Immune complex deposition within joints activates complement, triggering the complement cascade and activation of local macrophages/neutrophils. These release proteinases/elastases that destroy the local connective tissue matrix within the joint itself, resulting in mechanical breakdown of the joint. Macrophages and neutrophils are continually activated by ongoing release of inflammatory molecules into the joint fluid. Most important amongst these are a number of chemokines (molecules controlling cell migration into the inflamed joint) and cytokines that directly activate macrophages/neutrophils.

One of the key cytokines found at elevated levels in inflamed joints is TNF. TNF not only causes activation of inflammatory cells, it also alters (upregulates) expression of a number of so-called adhesion molecules (ICAM/LFA-1 etc) which play an important role in regulating migration of inflammatory cells to the joint synovium. One could speculate that treatments aimed at inhibiting inflammatory mediators, and/or molecules involved in cell recruitment, might prove beneficial.

Tests

Conventional tests affirm the diagnosis of rheumatoid arthritis as defined by the American Rheumatology Association (ARA). These include blood tests looking for generalized inflammation, including detection of C-reactive protein and rheumatoid factor (antibody to immunoglobulin itself). X-rays confirm the classical picture of joint derangement; and a physical exam confirms the presence of joint inflammation (effusions, tenderness and warmth).

Treatment

A series of clinical trials, particularly in patients who are not being adequately controlled using conventional therapy (anti-inflammatory drugs; steroids; methotrexate) have been initiated using anti-ICAMs to inhibit leukocyte recruitment to the inflamed synovium. One significant "downside" of this therapy is edema and other nonspecific toxicity caused by crosslinking of cell surface ICAM (on endothelial cells, leukocytes), with subsequent activation and production of cytokines/chemokines which themselves contribute to inflammation. There is more hope attached to clinical trials examining the possibility of using antibodies to TNF itself to "shutdown" the persistent stimulation of inflammatory cells within the rheumatoid joint by released TNF. Early studies appear to be quite promising.

Test Yourself

Multiple Choice Questions

1. Choose the incorrect statement.
   a. Activated NK cells secrete IFNγ.
   b. IFNγ enhances the cytotoxicity of macrophages.
   c. IFNγ inhibits cytokine production by Th1 cells.
   d. IFNγ receptors signal via the JAK/STAT pathway.
   e. Individuals with inactivating mutations in the IFNγ receptor should not be immunized with BCG.
2. Which one of the following cytokines is used in the treatment of hairy cell leukemia, genital warts, Kaposi's sarcoma, relapsing-remitting multiple sclerosis, and chronic hepatitis B/C infections?
   a. IL-10
   b. IL-12
   c. IFNγ
   d. IL-2
   e. IFNα/β
3. Most patients with XSCID carry a mutation in CD132. This defect impairs signal transduction initiated by all the following cytokines EXCEPT
   a. IL-3
   b. IL-4
   c. IL-7
   d. IL-2
   e. IL-9
4. All the following are biological functions attributed to TNF EXCEPT
   a. induction of chemoattractant secretion by endothelial cells
   b. induction of adhesion molecules on endothelial cells
   c. activation of neutrophils and monocytes
   d. impairment of macrophage cytotoxicity
   e. induction of IL-1 and IL-6 secretion by macrophages

5. Which one of the following cytokine receptors is an intrinsic serine/threonine kinase?
   a. TFGβ
   b. TNF
   c. INFγ
   d. IL-2
   e. IL-6

Answers 1c; 2e; 3a; 4d; 5a

Short Answer Questions
1. Which cytokine deficiency leads to uncontrolled proliferation of *Mycobacterium tuberculosis* in infected macrophages? Explain.
2. Why would a mutation/deficiency in CD132 manifest the same as a genetic deficiency in JAK 3?
3. What immunological changes are observed in patients to whom IFN α/β is administered for relapsing-remitting multiple sclerosis?
4. Compare and contrast signaling via IFNγ and TGFβ.
5. What is the rationale for using IL-12 in a clinical trial for patients with HIV infection?

Cells of Adaptive Immunity

Objectives	130
I. B Lymphocytes	130
B Lymphocyte Antigen Specific Receptor	130
Constructing an Immunoglobulin	131
B-cell Differentiation: Bone Marrow	134
Clinical Significance: B-cell Neoplasms	137
Summary	137
II. T Lymphocytes	137
T-lymphocyte Antigen-specific Receptor	137
Differentiation of Lymphoid Progenitor Cells in the Thymus	140
Transport of Lymphocytes from Primary to Secondary Lymphoid Tissues	146
Summary	146
Clinical Cases and Discussion	147
Test Yourself	151

Objectives

This chapter focuses on the structures of antigen specific receptors in B and T lymphocytes, and the mechanisms whereby diversity in the lymphocyte repertoire is established. In addition, the mechanisms by which lymphocytes that express potentially autoreactive receptors are deleted (i.e., tolerance induction) is also described. Relevant clinical vignettes are discussed.

I. B Lymphocytes

B-Lymphocyte Antigen-Specific Receptor

General features

B lymphocytes (B cells) express antigen recognizing receptors (antibodies) on their cell surface. The receptors, also referred to as membrane immunoglobulin (**mIg**), are expressed in association with a heterodimer, **CD79a/CD79b** (Igα-Igβ), which couples mIg to intracellular signaling pathways (Fig. 7.1). Immunoglobulin molecules are composed of two identical heavy chains and two identical light chains linked by disulfide bonds (Fig. 7.2). Each chain is made up of a variable region and a constant region. The **light chain variable region** is composed of segments designated "V" and "J", while the **heavy chain variable region** is composed of "V", "D", and "J" segments, where the letters "V", "D", and "J" refer to the **Variable, Diversity,** and **Joining** segments (Fig. 7.2). The constant regions are encoded by the same genes in all B cells.

Clinical Immunology, by Reginald Gorczynski and Jacqueline Stanley. 2001 Landes Bioscience

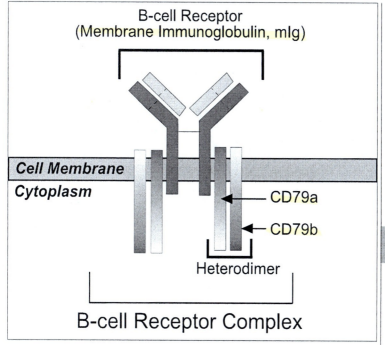

Fig. 7.1. Schematic illustration of the BCR in association with CD79a/CD79b heterodimer. Membrane Ig is expressed on the cell surface in association with the CD79a/CD79b heterodimer to form the B-cell receptor (BCR) complex.

CONSTRUCTING AN IMMUNOGLOBULIN

Unique variable region

Theoretically, in any given individual, it is possible to generate 10^9-10^{11} different B-cell clones each bearing mIg whose variable regions will differ from those present on other clones. Collectively, these clones represent the **B-cell repertoire**. This diversity is made possible because the V, D, and J gene segments, which encode the variable regions, are present as **multiple germline genes**. In the construction of a gene encoding the variable regions, the gene segments are recombined and so their sequence differs from that present in germline DNA. This process is termed **somatic recombination** (Fig. 7.3). The recombination process requires the activation of recombinases, nucleoprotein products of the **RAG-1** and **RAG-2** genes (recombination-activating genes).

For the **heavy chain**, these enzymes randomly select one "D" and one "J", to form a DJ gene segment, which then combines with a randomly selected "V" gene segment to form the variable region (VDJ) of that particular heavy chain (referred to as **combinatorial diversity**). Gene rearrangement of the variable **light**

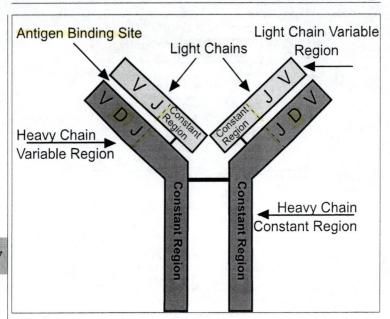

Fig. 7.2. Variable regions of both light and heavy chains are composed of segments. Variable regions of light and heavy chains are composed of distinct segments (V, J) and (V, D, J), respectively. Light and chain variable regions are ligated to a constant region.

chain region involves the selection and ligation of one "J", and one "V" to form a VJ segment. During the recombination process of either the light or heavy chain variable region, intervening unselected "Vs", "Ds" or "Js" are deleted. Additional DNA nucleotides may be deleted, or inserted at V, D, or J gene segment junctions in order to maintain (downstream) an open reading frame, thus generating **junctional diversity**. Incorporation of nucleotides at junctions is mediated by a template independent DNA polymerase, **terminal deoxynucleotidyl transferase** (Tdt).

The successful rearrangement of a heavy chain variable region from one chromosome inhibits the somatic recombination of the heavy chain variable region on the other member of the chromosome pair, a process known as **allelic exclusion**. The net effect of this is that all mIg present on the surface of any one B cell will have the same heavy chain variable region.

Entire immunoglobulin

In naive mature B cells, the heavy chain constant regions are mu (μ) and delta (δ), while the light chain constant regions are either kappa (κ) or lambda (λ). Light and heavy chains are not restricted in their association and so this provides more potential diversity for the B-cell repertoire. In summary, the construction of unique variable regions, leading to the construction of different mIg on B-cell

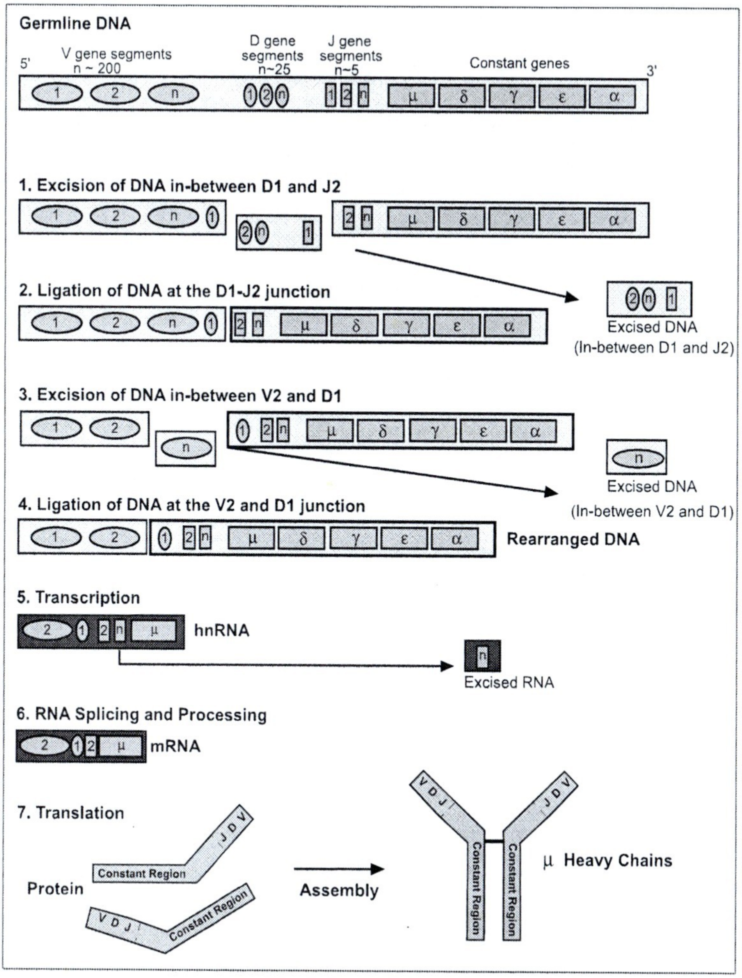

Cells of Adaptive Immunity

Fig. 7.3. Somatic recombination of a heavy chain variable region and generation of a mu (μ) heavy chain. In somatic recombination, a randomly selected "D" and "J" recombine to form a DJ gene segment which then combines with a randomly selected "V" gene segment to form the variable region of that particular heavy chain. The VDJ gene segment is subsequently joined to a constant region to generate the immunoglobulin heavy chain.

clones, is the result of: (i) multiple copies of germline V, D, and J gene segments; (ii) random selection and combination of V, D and J gene segments; (iii) junctional diversity generated by the addition or deletion of bases; and (iv) random assortment of light and heavy chains. However, the *random* selection of V, D and J gene segments generates B-cell receptors that may be **autoreactive**. Consequently, those B cells must be deleted or inactivated (below).

B-CELL DIFFERENTIATION: BONE MARROW

B-cell differentiation in the bone marrow occurs prior to any exposure to foreign antigen. It is characterized both by the expression and silencing of distinct sets of genes at discrete stages of development. The penultimate event of B-cell maturation is the generation of a B-cell repertoire that is nonautoreactive. Significant and discrete events that characterize the various stages of B-cell differentiation are illustrated in Figure 7.4.

Pro-B-cell stage
This stage is characterized by the transcription of multiple genes, including RAG-1 and –2, CD19, Tdt and CD79, required for differentiation of the B cell in the next developmental stage (Fig. 7.4).

Pre-B-cell stage
The pre-B-cell stage is characterized by the expression of a pre-B-cell receptor (pre-BCR) in association with the CD79a/CD79b heterodimer. The pre-BCR is composed of two rearranged μ heavy chains paired with two pseudo (ψ) light chains. Signaling via the pre-BCR complex, interacting with a ligand expressed in the stromal environment, directs proliferation and further differentiation of pre-B cells.

Immature B-cell stage
The immature B-cell stage is characterized by shifts in receptor expression from the pre-BCR to a BCR. The BCR is composed of the same two rearranged μ heavy chains, now synthesized for BCR expression, complexed with two identical light chains (described above). Specific inactivation of B cells expressing autoreactive mIg (tolerance induction) is accomplished by apoptosis (destruction) or induction of anergy (nonresponsiveness).

Mature B-cell stage
The mature B-cell stage is characterized by the coexpression of cell surface IgM and IgD, which is the consequence of alternative splicing (Fig. 7.5). Several cell surface proteins are expressed during the transition from the immature to mature B-cell stage (Fig. 7.4). Mature naive B cells leave the bone marrow, enter the blood stream, migrate to peripheral lymphoid tissues, and recirculate if they do not encounter antigen in a secondary lymphoid tissue. The exit from blood into peripheral lymph nodes is mediated by adhesive molecules (L-selectin) on B cells that interact with vascular addressin molecules present on high endothelial venules (HEV). Different addressins are expressed in peripheral lymph nodes versus intestinal mucosa HEVs. These molecules control the sites of "homing" for B cells. Entry into the spleen occurs at terminal branches of the central arterioles that end in the splenic lymphoid compartment. Failure to encounter antigen while transiting through secondary lymphoid tissues results in naive B cells entering the recirculating pool via efferent lymphatics, en route to the thoracic duct or right lymphatic duct.

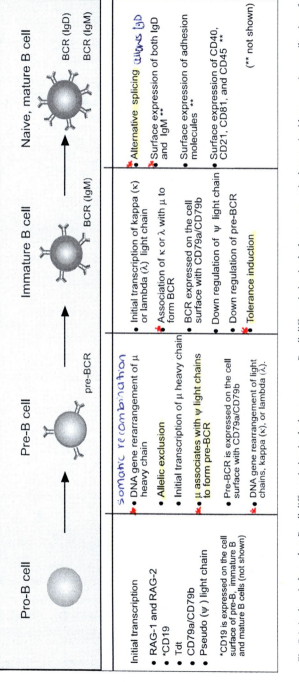

Fig. 7.4. Antigen independent B-cell differentiation in the bone marrow: B-cell differentiation in the bone marrow is characterized by expression or silencing of distinct sets of genes at discrete stages defined as "pro-B cell, pre-B cell, immature B cell, and mature B cell" stages.

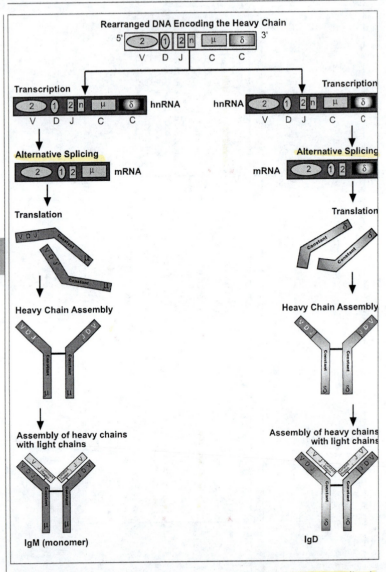

Fig. 7.5. Alternative splicing. Alternative splicing is a process in which the hnRNA encoding the variable region (VDJ) of the heavy chain is spliced to either a μ constant region or a δ constant region to form a heavy chain mRNA. This leads to the construction of both IgM and IgD expression on the same cell, each with the same specificity.

Clinical Significance: B-cell Neoplasms

Maturational arrest can occur at discrete stages of B-cell differentiation in the bone marrow. This arrest in maturation, accompanied by the uncontrolled proliferation of the progenitor, or mature naive B cells, is reflected as lymphoma and/or leukemia development. Phenotypically the malignant clones resemble the normal counterpart from the developmental stage at which arrest occurred, and are classified as "acute leukemia/lymphoma". Neoplasms arising from uncontrolled clonal expansion of mature B cells are termed "chronic lymphocytic leukemia" or "small lymphocyte lymphoma", while plasma cell neoplasms are termed "multiple myeloma" or "plasmacytomas".

Summary

B lymphocytes express antigen specific receptors, mIg, on their cell surface. These receptors are composed of two identical heavy chains, and two identical light chains, each of which is, in turn, composed of a variable region and a constant region. The variable regions define the antigen-binding site and are made up of variable segments, V (D) J whose encoding gene segments are brought together during a process of somatic recombination. The random selection of the V (D) J segments generates B-cell antigen receptors that are potentially autoreactive. The B cells that express these receptors are either inactivated or destroyed in a process termed tolerance induction. These processes occur in the bone marrow during B cell development. B-cell differentiation/development is characterized by the expression and silencing of distinct sets of genes at discrete stages of development. One of the main developmental features of B-cell maturation is the generation of a B-cell repertoire that is nonautoreactive. Mature naive B cells leave the bone marrow, enter the blood stream and migrate to peripheral lymphoid tissues where they establish "residence". Some naive B cells enter the recirculating pool of lymphocytes. Uncontrolled proliferation of cells at different stages of development results in leukemias/lymphomas.

II. T Lymphocytes

T-lymphocyte Antigen-specific Receptor

General features

T lymphocytes, or T cells, play a central role in immunity either by secreting cytokines (CD4+ T cells) or inducing osmotic lysis of infected cells (CD8+ T cells) (Fig. 7.6). T cells express unique receptors (TCRs) capable of recognizing antigenic fragments (e.g., viral or bacterial peptide) **only** when these peptide fragments are displayed in association with either a class I or a class II major histocompatibility cell molecule (MHC). Analogous to BCR expression (above), T cells express an array of different TCRs as a result of somatic recombination of the TCR variable genes, a process that occurs in the thymus.

Structure of the T-cell receptor complex

T-cell receptors (TCRs) are composed of two transmembrane polypeptide chains classified either as alpha/beta (α/β), or gamma/delta (γ/δ), as are the cells that bear them (Fig. 7.6). Most detail is available for α/β T cells, comprising more than 90% of the T cells in the body, and the discussion that follows focuses on them. Each heterodimeric TCR is expressed on the cell surface in association with five invariant polypeptides collectively termed CD3 (Fig. 7.7). CD3 serves to link the antigen binding receptor of the T cell with signaling pathways.

Each chain of the T-cell receptor consists of a variable and a constant region. Although most T-cell clones express T-cell receptors constructed with the same constant regions, each T-cell clone expresses receptors with unique variable regions. This apparent paradox occurs because variable regions are constructed from segments termed "variable (V)", "diversity (D)" and "joining (J)". More specifically, the TCRα variable regions are composed of a "V" and a "J" segment (VJ), while the TCRβ regions are composed of "V", "D", and "J" segments (VDJ).

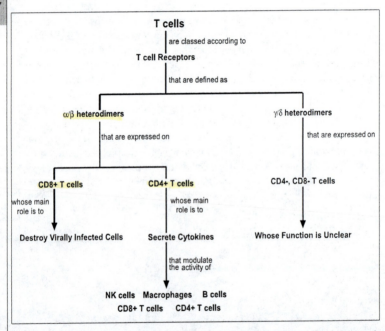

Fig. 7.6. Concept map depicting T-cell classes and T-cell subsets. T cells are defined phenotypically by the class of T-cell antigen receptor expressed on their cell surface. T cells are termed α/β T cells or γ/δ T cells depending on the T-cell receptor that they express. The α/β T cells are further classified by the coreceptor molecules, CD4 or CD8, expressed on the cell surface.

Constructing unique T-cell receptors

Theoretically, in any given individual, somatic recombination and diversification can create a repertoire of 10^{12}-10^{15} different TCRs, each potentially giving rise to a unique T-cell clone. There may be as many as 25,000 (identical) TCRs on any given cell. Collectively, the clones expressing these receptors represent the T-cell repertoire. This diversity is made possible because the V, D, and J gene segments, which encode the variable regions, are present as multiple germline genes. The processes that lead to the construction of TCRα and TCRβ are essentially the same as that described for B cells. Somatic recombination of the TCRβ variable region genes occurs prior to that of the TCRα chain. For the TCRβ chain, the variable region is constructed of a "V", "D", and a "J", whilst the TCRα, the variable region is constructed from a "V" and a "J" segment only (Fig. 7.8). For most T cells, all the TCRβ constant regions are the same, as are the TCRα constant regions.

Successful rearrangement of a TCRβ chain variable region leads to allelic exclusion of the other member of the chromosome pair. By analogy with B cells, the diversity in the T-cell repertoire is the result of: (i) multiple copies of germline V, D, and J gene segments; (ii) random selection and combination of V, D and J gene segments; (iii) junctional diversity generated by the addition or deletion of bases; and (iv) random assortment of TCRα and TCRβ chains. The *random* selection of V, D and J gene segments again leads to the generation of T cells expressing TCRs that may be autoreactive. Consequently, those T cells must be deleted during the screening process in the thymus (see below).

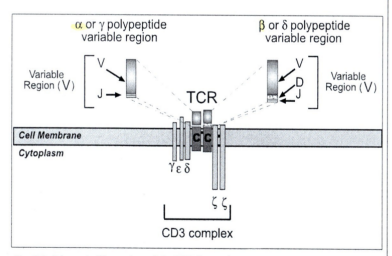

Fig. 7.7. Schematic illustration of the TCR heterodimer in association with CD3. Each heterodimeric TCR, (α/β) or (γ/δ), is expressed on the cell surface in association with five invariant polypeptides, collectively termed CD3.

DIFFERENTIATION OF LYMPHOID PROGENITOR CELLS IN THE THYMUS

General features

Progenitor cells originating in the bone marrow differentiate to naive mature T cells under the influence of the thymic microenvironment secreting the cytokine, IL-7 (Figs. 7.9, 7.10). Ideally, thymic maturation produces a diverse population of lymphocyte clones, each characterized by a unique T-cell receptor that recognizes foreign antigens, with none of those clones representing a population of T cells

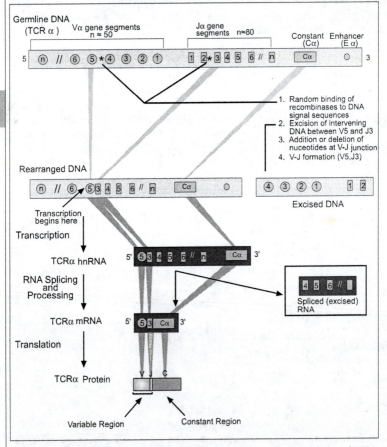

Fig. 7.8. Somatic recombination of TCRα variable region: transcription, translation of TCRα. Somatic recombination of TCRα occurs during T-cell development in the thymus (after somatic recombination of the TCRβ chain). In the construction of a TCRα chain variable region, one segment is selected from each of the V and J gene families. Excision of intervening DNA occurs between the selected V and J gene segments, as does either the deletion/insertion of a few nucleotides. Subsequent transcription and translation generates the TCRα polypeptide chain.

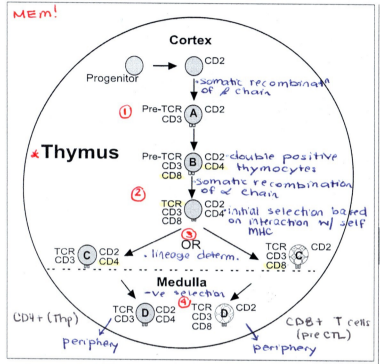

Fig. 7.9. T cells acquire cell surface molecules during differentiation in the thymus. T-cell progenitors undergo differentiation to mature T cells in the thymus. During this developmental process, T cells up- and down-regulate expression of a number of cell surface molecules, including CD4 or CD8, which determines both the biological role and subset to which the cell belongs.

whose receptors are self-reactive. The latter would, of course, result in autoimmunity. Paradoxically, this result is achieved, in separate stages of development, by first *selecting T cells to recognize self-MHC* in the thymus. The crux of the selection processes resides in the affinity by which self-MHC is seen.

Developmental phases

Phase I: Expression of the pre-TCR
Somatic recombination of the TCRβ chain variable region and subsequent cell surface expression of a pre-TCR complex characterizes phase 1. This pre-TCR complex is made up of a TCRβ polypeptide covalently linked to an invariant polypeptide chain, termed "pre-Tα" that associates with CD3. Signaling via the pre-TCR complex is thought to direct proliferation and further differentiation of thymocytes. In addition, cell surface expression of CD2 occurs and remains on all T cells, serving as a T-specific marker.

Great Chart

Fig. 7.10. Phases of intrathymic differentiation of α/β T cells.

	Phase I	Phase II	Phase III	Phase IV
Genes Expressed	+ CD2 TCRβ, Pre-Tα, CD3	+ CD2, CD4, CD8, TCRβ, TCRα and CD3	[CD4 or CD8],CD2,	[CD4 or CD8],CD2,
Somatic Rearrangement	TCRβ	TCRα	N/A	N/A
Genes Downregulated	N/A	Pre-Tα	CD4 or CD8	N/A
Cell Surface Expression	CD2 Pre TCR complex	CD2, CD4, CD8 TCR complex	CD2, CD4 or CD8 TCR complex	CD2, CD4 or CD8 TCR complex
Other	Allelic exclusion	N/A	Positive Selection Negative Selection Death by Neglect Lineage Selection	Negative Selection
Comments	Need thymic epithelium Cell proliferation	Need thymic epithelium Cell proliferation	Need thymic epithelium	Need APCs that are bone marrow derived (MHC/antigen)

Recombinase, bcl-2, RAG-1, RAG-2

Phase II: Double positive thymocytes and expression of α/β TCR
Cell surface expression of both CD4 and CD8 on the developing thymocyte occurs early in phase II. Somatic recombination of the TCRα chain and its covalent association with newly expressed TCRβ chains leads to the formation of a TCR that associates with the invariant CD3 to form the TCR complex. Downregulation of pre-Tα and the pre-TCR complex also occurs at this stage.

Phase III: Thymocyte selection
Phase III is a discriminating phase, in which screening of thymocytes occurs based on their expressed TCR. Double positive (CD4+, CD8+) thymocytes are selected to live or die depending on the interactive avidity of their TCR with self-antigen/MHC on thymic epithelial cells (Fig. 7.11). Interactive avidity depends on: (i) the intrinsic affinity of the TCR for self antigen/MHC complex; (ii) the density of TCRs; (iii) the density of self antigen/MHC complexes on the thymic epithelium; and (iv) the density of antagonistic peptide complexes (i.e., cell/cell molecular interactions that repel one another). In addition, contributing factors are the interaction of a variety of accessory molecules and adhesion molecules with their counterparts on the thymic epithelium (cognate ligands).

Insignificant interactive avidity with thymic epithelial cell results in **death from neglect**. If recognition exceeds a predetermined threshold, thymocytes are clonally eliminated or functionally inactivated by an *active* process termed **negative selection**. Finally, **positive selection** and preferential expansion of T cells occurs when the avidity of recognition is intermediate (i.e., between these two extremes). A more finely tuned process of negative selection occurs in the medulla.

Following this initial screening process, lineage commitment occurs, referring to the transition of a double positive thymocyte (CD4+, CD8+) to a single positive thymocyte expressing either CD4 or CD8, but not both. Silencing of either the CD4 or the CD8 gene occurs in each individual T cell. T-cell lineages are thus classified by their expression of CD4 or CD8, reflective of subsequent biological activity (cytokine secretion or cell killing, respectively).

Phase IV: Negative selection
Negative selection occurs whenever a *triggering threshold avidity* for T cells is exceeded, either in the thymic cortex or medulla (Fig. 7.11). The initial elimination of potentially self reactive T cells occurs in double positive cells in the thymic cortex, involving TCR-mediated contact with self antigen/MHC presented by thymic epithelial cells. Negative selection is a consequence of high avidity interactions of the TCR for self-antigen/self MHC, occurring in the absence of CD4/CD8 interaction with appropriate MHC.

Negative selection also occurs in the medulla, in a process acting on already positively selected single positive thymocytes. Selection conditions in the medulla are different from those in the cortex, with the antigen presenting cells now bone marrow derived, rather than thymic epithelium. Thus the nature of the peptide is not necessarily the same and the thymocyte is a single positive (either CD4 or CD8) cell.

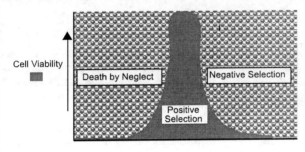

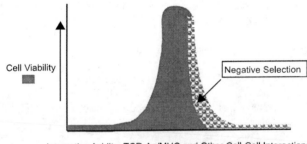

Fig. 7.11. Screening of thymocytes in the cortex and in the medulla. Thymocytes undergo a screening process in both the thymic cortex and medulla. In the cortex, screening occurs on double positive (CD4+, CD8+) thymocytes, interacting with thymic epithelial cells. Cells are selected to live, or die, based on the interactive avidity of their TCR with self-antigen/MHC on thymic epithelial cells. More finely tuned negative selection occurs in the medulla, acting on cells already positively selected in the cortex. Cells that survive this process exit the thymus.

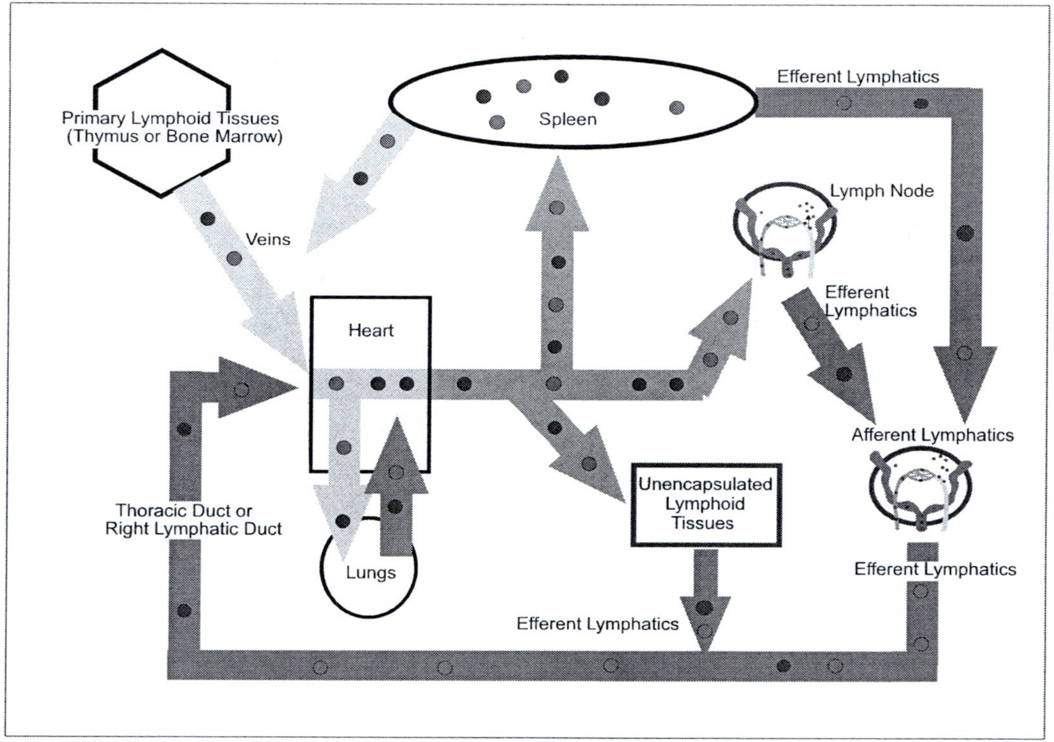

Cells of Adaptive Immunity

Fig. 7.12. Predominant pattern of naive lymphocyte trafficking during noninflammatory states. Naive lymphocytes leave primary lymphoid tissues via the circulation, ultimately leaving the blood circulation and entering secondary lymphoid tissues at postcapillary venules. In the absence of antigen encounter, lymphocytes mainly leave secondary lymphoid tissues via efferent lymphatics and join the major lymph circulation. En route to the thoracic duct (or right lymphatic duct) lymphocytes enter lymphatic nodes via afferent lymphatics and leave via efferent lymphatics.

At this stage, the interactive avidity of T cells with antigen presenting cells also includes the interaction of CD8 and CD4 with class I and class II MHC, respectively. Negative selection within the medulla is accordingly more finely-tuned than in the cortex, with multiple high avidity interactions, including TCR, CD4 (CD8) and class II (class I) MHC products all playing prominent roles.

Mature naive T cells

T cells exit the thymus as naive T cells, seeding secondary lymphoid tissues or entering the pool of recirculating lymphocytes.

Transport of Lymphocytes from Primary to Secondary Lymphoid Tissues

Blood and lymph vessels serve as *highways* for the movement of lymphocytes throughout the body. Lymphocytes leave their maturation sites via the blood, and either seed the secondary lymphoid tissues, or recirculate via immunosurveillance (Fig. 7.12). Migration of naive lymphocytes from the blood into lymph nodes occurs at specialized postcapillary venules, termed **high endothelial venules (HEV)** (Fig. 7.13). These cuboidal shaped endothelial cells feature a prominent filamentous layer (glycocalyx) on their luminal surface that traps molecules (Fig. 7.14). In addition, HEV express molecules that bind circulating lymphocytes.

Extravasation of naive lymphocytes into tissues at HEV requires: (i) interaction of **L-selectin** on lymphocytes with its ligand on endothelial cells to induce lymphocyte rolling; (ii) activation of **integrins**, (e.g., **LFA-1**) present on the lymphocytes, increasing their adhesiveness and allowing stable binding to HEV; (iii) lymphocyte secretion of **matrix metalloproteinases** that proteolytically degrade collagen to generate channels in the subendothelial basement membrane; and (iv) transendothelial migration of lymphocytes into the tissue.

If naive lymphocytes do not encounter antigen in the lymph nodes, they continue their immunosurveillance in the lymphatics (Figs. 7.12, 7.13). One cycle through the body takes approximately one to two days.

Summary

Alpha/beta T cells express a unique T-cell receptor (TCR) which consists of a variable region and a constant region. Gene segments termed "variable (V), diversity (D), and joining (J) regions, are randomly recombined in a process termed somatic recombination to encode variable genes. The recombined segments, along with the DNA encoding the constant regions, encode the TCRα and TCRβ polypeptides. Somatic recombination of the V, (D), or J segments is random and leads to the expression of TCRs that are potentially autoreactive, or ineffective. During a screening process in the thymus, cells expressing autoreactive TCRs are eliminated. T cells expressing TCRs that are not autoreactive are **positively selected** and undergo clonal expansion. Selection is based on the interactive avidity of the developing thymocyte with cells displaying a self-antigen/self MHC complex on their

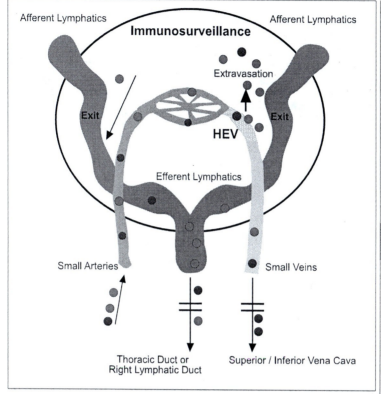

Fig. 7.13. Naive lymphocyte trafficking through a lymph node. Migration of naive lymphocytes from the blood into peripheral lymph nodes occurs at specialized postcapillary venules, termed high endothelial venules (HEV). In the absence of antigen recognition, lymphocytes exit via the efferent lymphatics and enter the main lymphatic circulation.

surface. T cells exit the thymus and seed the secondary lymphoid tissue or join the pool of recirculating T cells.

CLINICAL CASES AND DISCUSSION

Clinical Case #13

A patient on your transplant service, a recipient of a kidney graft last year, has complained of vague abdominal pain for several months. She has had multiple investigations to ensure her graft is functioning well with no evidence of rejection. A recent CAT scan of the abdomen suggests a mass in the liver. Biopsy reveals evidence for lymphoma. What further tests might you perform? What is a common finding in such a case?

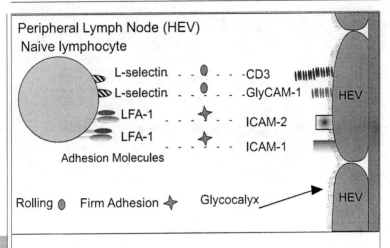
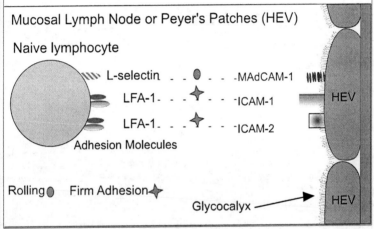

Fig. 7.14. Adhesive molecules on naive lymphocytes interact with ligands on HEV. Interactions of selectins with their cognate ligands mediate leukocyte rolling on HEV; interactions of integrins with their ligands mediate firm adhesion between leukocytes and the HEV. The expression of a specific contact ligand for L-selectin on endothelial cells in the HEV is different in different tissues.

Discussion Case #13
Background

This is a common problem in those patients known to be immunosuppressed for a variety of reasons. Presumably this abnormal growth of lymphocytes reflects a failure of normal growth control mechanisms. One of the first ways clinicians characterize lymphomas is to designate the cell of origin (B cell, T-cell lymphoma).

This is necessary because clinical trials have shown that these different histological tumors are susceptible to different anticancer drugs. In addition, even tumors within the B- (or T-) cell lineage, but from different developmental stages, have differential drug susceptibility. Our understanding of normal B- (and T-) cell development is such that we can pinpoint certain cell surface phenotypes of B- and T-cell classes/subclasses, which greatly improves diagnosis in comparison to older, more classical, morphological / histological classifications.

A lymphoma that expresses CD19 would be classified as a B-cell tumor. Subsequent analysis of surface (or intracytoplasmic) expression of Ig could help determine the development stage to which the tumor belongs. Finally, expression of other molecules characteristic of later stages of B-cell development (complement receptors, CD81, CD21) would characterize tumors arising at a late developmental stage. In the event that the cells also showed cytoplasmic features of cells engaged in active protein synthesis, along with sIg, one would consider the cell a terminally differentiated (plasmacytoid) one.

Infection of individuals in the Western world with Epstein Barr virus (EBV) is common with some 50% or more infected adults. Normally, infection (of B cells) is associated only with transient signs of viremia (fatigue, general malaise, etc.) which passes within days/weeks. More severe infections, lasting longer, characterize a disease referred to as mononucleosis. When the acute virus infection is cleared, however, some EBV genomes become stably integrated in host B cells as a latent infection. In the presence of immunosuppression, presumably also in association with other (unknown) stimuli to proliferate, the latently infected B cell begins to transcribe EBV DNA again. The virus is reactivated, infecting fresh B cells and stimulating their growth. If the body cannot control this growth a tumor results (EBV-induced B-cell lymphoma).

Tests

Firstly we need to classify the lymphoma as B cell or T cell, and then attempt subclassification of the stage of (B-) cell development affected. Measurement of CD19, CD21 and CD81, along with morphology, serves this purpose. In the later stages these lymphomas are associated with unique chromosomal translocations that help us understand why the cells are proliferating abnormally. Chromosomal translocations can be assessed by restriction enzyme analysis of the DNA.

Treatment

Because of the nature of the inciting events, in the early stages (virally induced proliferation of infected B cells) lymphomas often respond to conservative strategies. In the case of this transplant patient (where over-immunosuppression presumably was responsible for the inability to control the viral infection), decreasing immunosuppressive therapy often produces remission of the tumor. Presumably all of the normal "host control" mechanisms are still in place, but were temporarily "overridden" by over-immunosuppression. In the late stages (following gene translocation) such conservative strategies do not work, and chemotherapy must be employed.

Clinical Case #14

You are in the process of developing novel antibodies for use in autoimmune disorders. After extensive studies in patients with multiple sclerosis (MS), you conclude a major (unknown) antigen incites expansion of a family of Vβ8 T cells. How might this be of value? What might eventually limit the benefit from this form of therapy? (Note Vβ8 refers to a gene segment that encodes for "V" segment number 8 in the gene that encodes for the TCR β polypeptide).

Discussion Case #14

Background

Current treatment protocols for MS have been disappointing. This has fostered an incentive for medical research to develop novel therapies based on an improved understanding of the nature of the disease. MS is associated with T-cell mediated autoimmune reactivity. Unfortunately, nonspecific depletion of all T cells would leave the MS patient susceptible to opportunistic infections. Researchers have thus focused on how to develop reagents that might be used to eliminate specific groups of T cells.

T-cell recognition is a function of the TCR variable regions. Although numerous different copies of the "V" segments exist from which to construct TCR variable regions, not all are used equally, and some are used repeatedly. Construction of a TCR of unique specificity is not compromised by the repeated usage of a particular gene segment because different "Ds" and different "Js" are randomly selected as well. In addition, insertions/deletions at the segment junctions further ensures that each polypeptide chain will have a unique variable region. With this in mind, groups have been interested in determining which V regions are present on T cells expanded in disease (Vβ gene usage).

Tests

Commercial anti-Vβ subset antibodies are available that allow us to search for predominant Vβ usage in T cells present in particular diseases, compared to those present in the normal population. In addition, in vitro tests, culturing patient's T cells with "crude brain antigen", might indicate that unique populations, in this case Vβ8 T cells, are expanded in response to such stimulation.

Treatment

We are told that Vβ8 T cells are expanded in all MS patients. Presumably then, Vβ8 T cells recognize an antigen important in MS, regardless of the genetic background of the individual. Since the Vβ8 T-cell family only represents some ~ 8% of the total T-cell pool, deletion of Vβ8 might thus eliminate (or at least decrease) pathology in MS, without leaving the individual grossly immunodeficient. To do this, radioactive isotopes could be attached to antibodies that recognize amino acid sequences in the Vβ8, thus producing destruction of T cells expressing receptors with that particular Vβ(8) region. Note that there are some "downsides" to such forms of treatment.

Cells of Adaptive Immunity

The Vβ8 family of T-cell receptors also encodes recognition of antigens that are important common environmental pathogens (e.g., flu virus). Loss of Vβ8 T cells might then leave patients exquisitely susceptible to these common pathogens. In addition, there is the general problem associated with infusion of antibodies to deplete cells. Eventually the host begins to make antibodies to these antibodies, and they become less/noneffective. Finally, there is the theoretical problem that when Vβ8 T-cell subsets are depleted, another T-cell subset simply "takes over" as the dominant one to recognize the antigen, and the same pathology eventually ensues. Nevertheless, use of anti-Vβ antibodies is as yet an untried, but potentially promising, novel therapy for a number of human disorders.

TEST YOURSELF

Multiple Choice Questions
For questions 1-3, make the best match with a, b, c, or d. Use each answer once, more than once, or not at all.
  a. pro-B-cell stage
  b. pre-B-cell stage
  c. immature B-cell stage
  d. mature B-cell stage
1. expression of IgD
2. tolerance induction
3. somatic recombination of the μ heavy chain
4. Sam, a high school student, has been diagnosed with acute lymphocytic leukemia. Peripheral blood cells from the patient were incubated with anti-CD19 fluorescent antibodies. Flow cytometric analysis revealed a high intensity immunofluorescence, indicating enhanced expression of CD19, relative to controls. At what stage of B-cell development was the maturational arrest and unregulated clonal expansion?
  a. Mature B-cell stage
  b. Pre B-cell stage
  c. Immature B-cell stage
  d. Could be any of the above since CD19 is a pan marker at all stages of development.
5. Mechanisms which contribute to the generation of unique peptide/MHC binding sites on alpha/beta T-cell receptors include all the following EXCEPT:
  a. Multiple germline genes
  b. Alternative splicing
  c. Combinatorial association
  d. Random selection of alpha and beta chains
  e. Junctional diversity

Answers: 1d; 2c; 3b; 4d; 5b

Short Answer Questions

1. In general terms, what does somatic recombination entail? What is the consequence of constructing receptors whose components are randomly selected?
2. Compare and contrast tolerance induction in B cells and T cells.
3. What is alternative splicing? At which stage of B-cell differentiation is it initiated?
4. What is the consequence of allelic exclusion on the expression of antigen specific receptors?
5. Explain how determination of Vβ cell usage could potentially be useful in therapy.

Antigen Dependent B-cell Differentiation

Objectives	*153*
Antigen Dependent B-cell Differentiation	*153*
Fate of Activated B Cells in Germinal Centers	*155*
Primary versus Secondary Immune Responses	*159*
Clinical Significance	*159*
Model of Signal Transduction in B-cell Activation	*160*
Negative Signaling in B Cells	*161*
B-cell Responses to T-independent Antigens	*163*
Summary	*164*
Clinical Cases and Discussion	*164*
Test Yourself	*166*

Objectives

The events leading to B-cell differentiation following antigen-induced crosslinking of BCR are discussed. Key roles have been found for a number of phosphatases, kinases, and GTP binding proteins, as well as other signal transducing molecules. Activation signals are coupled to signals delivered via B-cell surface immunoglobulin (mIg) by ITAM (immune tyrosine activating motifs) sites on the intracellular tail of the CD79a/CD79b heterodimer expressed on the cell surface in association with mIg. Regulation of cell activation occurs in a number of ways, including delivery of negative feedback inhibition mediated by secreted immunoglobulins binding to low affinity FcγR present on B cells. This activates intracellular phosphatases, following phosphorylation of ITIM (immune tyrosine inhibitory motifs) sites on the intracellular region of the FcγR.

Antigen Dependent B-cell Differentiation

General features

Antigen-dependent B-cell differentiation is a process in which antigen encounter, in the presence of appropriate T-cell help, leads to isotype switching, affinity maturation (somatic mutation), differentiation to antibody secreting plasma cells, and memory B-cell formation (Fig. 8.1). Primary encounter with antigen occurs in secondary lymphoid tissues, producing *primary immune responses*. Primary immune responses may be initiated in *any* secondary lymphoid tissue, but the actual tissue involved depends on the manner of antigen penetration of host defense mechanisms (Chapter 1).

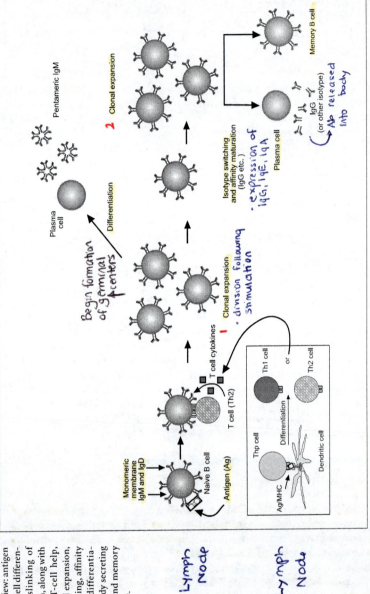

Fig. 8.1. Overview: antigen dependent B-cell differentiation. Crosslinking of mIg by antigen, along with appropriate T-cell help, leads to clonal expansion, isotype switching, affinity maturation, differentiation to antibody secreting plasma cells, and memory cell formation.

Antigen Dependent B-cell Differentiation

Activation of naive B cells

Secondary lymphoid tissues, regardless of location, contain regions predominantly populated by T cells or B cells. B cells predominate in **follicles**, while T cells are typically found in regions surrounding follicles (Fig. 8.2). Naive B-cell activation is initiated in the outer areas of follicles, where T-cell help is not limiting. The initiating stimulus for B-cell activation is antigen-induced crosslinking of the B-cell receptor complex, followed by its endocytosis in a cytosolic endosome. Lysosomes fuse with the endosome and in so doing release their enzymatic contents (lysosomal enzymes), that degrade any antigen present. When cytosolic endosomes containing class II major histocompatibility complex molecules (MHC) fuse with antigen bearing endosomes a peptide/class II MHC complex is formed, which translocates to the B-cell surface (Chapter 3). This complex is recognized by differentiated, activated CD4+ T cells and leads to T-cell/B-cell conjugate formation, which is further stabilized by adhesion molecules (e.g., I-CAM I/LFA-1; LFA-3/CD2). Conjugate formation facilitates several membrane bound ligand interactions (e.g., **B7/CD28; CD40/CD40 ligand**) that together encompass B cell costimulatory signals. Activated naive B cells undergo clonal expansion that is detectable within 24 hours of immunization. Following the initial burst of proliferation, activated B cells and T cells migrate to **primary follicles** where enhanced proliferation of B cells leads to the formation of **germinal centers**, the hallmark of **secondary follicles**.

FATE OF ACTIVATED B CELLS IN GERMINAL CENTERS

General features

Germinal centers are associated with B cell clonal expansion, isotype switching, affinity maturation, differentiation to plasma cells, and differentiation to memory B cells (Fig. 8.2). **CD40/CD40 ligand interaction** is thought to deliver an essential signal. In support of this notion, disruption of the T-cell gene for the CD40 ligand, or injection of CD40 neutralizing antibodies during immunization, prevents the formation of germinal centers and associated B-cell differentiation.

Differentiation to Ig secreting plasma cells

B cells express antigen specific antibodies as cell surface receptors, while plasma cells secrete antibodies (Fig. 8.1). Secreted antibodies lack carboxy terminal cytoplasmic sequences and the transmembrane domain required for anchorage into the plasma membrane, though they have identical antigen specificity to that of the cell surface Ig on the precursor B cell. Differentiation to the plasma cell stage occurs four days after immunization and is marked by secretion of IgM antibodies. Later in the response, naive B cells undergo isotype switching (below) and B-cell differentiation to the plasma cell stages is characterized by the secreted antibody isotype to which class switching occurred. IgD is not secreted, however.

Isotype switching

Isotype switching refers to the process by which cells expressing IgM and IgD are modified at the genomic level such that they produce antibodies of different

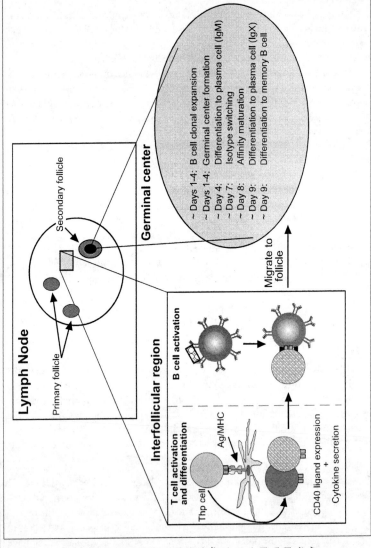

Fig. 8.2. Antigen dependent B-cell differentiation in a lymph node. Naive B-cell activation commences at the outer regions of T-cell defined zones in secondary lymphoid tissues. Following antigen binding and appropriate signals from T cells, naive B cells undergo clonal expansion, detectable within 24 hours of immunization. After this initial burst of proliferation, activated B cells and T cells migrate to the lymphoid follicles where increased proliferation of B cells leads to the formation of germinal centers. Germinal centers are associated with B-cell clonal expansion, differentiation to plasma cells and memory B cells, isotype switching, and affinity maturation.

isotypes (IgA, IgE, or IgG). As expected, since the constant region determines the antibody isotype, it is the gene encoding the heavy chain constant region that is modified (Fig. 8.3). DNA encoding the μ and the δ constant regions is excised, resulting in the juxtaposition of the heavy chain variable region to either an α, ε, or γ heavy chain constant region (isotype switching). Isotype switching, also known as **switch recombination**, occurs at unique switch regions, located between each gene encoding a constant segment of heavy chains. This phenomenon occurs in the germinal centers approximately one week after initial B-cell activation by T-dependent antigen. Specificity is maintained because only the constant region of the immunoglobulin heavy chain is altered.

The segment of DNA that is downstream (3') of the variable region genes, but upstream (5') of the "new" switch region, is deleted from the genome. Thus, isotype switching is irreversible. The selection of one heavy chain constant region over another during switch recombination is a function of signals generated during B-cell/T-cell conjugation, as well as of certain T-cell derived cytokines present in the microenvironment. Thus, disruption of the IL-4 gene in mice inhibits switch recombination to IgE.

Affinity maturation

Affinity maturation, or somatic mutation, is a process that leads to the gradual accumulation, with time after immunization, of higher affinity antibodies for the immunizing antigen (Fig. 8.1). Production of an antibody with increased affinity for the immunizing antigen occurs randomly, as a result of random **somatic mutation**, which gives rise to point mutations. These point mutations occur in the rearranged immunoglobulin "VDJ" gene region of both light and heavy chains. Somatic mutation (affinity maturation) occurs in germinal centers 7-10 days following B-cell activation. (Fig. 8.2).

Generation of memory B cells

Differentiation of activated B cells to **memory cells** occurs in germinal centers, beginning approximately one week after antigenic challenge with a T dependent antigen (Fig. 8.1). Because this event occurs within the same time frame as isotype switching and affinity maturation, memory B cells usually express high affinity immunoglobulin, and isotypes other than IgM. The unique signals that determine whether a naive B cell will differentiate to a plasma cell or a memory cell are not known.

Some memory B cells colonize the secondary lymphoid tissues. However, most join the pool of recirculating B cells that circulate from blood, lymph, and tissues that were the primary sites of previous antigen encounter. Entry of memory B cells into lymph nodes occurs via afferent lymphatics rather than high endothelial venules (HEVs), because memory B cells have reduced expression of L-selectin, the molecule that facilitates extravasation of naive B cells from the blood to the lymph node at the HEVs (Chapter 7). Memory B cells survive for weeks or months without further stimulation, and are not in cell cycle. Nonetheless, there is some evidence that antigen trapped as antigen-antibody complexes on the surface of

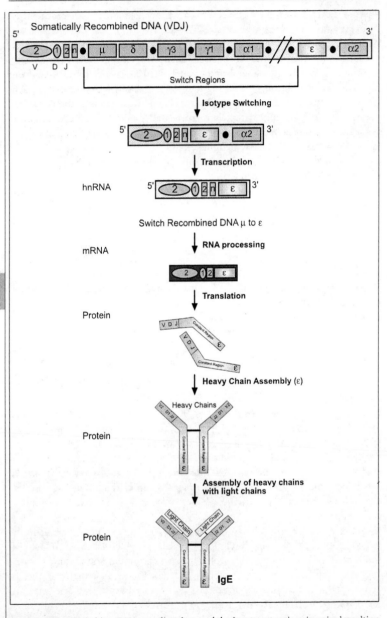

Fig. 8.3. Isotype switching. DNA encoding the μ and the δ constant regions is excised resulting in the juxtaposition of the heavy chain variable region to either an α, ε, or γ heavy chain constant region. Switch recombination occurs at unique sites, located between each gene encoding a heavy chain constant region.

follicular dendritic cells in follicles are important for stimulating long term memory B cell renewal.

An alternative hypothesis explaining persistence of memory cells suggests that, because the generation of antibody specificity is a random event, at least some sIgs are complementary to the surface Igs on other B cells, that is, they recognize the unique idiotype of another B cell sIg as antigen. These anti-idiotypes then, themselves, serve as "internal" (to the immune system) representations of antigen, capable of continually stimulating B cells by idiotype-anti-idiotype interactions. Initially proposed by Jerne, this hypothesis constitutes the so-called network theory (of regulation) of the immune system.

PRIMARY VERSUS SECONDARY IMMUNE RESPONSES

Primary exposure to antigen leads to antigen dependent B-cell differentiation as described above. Secondary exposure to the same antigen induces the activation and differentiation of memory B cells (Fig. 8.4), generating a **secondary immune response**. During secondary responses, B-cell proliferation is detected much sooner, and the number of progeny is nearly one log greater than that generated in a **primary immune response**. Migration to follicles occurs sooner, as does affinity maturation and differentiation to plasma cells (Fig. 8.4).

CLINICAL SIGNIFICANCE

Hyper IgM syndrome
Hyper IgM syndrome is a disorder that presents as recurrent pyogenic infections, pneumonia and sepsis, particularly in response to infection with extracellular bacteria. Hyper IgM syndrome is characterized by an increased level of IgM and an associated decrease in IgG and IgA, suggesting that the disorder results from an inability to undergo isotype switching. Isotype switching occurs after naive B cell activation by antigen induced crosslinking of mIg, along with T-cell signals generated following conjugate formation with T cells. T cells from patients diagnosed with hyper IgM syndrome lack expression of CD40 ligand, as indicated by flow cytometry. This implies that the CD40/CD40 ligand interaction between B cells and T cells is required for isotype switching.

Hypogammaglobulinemia
Hypogammaglobulinemia is a term describing disorders characterized by a deficiency in the production of immunoglobulins (i.e., gammaglobulins). Patients suffer from chronic severe bacterial infections. Hypogammaglobulinemia may be caused by the absence or severe reduction in the number of B cells (X-linked infantile hypogammaglobulinemia); by a maturational delay in the ability of B cells to differentiate to antibody secreting plasma cells (transient hypogammaglobulinemia of infancy); or by an acquired hypogammaglobulinemia which can affect males and females at any age (common variable hypogammaglobulinemia). The treatment for most of these immunodeficiencies is prophylactic administration

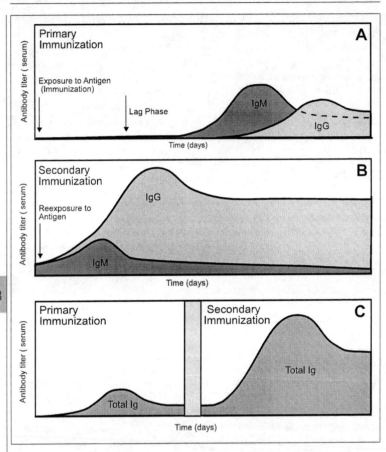

Fig. 8.4. Relative concentration of antibody serum titers. (A) IgM and IgG levels during a primary immune response. (B) IgM and IgG levels during a secondary immune response. (C) Comparison of total Ig levels during a primary and a secondary immune response. Primary and secondary immunization with antigen leads to different antibody responses with respect to latency, magnitude, and isotype.

of gammaglobulins and antibiotics, though replacement of the lymphoid stem cell pool (by bone marrow transplantation) is a (more aggressive) option.

MODEL OF SIGNAL TRANSDUCTION IN B-CELL ACTIVATION

Role of mIg and the CD79a/CD79b heterodimer

The BCR is composed of **mIg** complexed with the **CD79a/b heterodimer**, each with distinct roles in B-cell activation. Whereas mIg is the antigen recognition moiety, CD79a/CD79b serves to link mIg to signaling pathways. An emerging model of B-cell activation suggests that one of the earliest events following crosslinking of mIg is the activation (by **CD45** mediated dephosphorylation) of src family kinases. Subsequently, the **src family kinases** are auto/trans phosphorylated, as are other substrates including the tyrosine residues in the **ITAM** (immunoreceptor tyrosine based activation motif) in the CD79a/CD79b heterodimer. ITAM (sequence: YxxL/IxxxxxxxYxxL/l where Y is tyrosine, x any amino acid, L, leucine, and l is isoleucine) motifs represent sequences of amino acids containing two strategically located tyrosine residues, whose phosphorylation confers "docking" sites for proteins with **SH2 (Src homology 2) domains** (Fig. 8.5).

Role of phosphorylated ITAMs in linking BCR to signaling pathways

Tyrosine phosphorylated ITAMs contain docking sites for src family kinases, the Syk tyrosine kinase, and some adapter molecules, all of which bind the phosphorylated ITAMs via their SH2 domains. Based on in vitro studies of **Syk** substrates, it is proposed that **phospholipase Cγ (PL-Cγ)** is activated by Syk mediated phosphorylation. PL-Cγ hydrolyzes phosphatidylinositol bisphosphate (PIP2), whose products, inositol trisphosphate and diacylglycerol, bind to their respective receptors and initiate distinct biochemical changes, leading to increases in the concentration of cytosolic calcium and activation of protein kinase C, respectively. Many of the adapter proteins that bind to phosphorylated ITAMS also possess an **SH3 domain**. SH3 domains recognize and bind to motifs bearing *proline* residues. Proteins that possess both SH2 and SH3 domains can function in protein/protein interactions because binding of one "face" to ITAMs still allows for binding to proline rich proteins that directly or indirectly link the B-cell receptor to other signaling molecules. Thus some adapter molecules can connect the B-cell receptor to a **guanine exchange factor (GEF)**, via SH3 domains. GEF activates p21 ras by exchanging the bound GDP for GTP. Ras (p21) is known to mediate signaling events that lead to the activation of a kinase cascade that modulates the activity of transcription factors, and hence de novo protein synthesis.

Other molecules required for optimal activation of B cells

Costimulatory signals from ligated **CD19** are required for optimal B-cell activation, as is stimulation of **CD40** by the **CD40 ligand** present on activated T cells. Signaling via CD40 activates another family of molecules, the so-called **TRAF (tumor necrosis factor associated factors)** molecules. The end result of this signaling cascade is activation of the transcriptional regulator NFκB, and increased transcription of a number of developmentally important genes. **Another tyrosine kinase significant in B-cell activation is the Btk kinase.** Mutations in any of the Btk domains leads to a disorder **X-linked agammaglobulinemia** which is characterized by a reduction in the number of mature B cells and in circulating antibody.

NEGATIVE SIGNALING IN B CELLS

Negative signaling refers to the inhibition of B cells following antigen induced activation. Negative signaling occurs when secreted IgG crosslinks the antigen

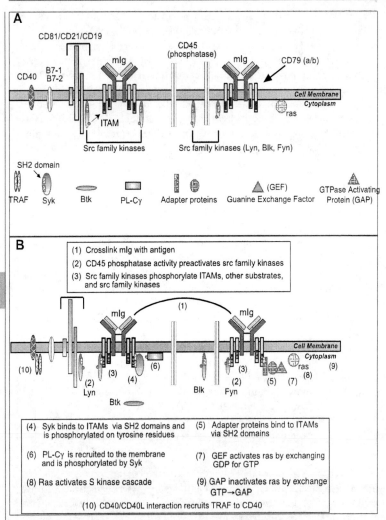

Fig. 8.5. Initial molecular interactions in B-cell activation. A number of coreceptor signals synergize with signals generated following crosslinking of mIg by antigen. Phosphorylation of tyrosine residues within the ITAM regions of the CD79a/CD79b heterodimer, produces docking sites for proteins that will link the B-cell receptor to signaling pathways.

Antigen Dependent B-cell Differentiation

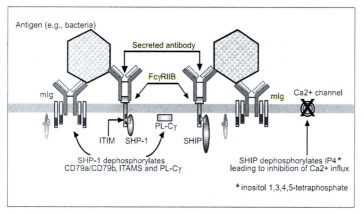

Fig. 8.6. Negative signaling in B cells. Following crosslinking of the BCR with FcγRIIB, phosphatases (SHP-1 and SHIP) are activated after binding via SH2 domains to FcγRIIB ITIM sequences. SHP-1 dephosphorylates PL-Cγ and CD79a/CD79b, leading to a decrease in the activity of protein kinase C, and the release of calcium from intracellular stores. The main effect of crosslinking BCR and FcγRIIB is inhibition of extracellular calcium influx. Ca^{2+} channel opening is induced by inositol 1,3,4,5-tetraphosphate (IP4), and IP4 is a known substrate for SHIP, which thus regulates Ca^{2+} channel activity.

bound mIg and integral membrane receptor, **FcγRIIB**, a low affinity receptor (Fig. 8.6). In this way secreted immunoglobulin serves as a negative feedback regulator to inhibit further secretion of antibody. This process is thought to involve tyrosine phosphorylation of **ITIMs** (**i**mmunoreceptor **t**yrosine-base **i**nhibition **m**otif) in the intracellular cytoplasmic tail of FcγR11B. The ITIM consensus sequence is V/IxYxxL/V where V is valine, x any amino acid, Y is tyrosine, and L is leucine.

The present model of negative signaling following crosslinking of the BCR with FcγRIIB suggests that the activated src family kinase, lck, phosphorylates the ITIMs, creating docking sites for binding (via SH2 domains) and activation of **phosphatases** (SHP-1 and SHIP). The main effect of crosslinking the B-cell receptor with FcγRIIB is inhibition of extracellular calcium influx. As discussed earlier, because inositol 1,3,4,5-tetraphosphate (IP4) activates an endothelial membrane Ca^{2+} channel, and IP4 is also a substrate for SHIP, it is thought that SHIP regulates the plasma membrane calcium channel.

B-CELL RESPONSES TO T-INDEPENDENT ANTIGENS

T-independent (T-indep) antigens are antigens that can induce naive B-cell activation in the absence of T-cell "help". T-indep antigens are divided into two categories, Type I or Type II. B-cell activation, in response to T-indep antigens, leads mainly to IgM production. However, for Type II T-indep antigens, some isotype switching has been detected, in the presence of appropriate cytokines. In contrast to T-dependent (T-dep) antigens, differentiation to memory cells does not occur in response to either Type I or Type II T-indep antigens. The prototypic **Type I T-independent antigen** is the bacterial cell wall component, **lipopolysaccharide (LPS), when used at low concentrations**. At high concentrations LPS is mitogenic. The prototypic **Type II T-independent antigen** is **pneumococcal polysaccharide**.

SUMMARY

The initiating stimulus for naive B-cell differentiation is antigen-induced crosslinking of BCR, in the presence of costimulatory signals arising from conjugate formation with activated T cells and their cytokines. The proliferation of B cells following these triggering signals leads to the formation of germinal centers in the follicles, the site of isotype switching, affinity maturation (somatic mutation), and differentiation to antibody secreting plasma cells and memory B cells.

Antigen-induced cross linking of B-cell antigen receptors leads to the activation of phosphatases, kinases, and GTP binding proteins, as well as other signal transducing molecules required for B-cell differentiation and proliferation. Although crosslinking of membrane immunoglobulin is the initiating stimulus for B-cell activation, coupling of mIg to signal transducing molecules is mediated via the CD79a/CD79b heterodimer expressed on the cell surface in association with mIg. Negative feedback inhibition is in part mediated by secreted immunoglobulins that bind to low affinity FcγR present on the B cell, an interaction that delivers a negative signal to the B cell.

During secondary responses, B-cell proliferation is detected much sooner than that observed for primary responses, and the antibody titer is much greater.

CLINICAL CASES AND DISCUSSION

Clinical Case #15
E.D. is a 33 year old male, who has a history of "globe-trotting" since the age of 18, and has recently returned from a 4-month trip to Indonesia. E.D. had no vaccinations before travel, with the exception of those (e.g., yellow fever), demanded by the immigration authorities of the host countries. Three weeks after his return from Indonesia his family noticed he was "yellow" in the face, and he felt listless and nauseous. His family physician ordered a variety of blood tests, which suggested acute hepatitis. Serology was negative for hepatitis C (HepC), hepatitis A (HepA) and hepatitis E (HepE), but results were positive for hepatitis B (HepB). Which tests should you now request from the laboratory, and why?

Discussion Case #15
Background
Determine first if E.D. is a carrier of HepB (infected a long time ago) or whether this is a new infection. Because primary antibody responses are of the IgM isotype, while memory responses are of the IgG isotype, measurement of anti-HepB antibody isotype should be a first step. Because different antibody specificities exist at

different stages of infection with HepB, you should assess this infection by determining the antibody specificity. For HepB, analysis would be as follows:

Antibody	HepB Viral Antigen	Interpretation
IgG	core antigen "c"	confirms new or old infection with Hep B
IgG	core antigen "Be"	suggests chronic infection, with low virulence
IgM	surface antigen "s"	strongly suggests new infections, though persistence suggests a chronic carrier state

Similar analyses of IgG and IgM antibodies are applied to assess recurrent/novel infection with HepA. There are other less common hepatitis viruses that we should be concerned with, including HepG (acute-like Hep A, and thus self-limiting); delta (coinfection with HepB, leads to chronic hepatitis and cirrhosis); and HepC (chronic infection).

Tests
As described above

Treatment
There is currently no cure for HepB infection once this occurs. A number of pilot studies are testing newer antiviral agents (synthetic inhibitors of viral DNA synthesis, e.g., ribavirin) and/or potential physiologic antiviral agents (e.g., IFNα). Long term, complications of HepB infection include cirrhosis and liver failure, or (particularly in the oriental population) hepatocellular carcinoma. This case underlines the need to stress vaccination where possible.

Clinical Case #16
HJ is a young (4 year old) boy with recurrent sinus infections over the last few years. In preparation for a planned trip to the Far East he began a series of vaccinations with recombinant HepB vaccine. Before the third vaccination, you test his titer of IgG antibody (from the previous immunizations) to assess the efficacy of the vaccination and find he has extraordinarily low titers (barely above the nonimmune level), with relatively high IgM titers. What might be going on here? How would you proceed?

Discussion Case #16
Background
Questions to address include, "What is the significance of the sinus infections?" "Why is there such a poor IgG response to vaccination?" "Are these issues related?"

Immunodeficiencies related to B lymphocyte lineage defects are not uncommon (Chapter 15). Severe deficiencies (with no or little endogenous production of Ig) often present early in life, following that period of time when passive Ig protection (from the mother) wanes (generally approximately 6 months of age). This is unlikely to be the case here. Another later manifestation of immunoglobulin deficiency is so-called **transient hypogammaglobulinemia of infancy** (thought to be due to inadequate cytokine-mediated promotion of B-cell differentiation), in which all antibody isotypes are affected. The immunodeficiency, **selective IgA deficiency** (the Ig most needed for protection at mucosal surfaces), can lead to recurrent infection at these sites, with repeated sinus infections (upper respiratory tract). Given the additional evidence for both repeated sinus infections AND poor IgG production after vaccination, a selective IgA deficiency does not explain all of the disease manifestations in this boy. There is not a generalized B-cell defect in differentiation to plasma cells *per se*, because IgM levels are very high.

T lymphocytes contribute to class switching during differentiation of B cells, by virtue of signals delivered to B cells by engagement of CD40 (on the B cell) with CD40 ligand (on the T cell). In the absence of the latter, there exists a malfunction in the final stages of B-cell differentiation/development, and a so-called **hyper IgM syndrome** ensues. All Ig isotypes (other than IgM) are affected, with low to absent IgG and IgA, IgE. This is the most likely explanation of the clinical findings described.

Tests

We should measure (quantitatively) the levels of IgM, IgG and IgA in this fellow, predicting that only the former levels would be normal/high. Next we might look for evidence for expression of CD40 ligand on this boy's T cells. Greatest levels are expressed on activated cells, so one test would stimulate T cells with a mitogen (concanavalin A) and then stain with a fluorescein conjugated antibody to CD40 ligand. We would expect low/negative staining compared with control subjects. Finally, we might examine the effect of artificially including cells expressing CD40 ligand in cultures of this boy's B cells, which are then stimulated with a B-cell mitogen (lipopolysaccharide). In the presence of exogenous CD40 ligand class switching will occur so that the cultures might now produce some IgG and IgA. This would indicate that the B cells in this patient are not intrinsically abnormal.

Treatment

The only simple treatment here is passive administration of pooled immunoglobulin. In the future, as biotechnology develops and clinical applicability of our current knowledge becomes the norm, we may be able to offer gene transfer technology (giving this child back the defective CD40 ligand gene). For now, as he prepares to travel to an area of HepB endemicity, he should certainly receive passive HepB immune globulin for protection!

TEST YOURSELF

Multiple Choice Questions

For questions 1-3 make the best match with one of the following. Use each choice once, more than once, or not at all.

    a. CD79a/CD79b
    b. Btk
    c. ITAM
    d. ITIM
    e. mIg

1. Mutations in this protein leads to X-linked aggamagobulinemia
2. Activation motif
3. Present on FcγRIIB
4. All the following occur in germinal centers EXCEPT
   a. differentiation to plasma cells
   b. affinity maturation (somatic mutation)
   c. isotype switching
   d. memory cell formation
   e. somatic recombination
5. Mrs. L, a 37-year-old housewife with no history of childhood illness, has had recurrent chest and pyogenic infections over the last 18 months. She appears unwell and is found to be anemic. Tests indicate low levels of circulating immunoglobulins and she failed to produce specific antibodies to a booster dose of tetanus toxoid given one month previously. What is the most likely diagnosis?
   a. x-linked hypogammaglobulinemia
   b. common variable hypogammaglobulinemia
   c. transient hypogammaglobulinemia of infancy
   d. selective IgA deficiency
   e. could be any one of the above

Answers: 1b; 2c; 3d; 4e; 5b

Short Answer Questions
1. What are ITAMS, and what is their role in signal transduction?
2. Compare B cells and plasma cells with respect to phenotype and function.
3. How and when does isotype switching occur? Why is it irreversible?
4. Define affinity maturation. What is the stimulus for affinity maturation?
5. Compare and contrast primary and secondary B-cell responses.

T Lymphocytes

Objectives	168
CD4+ T Cells: Antigen Induced Differentiation	168
Memory CD4+ T Cells	174
Clinical Relevance of Type 1 versus Type 2 Cytokines	175
CD8+ T Cells: Antigen Induced Differentiation	177
Memory CD8+ T Cells	179
Clinical Relevance CD8+ T Cells	179
Model of Signal Transduction in T-cell Activation	180
Negative Regulation of T-cell Signaling	182
Memory Lymphocytes in Immunosurveillance	184
Gamma/Delta T Cells	184
Summary	185
Clinical Cases and Discussion	186
Test Yourself	189

Objectives

After reading this chapter the reader will first understand the functional significance of classifying T cells into CD4+ and CD8+ T-cell subsets; the manner in which both CD4+ and CD8+ T cells differentiate into effector cells following encounter with antigen; and how CD4+ T cells may be characterized by the various factors (cytokines) they produce. The role of cytokines, in the extracellular milieu, in regulating T-cell differentiation, and the role of different T-cell subsets in immune responses will be discussed next. This leads to a consideration of how alterations in T-cell differentiation can lead to pathological processes, particularly when the effects of various cytokines on immune processes are considered.

The discussion on T-cell biology concludes with a review of T-cell signaling, and the various intracellular signaling pathways that are activated and involved in delivering signals (to the nucleus) to regulate transcription of functionally important genes. Finally the reader will find a brief discussion on the properties and potential importance of another distinct class of T cells, bearing unique γδ T-cell receptors.

CD4+ T Cells: Antigen Induced Differentiation

General features

CD4+ T cells are a subset of T cells whose primary biological function is the secretion of cytokines. CD4+ T cells that survive the screening process in the thymus are still termed *naive* because they are unable to perform their biological function without a further differentiation stage. This differentiation stage occurs outside the thymus and is induced by high avidity interaction with peptide/class II MHC, in the presence of appropriate costimulatory signals. The process occurs in secondary lymphoid tissues and leads to the generation of T-cell subsets (Th1 and Th2) that secrete distinct patterns of cytokines. Some of the Th1 and Th2 cells differentiate to memory cells while others undergo apoptosis (Fig. 9.1A). Subsequent exposure to the same peptide/class II MHC induces the reactivation of these memory cells (Fig. 9.1B).

Regardless of the secondary lymphoid tissue where contact with antigen occurs, activation of T cells requires that the antigen be displayed on the surface of an **antigen presenting cell** in association with class II MHC (peptide/class II MHC). The most efficient antigen-presenting cell is the **dendritic cell**. This cell constitutively expresses both class II MHC and various costimulatory molecules whose counter-ligands (see below) are present on the T cell. When a T cell interacts with peptide/MHC complexes in the **absence** of these costimulatory interactions the T cell becomes unresponsive (**anergic**).

Cell surface interaction for Thp cell activation
Naive CD4+ T-cell activation is a stringently controlled process and occurs optimally when the T cell receives several signals delivered by an antigen-presenting cell. These signals arise from the interaction of: (i) peptide/class II MHC with TCR, (ii) class II MHC with CD4; (iii) the B7 family of costimulatory molecules with their counter ligands, CD28/CTLA4; (iv) CD40 with its counter ligand CD40L; and (v) various **adhesion molecules** on the T cell interacting with counter molecules on the antigen presenting cell. The molecular interactions occurring during conjugate formation enhance the avidity of peptide/MHC interactions with the TCR (Fig. 9.2).

Progression from CD4+ naive T cell (Thp) to Th1 or Th2 subsets
In the presence of TCR interaction with peptide/MHC and appropriate costimulatory molecules, naive CD4+ T cells, (Thp), express IL-2 receptors and secrete the cytokines, interleukin-2 (IL-2). Interaction of IL-2 with the IL-2 receptor (cognate interaction) induces clonal expansion of antigen stimulated T cells (Fig. 9.3), increasing the number of T cells with a specificity uniquely recognizing the peptide/class II MHC complex that induced the initial differentiation.

Antigen-induced differentiation of a Thp proceeds via a Th0 intermediate to either a Th1 or Th2 subset (Fig. 9.4). These latter subsets have been defined by the pattern of cytokines that they secrete. Th0 cells secrete cytokines common to both subsets. There is some evidence that the cytokines present in the microenvironment contribute to polarization of Th0 to either a Th1 or Th2 subset. Thus, in the presence of IL-4, the Th0 populations are driven towards the Th2 profile and Type-2 cytokine secretion. Both mast cells and Th0 cells may serve as the source of IL-4 in the early phase of the response. This is in accord with the evidence that conditions of mast cell stimulation (chronic mucosal antigen challenge) are often associated with Th2 development (e.g., gastrointestinal parasitic infestation, asthma, etc.).

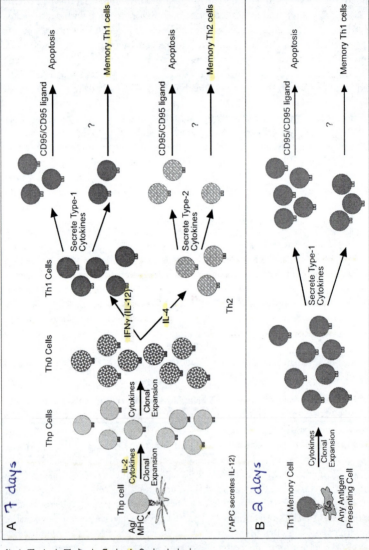

Fig. 9.1. Overview: A. Fate of activated Th1/Th2 subsets; B. Fate of activated memory cells. A. Upon exposure to an antigenic peptide/MHC complex and appropriate costimulatory signals Thp undergo a series of differentiation stages to cytokine producing Th1 and Th2 cells. Some of these undergo apoptosis while some differentiate to memory cells. B. Memory cells are similarly triggered, without requiring differentiation.

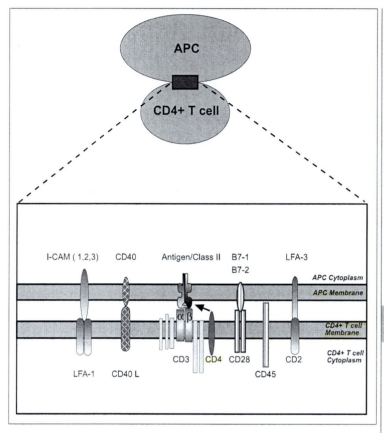

Fig. 9.2. Cell surface interactions during conjugate formation of a T cell and an antigen presenting cell. Several cell surface interactions, in addition to TCR/class II MHC, contribute to high affinity conjugate formation between the T cell and the antigen presenting cell.

IL-12 and IFNγ, in contrast, selectively drive Th0 cells towards the Th1 developmental state and Type-1 cytokine secretion. IFNγ is produced by Th0 cells and by IL-12-activated natural killer cells. Because activated dendritic cells and/or macrophages secrete IL-12, the influence of IL-12 on development may thus be indirect. It is likely that so-called Th1 and Th2 subsets actually merely reflect two extremes of Th cell differentiation because many T-cell clones have been identified that secrete different intermediate combinations of cytokines other than the patterns associated with either Th1 or Th2 subsets.

Controlling the response

Control of the immune response requires dampening of cytokine secretion. This is achieved in two ways: (i) loss of T-cell stimulation because the infectious

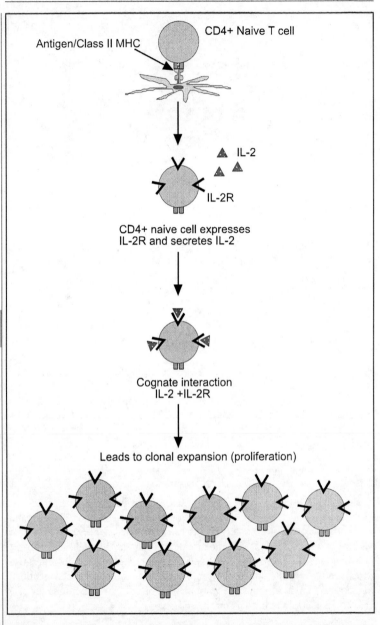

Fig. 9.3. Interaction of IL-2 with IL-2 receptors leads to clonal expansion of T cells. T-cell activation leads to the expression of high affinity IL-2 receptors and secretion of IL-2. Interaction of IL-2/IL-2R leads to clonal expansion of the T cell.

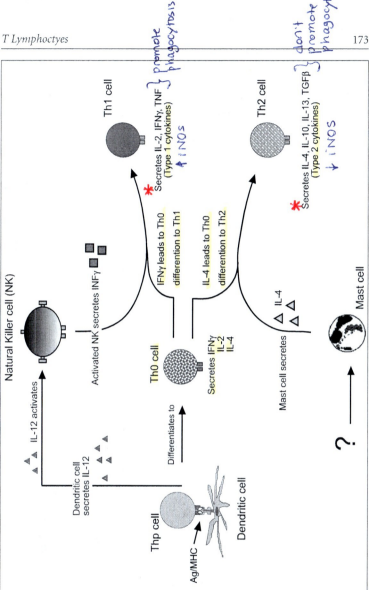

Fig. 9.4. Antigen induced Thp differentiation. Antigen processing by dendritic cells leads to secretion of IL-12. Antigen presentation to Thp by these activated dendritic cells can bias the differentiation of the Thp to that of a Th1 phenotype through IL-12 mediated activation of NK cells and subsequent IFNγ production. In contrast, the presence of IL-4 biases the response to that of a Th2 phenotype.

agent has been eliminated, and so peptide/MHC complexes are no longer being presented to T cells; and (ii) reciprocal regulation of cytokine secretion by Th1 and Th2 cells. IL-4 and IL-10, produced by Th2 clones, dampen the Th1 response. IFNγ produced by Th1 cells correspondingly dampens the Th2 response (Fig. 9.5). IL-10 inhibition is believed to be mediated by inhibiting the function of antigen presenting cells, and may involve inhibition of IL-12 secretion (and in turn inhibition of IFNγ production). Following resolution of infection, Th1 and Th2 clones die by apoptosis or become memory cells (Fig. 9.1A).

MEMORY CD4+ T CELLS

Memory cells (Th1 and Th2 clones) can serve an immunosurveillance role, having been *presensitized* to the immunizing agent that induced their differentiation (Fig. 9.1B). Memory cell formation serves a crucial role in immune responses because subsequent re-exposure to the initiating agent results in a rapid (1-2 days) response, unlike the seven days required for Thp differentiation to Th1 and Th2 cells. The conditions for memory T-cell activation are less stringent than for naive cells regarding requirements for adhesion and costimulatory molecules. Consequently, antigen presenting cells, other than dendritic cells, can serve in this capacity early in response to antigen re-exposure. In addition, memory cell activation can occur at the site of antigen contact, rather than in secondary lymphoid tissues. Memory CD4+ T cells secrete cytokines.

GREAT SUMMARY FIGURE

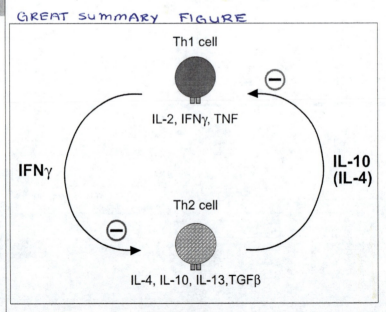

Fig. 9.5. Reciprocal regulation of Th1 and Th2 cells. Cytokines produced by Th1 cells dampen Th2 responses, while cytokines produced by the Th2 cells dampen Th1 responses.

CLINICAL RELEVANCE OF TYPE 1 VERSUS TYPE 2 CYTOKINES

Cellular and humoral immunity
Whether a Type 1 or a Type 2 cytokine profile predominates in response to antigenic stimulation has significant consequences because the cytokines produced by Th cells preferentially activate distinct branches of adaptive immunity. Th1 cytokines, more appropriately referred to as Type 1 cytokines, support cell mediated immune responses in which macrophages, natural killer cells, and cytotoxic T cells are effector cells. Other responses associated with Type 1 cytokines include isotype switching to IgG2a and delayed type hypersensitivity (DTH) responses. DTH responses are delayed (24-48 hrs) reactions of (CD4) memory T cells following activation by antigen, in which Type 1cytokines (including TNF) are produced. The latter leads to nonspecific inflammatory tissue reactions, including altered blood vessel permeability and tissue accumulation of macrophages. The DTH reaction is the *sine qua non* of Th1 cell activation. In contrast, Th2 cytokines, more appropriately referred to as Type 2 cytokines, induce B-cell activation, isotype switching to IgG1 and IgE, and the differentiation of activated B cells to plasma cells (Fig. 9.6).

N.B. The rationale for now using Type 1 (or Type 2) cytokines, rather than the (older) Th1 (or Th2) cytokines, as a nomenclature is that is has now become apparent that CD8+ T cells (not merely Th, CD4+, T cells) can also be subdivided into separate classes of cells (Tc1 and Tc2), which similarly produce one or the other panel of cytokines.

Microbial immunity
The importance of polarized Th responses becomes evident as one considers the immune mechanisms that are optimal in protection against different pathogens. Cell mediated responses (Th1 cells and Type 1 cytokines) are most efficient for protective immunity against viruses, parasites, fungi, and intracellular bacteria, while, in general, humoral responses (Th2 cells and Type 2 cytokines) occupy this niche for responses to extracellular bacteria and parasites. Because the cytokine microenvironment at the time of infection can regulate development of Th1 vs Th2 cells (see above), it thus becomes apparent that this same environment may alter the course of infection and disease progression.

There are clinical scenarios where the differential development of polarized Th subsets is correlated with pathology. Spontaneous resolution of infection with *Leishmania major* or *Mycobacterium leprae*, versus the development of persistent nonhealing lesions, is associated with the presence of Type 1 vs. Type 2 cytokines, respectively. This probably reflects the important role for intracellular macrophage activation, by IFNγ produced by Th1 cells, as a precursor to the clearing of these infections. In the relative absence (or paucity) of IFNγ production, with Type 2 cytokines instead predominating, infected macrophages are unable to eradicate the organism(s). In consequence, the infected individual develops a pathology typical of a persistent chronic infection.

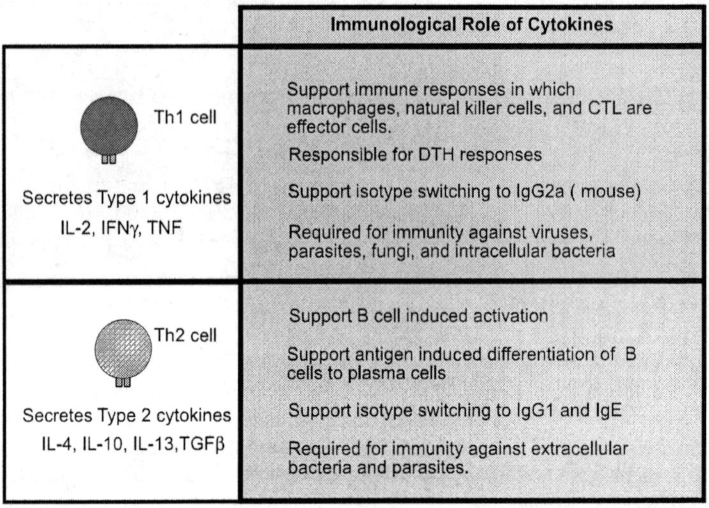

	Immunological Role of Cytokines
Th1 cell Secretes Type 1 cytokines IL-2, IFNγ, TNF	Support immune responses in which macrophages, natural killer cells, and CTL are effector cells. Responsible for DTH responses Support isotype switching to IgG2a (mouse) Required for immunity against viruses, parasites, fungi, and intracellular bacteria
Th2 cell Secretes Type 2 cytokines IL-4, IL-10, IL-13, TGFβ	Support B cell induced activation Support antigen induced differentiation of B cells to plasma cells Support isotype switching to IgG1 and IgE Required for immunity against extracellular bacteria and parasites.

Fig. 9.6. Immunological relevance of Type 1 and Type 2 cytokines. Whether a Type 1 or a Type 2 cytokine profile predominates in response to antigenic stimulation has profound consequences since the cytokines produced by Th cells preferentially activate distinct branches of adaptive immunity.

Autoimmune disorders

In many patients with a variety of autoimmune disorders (multiple sclerosis, insulin-dependent diabetes, Hashimoto's thyroiditis), pathology is associated with the existence of a Th1 response to the relevant autoantigen. This underlies the scientific rationale for attempting to identify the factors that skew the Th profile in these scenarios, in order to develop immunotherapeutic strategies that would alter the relative balance of antigen specific Th 1 versus Th2 subsets. As one example of such a strategy, it has been found that oral administration of antigen preferentially induces Th2 subsets, perhaps by stimulating TGFβ production (a cytokine believed to promote Th2 development). Thus, patients with multiple sclerosis have been fed myelin extracts with the expectation that this might favor Th2 development at the expense of Type 1 cytokine production, with a concomitant beneficial effect on their disease status. While the results were not as dramatic as had been hoped, there were some clinical benefits observed, more apparent in men than in women. These sex-related differences may be taken to imply that endogenous hormones contribute to the microenvironment that regulates the cytokine profile induced in response to antigenic stimulation.

Transplantation

There has been interest within the field of transplantation in the possible role for manipulation of Type 1 vs Type 2 cytokine production as a means to regulate graft rejection (Chapter 17). There seems to be a consensus that T cells isolated from patients undergoing active graft rejection produce IL-2 and IFNγ (Type 1 cytokines). However, controversy exists concerning the production of IL-4 and IL-10 (Type 2 cytokines) by T cells isolated from nonrejecting patients. It is not clear if this inconsistency is related to: (i) the type of organ/tissue graft studied; (ii) the tempo of rejection (perhaps Th1 development merely correlates with faster rejection than Th2 development); or (iii) the existence of other cytokines that are more important in immunoregulation, but which have yet to be examined. Amongst these, some combination of TGFβ and IL-10 is thought to be important.

CD8+ T CELLS: ANTIGEN INDUCED DIFFERENTIATION

Activation of pCTL

Interaction of pCTL with an autologous cell expressing peptide/class I MHC, in the presence of CD4+ T cell derived IL-2, provides the initiating stimulus for antigen induced differentiation of pCTL to CTL, a process requiring about seven days (Fig. 9.7). CD8+ T cells do not require a special microenvironment, such as a secondary lymphoid tissue, for antigen induced differentiation. They can develop within a site of infection. Although TCR engagement with antigen/MHC is a prerequisite for T-cell activation, it is insufficient to trigger optimal T-cell activation. Costimulatory molecules and other accessory molecules stabilizing interactions with the target cells are required. Conjugate formation between the target cell and the pCTL is stabilized by high avidity interaction of adhesion molecules CD2 and LFA-3, LFA-1 and ICAM (1-3). Optimal activation of the pCTL also requires that CD8 bind to class I MHC at a site distinct from that which binds to the TCR.

Progression from pCTL to CTL

One of the early signals detected in the progression from pCTL to CTL (cytotoxic lymphocyte) is IL-2 receptor expression. Differentiation of most pre-CTLs requires auxiliary activation of Th1 cells to provide a source of IL-2, which in turn functions in a paracrine manner to induce proliferation and clonal expansion of those pCTLs that express IL-2 receptors (Fig. 9.7). Some *helper independent* CTLs have been identified that themselves secrete enough IL-2 to support their own clonal expansion in the absence of auxiliary CD4+ cells. The progression from pCTL to CTL occurs over one week. Circulating mature CTLs (hereafter termed CTLs) function in immune surveillance by destroying cells infected with the virus that initiated their differentiation.

Delivering the lethal hit

CTL-mediated lysis of the target cell is commonly referred to as delivery of the "lethal hit", and is initiated following formation of a high affinity conjugate of the mature CTL with the target cell (Fig. 9.7). Conjugate formation triggers the localization of lytic granules to the CTL membrane where the two cells are in contact, with polarization of granule release directed "outward" towards the target cell. This polarized release of lytic granules ensures specificity of killing (i.e., killing of target cells but not the CTL itself). The CTL is unimpaired by the lytic process and

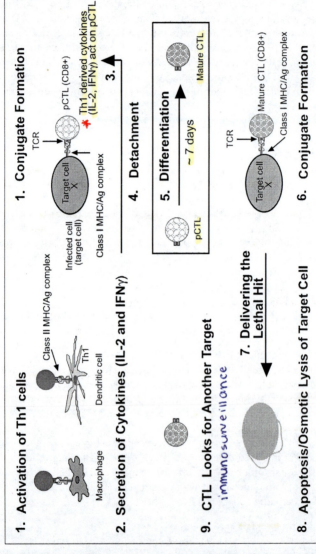

Fig. 9.7. Antigen-induced differentiation of pCTL and subsequent killing of virally infected cells. Interaction of pCTL (TCR) with peptide/class I MHC in the presence of IL-2 triggers the differentiation of pCTL to CTL. Mature CTL lyse infected cells expressing the same peptide/class I MHC as that which triggered their production. The polarized release of lytic granules apparently ensures specificity of killing (i.e., killing of target cells but not the CTL itself). The CTL is unimpaired by the lytic process and, once it has delivered its lethal hit, detaches and continues its function of surveillance and killing.

once it has delivered its "lethal hit", detaches and continues its function of immunological surveillance.

Death of the target cell occurs by either osmotic lysis or apoptosis. Osmotic lysis is induced when the CTL exocytoses specialized secretory granules containing perforin into the target cell contact zone. **Perforin is a pore forming protein whose insertion into the target cell membrane leads to colloidal swelling and osmotic lysis.** There is evidence that destruction of target cells by CTLs occurs by both calcium dependent and calcium independent mechanisms. Because release of perforin, and its lytic actions, depend on the presence of calcium, some other mechanism must also be capable of inducing DNA fragmentation, characteristic of cells that have undergone apoptosis (see below).

Memory CD8+ T Cells

As elimination of virally infected cells occurs, the antigenic stimulus for expansion of the specific CD8 T-cell pool disappears. In the process of antigen induced differentiation, CTL clones have been generated with TCRs specific for the inciting viral peptide/class I MHC complex. Following resolution of infection many activated T cells will die. Others will become dormant and are referred to as memory cells. Memory cells serve a crucial role in immune responses because host defenses to subsequent infections are activated immediately instead of after seven days, the time period for pCTL differentiation to CTL. As discussed earlier for CD4+ T cells, activation of CD8+ T cells requires less *costimulation* than for primary responses.

Clinical Relevance CD8+ T Cells

As expected from what we know of their biological properties, a clinical role for CD8+ cells becomes most apparent when we examine pathology in at least two kinds of patient populations, namely those suffering from viral infections (Case #18) and those undergoing tissue transplantation.

Recipients of solid organ grafts (heart, kidney, and liver) receive nonspecific immunosuppressive drugs to counter the immune attack of the host (recipient) against the graft (organ). Unfortunately this nonspecific immunosuppression often leads to an increased incidence of cancers and/or opportunistic infections (e.g., with cytomegalovirus (CMV); pneumocystis carinii, (PCP)). To combat these side effects it often becomes necessary to decrease the dose of nonspecific immunosuppressive drugs used. When this is done, there now often occurs an immunological *attack* against the grafted organ, involving both direct cytotoxicity (CD8-cell mediated), as well as cytokine-mediated reactivity (CD4 mediated). Balancing this line between avoiding graft rejection, but not leaving the recipient an immunological cripple, has become a major issue in clinical transplantation (Chapter 17).

To counter the problem of CMV infection in the special case of bone marrow transplantation it has been proposed that clonally expanded **recipient** CD8+ T cells be infused along with the graft. These CD8+ T cells would be specific for the host

CMV peptide/ class I MHC complex (not the donor graft antigens). When in the face of the immunosuppressive effects of antirejection drugs CMV begins to replicate in the recipient, the infused cytotoxic T cells would attack the virally infected cells. Because mature, clonally expanded CTL are used, the lack of IL-2 needed for differentiation of the pCTL to CTL (see above) does not impair the killing of virally infected cells. (One of the effects of immunosuppression with the commonly used agent, cyclosporin A, is to decrease IL-2 production).

MODEL OF SIGNAL TRANSDUCTION IN T-CELL ACTIVATION

Role of TCR and the CD3 complex

The TCR is comprised of α/β polypeptides complexed with the CD3 invariant chains, each having distinct roles in T-cell activation. Whereas the α/β polypeptides represent the antigen recognition moiety, CD3 serves to link these polypeptides to signaling pathways. An emerging model of T-cell activation suggests that one of the earliest events following antigen/MHC interaction with the TCR, and high affinity conjugate formation of the T cell with an antigen presenting cell, is the activation (by **CD45** mediated dephosphorylation) of src family kinases, lck and fyn. Subsequently, these kinases are auto/trans phosphorylated, as are other substrates, including the tyrosine residues in the **ITAM** (**i**mmunoreceptor **t**yrosine based **a**ctivation **m**otif) of the CD3 molecules. ITAM (sequence: YxxL/ IxxxxxxxYxxL/l where Y is tyrosine, x any amino acid, L, leucine, and l is isoleucine) motifs represent sequences of amino acids containing two strategically located tyrosine residues, whose phosphorylation confers "docking" properties for proteins with **SH2 (Src homology 2) domains** (Fig. 9.8). The collection of proteins recruited to CD3 serve as the focal points for the construction of a molecular scaffold that links the TCR to signaling pathways.

Role of phosphorylated ITAMs in linking TCR to signaling pathways

Tyrosine phosphorylated ITAMs serve as docking sites for src family kinases, the ZAP 70 tyrosine kinase, and some adapter molecules. All of these molecules bind to phosphorylated ITAMs via their SH2 domains. Based on in vitro studies of **ZAP 70 kinase** substrates, it is proposed that **phospholipase Cγ (PL-Cγ)** is activated by ZAP 70 mediated phosphorylation. PL-Cγ hydrolyzes phosphatidylinositol bisphosphate (PIP2) whose products, inositol trisphosphate and diacylglycerol, bind to their respective receptors, initiating distinct biochemical changes that lead to increases in the concentration of cytosolic calcium and activation of protein kinase C, respectively. Many of the adapter proteins that bind to phosphorylated ITAMS also possess an **SH3 domain**. SH3 domains recognize and bind to motifs bearing proline residues. Proteins that possess both SH2 and SH3 domains can function in protein/protein interactions because binding of one "face" to ITAMs still allows for binding to proline rich proteins that directly, or indirectly, link the TCR to signaling molecules. As an example, one adapter molecule binds a guanine exchange protein (GEF) that activates p21 ras by exchanging the bound GDP for GTP. Ras (p21) is known to mediate signaling events that

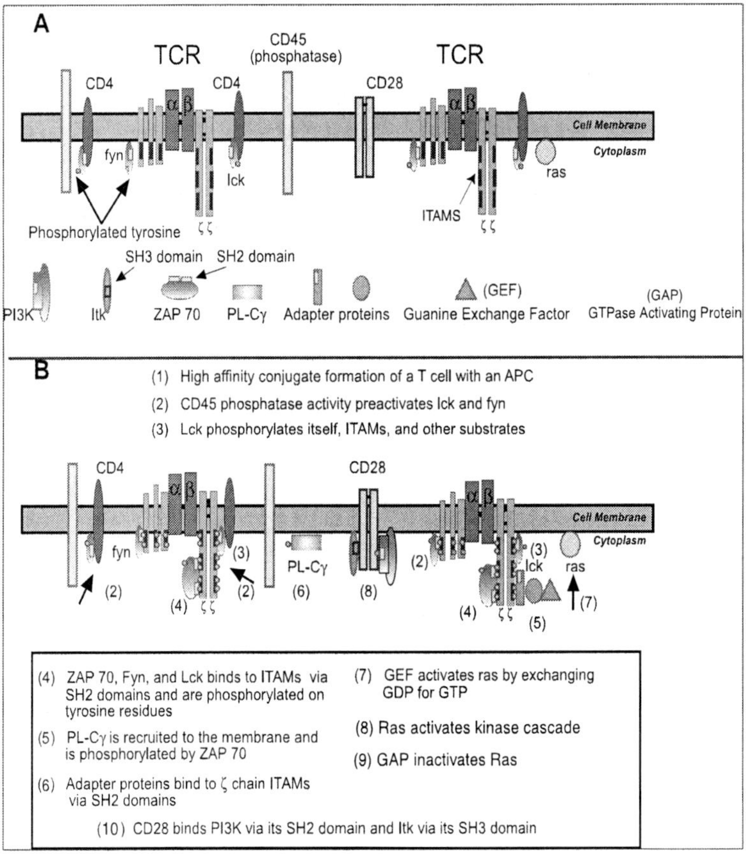

T Lymphoctyes

A

[Diagram showing resting T cell molecular interactions with labels: TCR, CD4, CD45 (phosphatase), CD28, TCR, fyn, lck, ras, ITAMS, Cell Membrane, Cytoplasm, Phosphorylated tyrosine, SH3 domain, SH2 domain, PI3K, Itk, ZAP 70, PL-Cγ, Adapter proteins, (GEF) Guanine Exchange Factor, (GAP) GTPase Activating Protein]

B

(1) High affinity conjugate formation of a T cell with an APC
(2) CD45 phosphatase activity preactivates lck and fyn
(3) Lck phosphorylates itself, ITAMs, and other substrates

[Diagram showing activated T cell with labels: CD4, CD28, fyn, PL-Cγ, lck, ras, Cell Membrane, Cytoplasm, with numbered steps (2), (3), (4), (5), (6), (7), (8)]

(4) ZAP 70, Fyn, and Lck binds to ITAMs via SH2 domains and are phosphorylated on tyrosine residues
(5) PL-Cγ is recruited to the membrane and is phosphorylated by ZAP 70
(6) Adapter proteins bind to ζ chain ITAMs via SH2 domains
(7) GEF activates ras by exchanging GDP for GTP
(8) Ras activates kinase cascade
(9) GAP inactivates Ras
(10) CD28 binds PI3K via its SH2 domain and Itk via its SH3 domain

Fig. 9.8. Molecular interactions in (A) resting T cells and (B) activated T cells. High affinity interaction between a T cell and an antigen presenting cell leads to the activation of biochemical signaling pathways mediated via kinases, phosphatases, phospholipases, and G proteins.

lead to the activation of a kinase cascade required for production of IL-2 and T-cell proliferation.

Other molecules required for optimal activation of T cells

T-cell activation requires costimulatory signals transduced via T-cell counter ligands for the B7 family of molecules, and CD40, both of which are expressed on antigen presenting cells. These counter ligands (on T cells) are CD28, CTLA4 and CD40L respectively. In the absence of costimulatory signals, initiation of T-cell activation leads to anergy rather than activation. Following T-cell activation expression of CD28 initially increases, then is transiently down regulated before returning to its constitutive level. B7, the ligand for CD28, exists in two distinct forms, B7-1 and B7-2. Both forms are constitutively expressed on dendritic cells and peritoneal macrophages, but induced on activated B cells, monocytes, and Langerhans cells. CD28/B7 interactions lead to enhanced transcription and stabilization of IL-2 mRNA. Costimulatory signals from ligation of **CD4 (or CD8) with class II MHC (or class I MHC)** are also required for optimal T-cell activation.

Role of CTLA-4

The identification of a second receptor on T cells, **CTLA-4**, that also binds the B7 family members, has spurred investigations designed to unravel the relative roles of CD28 and CTLA-4 in T-cell activation. In contrast to CD28, CTLA-4 is not expressed constitutively. Rather, its expression peaks some two days after the initial T-cell activation and it disappears from the T-cell surface by day four. CTLA-4 has a higher affinity for both B7-1 and B7-2 than does CD28.

Although the role of CD28 as a costimulatory molecule is well established, the role of CTLA-4 is controversial. One proposed model envisages CTLA-4, under normal circumstances, to operate as a negative regulator of T-cell activation (triggered by TCR/CD28 signaling). In support of this idea, it has been shown that CTLA-4 knockout mice show an increase in the number of activated lymphocytes. This model is based on the temporal expression of CTLA-4, the temporal level of CD28 expression, and the greater avidity of CTLA-4 for the B7 molecules. In this model the interaction of CD28 with B7 serves as a costimulatory molecule leading to enhanced expression of IL-2 and bcl-x which allows T cells to proliferate. Expression of CTLA-4 and down regulation of CD28 follow this activation. Because expression of CD28 is decreased, and because B7 has a greater avidity for CTLA-4, the dominant interaction will be CTLA-4/B7 delivering an apoptotic stimulus.

NEGATIVE REGULATION OF T-CELL SIGNALING

SHP-2 Phosphatase

Recent studies have implicated the tyrosine phosphatase SHP-2 as a negative regulator of T-cell activation. In addition, reports that SHP-2 immunoprecipitates with CTLA-4 has fueled speculation that recruitment of SHP-2 to CTLA-4 inactivates T cells. However, direct evidence that this is an important regulatory mechanism for negative signaling in T cells is lacking.

Apoptosis

Apoptosis refers to a phenomenon of programmed cell death, which is characterized by fragmentation of DNA into units (nucleosomes) of 200 base pairs or its multiples. Although proliferation of activated T cells represents *rescue* from **programmed cell death**, T-cell activation also leads to the expression of fas ligand and fas receptor whose interaction *leads to* programmed cell death. Both membrane bound and soluble forms of fas ligand are produced by activated T cells. Therefore, activation induced T-cell apoptosis may occur following interaction of the **fas receptor** with membrane bound **fas ligand** on a neighboring cell or following interaction with soluble fas ligand in an autocrine manner (Fig. 9.9).

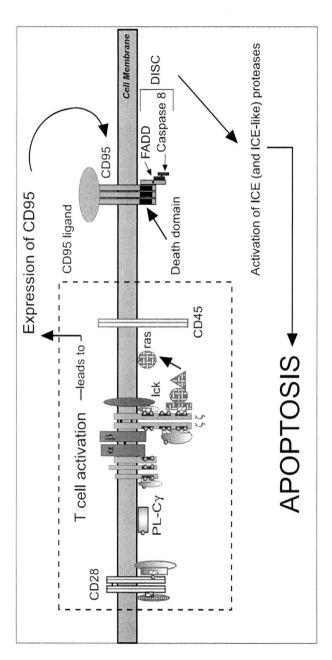

Fig. 9.9. T-cell activation is followed by CD95 expression, ligand binding and apoptosis. T-cell activation leads to the expression of fas (CD95), an integral transmembrane protein whose cytoplasmic tail has a characteristic "death domain". Interaction of CD95 with its cognate ligand serves as the stimulus for the formation of a "death domain inducing signaling complex" (DISC) in which FADD (fas associated death domain) and caspase 8 proteins are recruited to the death domain. This protein complex induces the activation of ICE (and ICE-like) proteases and apoptosis.

Fas receptor, also referred to as **Apo-1**, or **CD95**, is an integral transmembrane protein whose cytoplasmic tail has a characteristic *death domain*. Interaction of CD95 with its cognate ligand, fas, serves as the stimulus for the formation of a *death domain inducing signaling complex (DISC)* in which *FADD (fas associated death domain)* and caspase 8 proteins are recruited to the death domain. This protein complex induces the activation of the interleukin-1b converting enzyme (ICE), and ICE-like proteases that, in turn, promote apoptosis. ICE (and ICE-like) proteases cleave a number of proteins, including an enzyme involved in DNA excision repair and the retinoblastoma protein (Rb) that controls cell proliferation. T cells stimulated only by peptide/MHC in the absence of suitable costimulation become anergic or undergo programmed cell death. One of the mechanisms by which CD28/B7 interaction rescues T cells from programmed cell death is now becoming clear. It seems that engagement of CD28 and B7 enhances the expression of bcl-x, a molecule important in protecting T cells from *fas* mediated apoptosis.

Preliminary studies to resolve the signaling mechanisms associated with CD28/B7 interaction have shown that this interaction leads to the association of CD28 with two cytoplasmic tyrosine kinases, Itk and the phosphatidylinositol 3' kinase, PI3K. The functional significance for recruitment of these two kinases to CD28 remains unresolved.

MEMORY LYMPHOCYTES IN IMMUNOSURVEILLANCE

Memory lymphocytes are long lived and play an important role in immunosurveillance. However, unlike naive cells, memory cells do not preferentially home to the lymphoid tissues by exiting at high endothelial venules because, in general, memory cells do **not** express **L selectin**. Therefore, memory lymphocytes enter lymph nodes primarily via the afferent lymphatics. Memory lymphocytes preferentially *home* to the anatomical site of initial antigen encounter by exiting at the postcapillary venules of the tissue. The tendency of memory cells to home to the anatomical site of initial antigen encounter is a reflection of the unique molecules which are expressed by them (counter-ligands for the respective tissue sites) as a function of the site where the initial immune response occurred.

GAMMA/DELTA T CELLS

General properties

Thymus derived gamma/delta ($\gamma\delta$) T cells are the first T cells to appear during embryonic development. There is evidence that different subsets of $\gamma\delta$ T cells, using different combinations of V-J-C genes, appear at different times during ontogeny, and are restricted to different anatomical locations in the adult. Thus, $\gamma\delta$ T cells appearing early in ontogeny migrate to skin epithelia, the mucosal associated lymphoid tissues of the intestine, and to the reproductive tract. In each site distinct $\gamma\delta$ T cells expressing unique rearranged $\gamma\delta$ TCRs are found. Thus, the skin $\gamma\delta$ TCR+ T cells use predominantly genes from the Vγ3,Vδ1 family, while in the gut γδ TCR+ cells using Vγ5,Vδ(4,6) predominate. γδ T cells that appear later in development will express a vast array of heterogeneous TCRs, and seed peripheral lymphoid tissues. The relationship between TCR gene usage and the site of γδ T-cell development (intra- or extra-thymic) has not been studied extensively. Nor indeed is it clear whether γδ chain rearrangement is a necessary first step in the development of αβ T cells.

Antigen recognition by gamma/delta cells

In contrast to αβ T cells that recognize processed antigen (peptide) presented in the groove of MHC (class I or II) in association with CD4 or CD8, γδ T-cell recognition of antigen is not uniform. Some γδ T-cell clones recognize nonprocessed antigen like immunoglobulin receptors, "seeing" the topography of the antigen, rather than unique determinants. Other γδ T cells recognize processed antigen. Often these processed antigens are recognized in association with non-classical MHC molecules (Qa loci, etc.) MHC-like molecules (CD1 etc.), or other molecules such as heat shock proteins.

Role of gamma/delta T cells

The role of γδ T cells in immunity remains unclear. There is some evidence that these cells play an important role, alone or in concert with αβ T cells, in immunity to parasitic infection. In addition, clonal expansion of γδ T cells recognizing heat shock protein (hsp) related antigens (or antigens expressed with hsp) are observed in malignancy, autoimmune diseases, and transplantation. Whether this expansion of these cells represents an epiphenomenon or a functional role for γδ T cells in these situations is unknown.

Summary

T cells exit the thymus as *naive cells* and may either seed the peripheral organs or enter the pool of recirculating T cells. Naive T cells must be activated by antigen encountered in secondary lymphoid tissues in order to express their effector function, a process termed antigen-induced differentiation. Antigen induced differentiation of CD4+ T cells leads to clonal expansion and gives rise to at least two subsets of Th cells, Th1 and Th2, classified according to the pattern of cytokines that they secrete. A reciprocal regulatory relationship exists whereby cytokines secreted by one Th subset regulate the activity of the other Th subset. Whether a Th1 or Th2 cytokine profile predominates in response to antigenic stimulation has significant consequences because cytokines produced by Th cells preferentially activate distinct branches of adaptive immunity. Following eradication of antigen, Th1 and Th2 clones are eliminated by apoptosis, or become dormant memory cells. Different branches of immunity are required for immunity to different classes of microbes. In addition, different cytokine profiles predominate in autoimmune disorders and in transplant graft rejection/nonrejection.

Antigen induced differentiation of naive CD8+ T cells, pCTL, to mature CTL requires conjugate formation with an infected cell expressing antigenic peptide/ class I MHC complexes on its cell surface and also requires the presence of IL-2.

Additional signals arising from the interaction of molecules on the two conjugated cells are also needed. Following the delivery of these signals the conjugate dissociates, giving rise some one week later to mature CTL. CTL circulate in immunosurveillance in search of target cells expressing the same peptide/class I MHC complex as that which induced their differentiation. Conjugate formation between the target cell and the CTL leads to the polarization of lytic granules to the CTL membrane region that is in contact with the infected cell. Release of the polarized granules ensures that the damage is localized to the contact site. This is referred to as delivery of the *lethal hit*. The lytic granules kill the infected cell, but not the CTL. CTLs dissociate from the conjugate and continue their role in immunosurveillance and destruction of the relevant target cells. Following resolution of infection, CTL clones again either die by apoptosis or become dormant memory cells.

It is now known that antigen encounter alone is insufficient to trigger optimal T-cell activation. The TCR recognizes antigen in association with a unique cell surface molecule, the major histocompatibility molecule. However, it is the CD3 complex that couples the TCR, the ligand (antigenic) binding moiety of the complex, with intracellular signaling molecules. In addition, signals arising from costimulatory molecules and other accessory molecules contribute to the orchestra of stimuli that lead to T-cell activation. These interactions trigger events which include the activation of kinases and phosphatases specific for tyrosine, serine, or threonine, as well as the activation of G proteins and phospholipases resulting in the transition from G_0-G_1 of the cell cycle, clonal expansion and differentiation of the T cell to express its effector function.

CLINICAL CASES AND DISCUSSION

Clinical Case #17

MB recently received an HLA-matched bone marrow transplant for treatment of acute leukemia. While initial blood work following transplantation suggested a good reconstitution of the T-cell component of his immune system, over the past several weeks he has developed a general lethargy, some jaundice, and a significant desquamating skin rash. You are unsure whether you are dealing with a so-called acute graft-vs-host disease(GvHD) reaction or a more chronic GvHD. One of your colleagues suggests that the former is more associated with Type 1 cytokine production, while Type 2 cytokines are more associated with chronic graft-vs-host disease. Why might this be the case?

Discussion Case #17
Background

Type 1 cytokines include IL-2, TNF and IFNγ. TNF and IFNγ are major inflammatory cytokines. *Acute* graft versus host disease (GvHD) is correlated with nonspecific inflammation in many sites, often along with IFNγ activated "angry" macrophages, and CTL differentiation following IL-2 release. These reactions are understandable in terms of the cytokine milieu that predominates. *Chronic* GvHD, in contrast, exhibits many of the features of systemic sclerosis, with "smouldering" immune stimulation associated with hypergammaglobulinemia and fibrotic reactions.

Type 2 cytokines (IL-4, IL-5, IL-10, IL-13, and TGFβ) are a predominant feature of *chronic* GvHD. Interleukin-4 and IL-5 cytokines are known to be major B cell stimulating factors, while IL-10 and TGFβ "turn off" Type 1 cytokine production. This action is indirect and likely occurs by altering the functional state of those antigen presenting cells needed to bias the differentiation of Thp to a Th1 phenotype, secreting Type 1 cytokines. Within this cytokine milieu macrophages and T cells also secrete fibroblast growth factor (FGF), which is associated with nonspecific connective tissue cell growth.

Following transplantation, there is evidence that the first "wave" of acute rejection phenomena is associated with activation of T cells producing predominantly Type 1 cytokines. Not surprisingly, in a number of cases, both clinically and experimentally, it has been observed that immunoregulation in this first phase of rejection, with stabilization of the graft (and graft acceptance), is often associated with reduced Type 1 cytokine production and increased Type 2 cytokine production. It is not clear if this is necessarily indicative of true tolerance (of the graft) however, or merely a slower, and qualitatively different rejection (induced by Type 2 cytokines). There are data to suggest that the chronic proliferation and fibrotic changes associated with slow, chronic, rejection are functionally related to the polarization to Type 2 cytokines.

Tests

Determine if the cytokine milieu is more indicative of an acute or chronic immune rejection process. Based on the discussion above, measurement of serum cytokines (and/or intracellular cytokines in isolated CD4+ T cells by FACS, (fluorescence activated cell sorting)), could be of use. In particular, high levels of IL-2 and IFNγ, rather than of IL-4, IL-5, TGFβ etc. would suggest a pattern of acute GvHD.

Treatment

Acute rejection, (both in solid organ grafts (e.g., heart/liver/kidney etc.) and bone marrow transplants) is generally treated by increasing the levels of nonspecific immunosuppressive therapy. This is associated with some risk (e.g., of opportunistic infection, cancer etc.). In contrast, chronic rejection, while a slower process, has proven to be a more difficult entity to treat satisfactorily. As a general rule one would be more inclined to treat the symptoms rather than introduce more aggressive immunosuppression. In part, this reflects our acknowledgement that there are likely other factors (besides immunological) which have a profound importance in the pathophysiology of this condition.

Clinical Case #18

A vaccine is being developed for trials in HIV infection. In recent studies it is found that a novel molecule isolated from the viral coat protein stimulates CD4+ Th2 production in monkeys and in human volunteers. However, when immunized animals are challenged they remain fully susceptible to infection, and the "leader" of the clinical trials group concludes this molecule will not be valuable. Why are the animals not protected and does this explain the lack of enthusiasm for this approach?

Discussion Case #18

Background

HIV infects CD4+. Slow declines in the numbers of CD4+ T cells leads eventually to the phenotypic presentation of acquired immunodeficiency syndrome (AIDS). Studies of individuals in the late stages of HIV infection have suggested evidence for an alteration in cytokine production profiles (from Type 1 to Type 2 cytokines). Type 1 cytokines, IL-2 and IFNγ are crucial for cell mediated immune responses, while Type 2 cytokines (IL-4, IL-10, IL-13) are more important for the development of humoral immunity. However, it should be borne in mind that our current dogma suggests that the primary means by which the immune system deals with viral infections is through the activation and expansion of CD8+, cytotoxic killer T cells.

Analysis of long-term survivors from HIV infection (e.g., in Thailand, with studies of sex workers engaging in unprotected intercourse) has suggested an important role for CD8 cells in this disease. Some individuals have been described who, though seropositive (i.e., have circulating anti-HIV antibodies), are nevertheless completely symptom free and are also apparently free of recirculating virus. When cells from the peripheral blood of these individuals were studied, they were found to show significant CD8 reactivity (lytic capacity) for HIV infected target cells. Such data has spurred interest in understanding how best to develop a vaccine that would induce protective (CD8) immunity from HIV infection.

While IL-4 can be a growth factor for T cells (particularly Th2 CD4+ cells), the key growth factor for CD8+ CTL is IL-2. Hence a decline in production of IL-2 would not favor expansion of CTL. Humoral immunity, particularly in the late stages of HIV, does not seem to offer protection (see above). These features take on crucial importance in trials designed to investigate a suitable vaccine. Ideally, it would seem, we need one that will induce strong CTL responses by first priming Th1 CD4+ cells (to "help" CTL expansion). Developing (and monitoring) a vaccine that induces humoral immunity might already be a protocol "doomed" to failure in clinical practice.

Tests

First, determine whether the cytokines produced from the cells of individuals receiving the vaccine are Type 1 or Type 2. In addition, it is important to ask whether the vaccine induced any CD8 killing activity. To test for CD8+ killing activity in these monkeys, one needs to use virally infected monkey cells (not infected human targets) and vice versa. (CD8+ T cells only kill infected cells that express the same class I MHC as themselves) Finding that the molecule stimulates only CD4+ T cells, and only type 2 cytokine production, despite good evidence for anti-HIV antibody formation, would help explain the negative findings after challenge infection.

Treatment

How to select a vaccine that induces both Type 1 cytokine producing CD4+ cells and CD8+ killer cells remains an enigma. Nevertheless, understanding the mechanism of immunity for the disease in question is clearly of paramount importance before we can begin a rational attempt at vaccine development.

TEST YOURSELF

Multiple Choice Questions
For questions 1-5 make the best match with a, b, c, d or e. Use each answer once, more than once, or not at all.
- a. Th1 cells
- b. Th2 cells
- c. Both Th1 and Th2 cells
- d. CTL
- e. All of the above

1. Kill virally infected cells
2. Secrete cytokines required for activation of macrophages
3. Activation via the TCR complex leads to the phosphorylation of ITAMS
4. Secrete cytokines that inhibit IL-12 production by dendritic cells
5. May differentiate into memory cells

Answers: 1d; 2a; 3e; 4b; 5e

Short Answer Questions
1. What type of immune responses do Th1 cytokines support? Th2 cytokines?
2. What cytokines are required for spontaneous resolution of infection with *Mycobacterium leprae*, the causative agent of leprosy?
3. What is the rationale for feeding bovine myelin to patients with multiple sclerosis?
4. Which Th cytokines do cells, isolated from patients undergoing allograft rejection, produce?
5. Define apoptosis and its "fingerprint". Which family of proteases is activated during apoptosis?

Inflammation

Objectives 190
Inflammation 191
General Features 191
Vasodilatation, Increased Vascular Permeability and Edema 191
Recruitment of Neutrophils and Monocytes to the Site of Inflammation 195
Adaptive Immune Responses in Inflammation 202
Role of Innate and Adaptive Immunity in Inflammation 203
Clinical Relevance 205
Summary 205
Clinical Cases and Discussion 206
Test Yourself 209

Objectives

The primary purpose of this chapter is to introduce the reader to an understanding of the multiple facets of an inflammatory response, and to integrate the understanding of these events within the context of what he/she will already know from previous chapters. The term inflammation, we will see, encompasses a myriad of events occurring after trauma or infection, which have as a common denominator the activation of macrophages, the complement system and the blood coagulation system, resulting eventually in the release of a number of chemical mediators, cellular chemoattractants, and many systemic physiological changes.

We will find that many of the changes seen occur as a result of altered permeability in blood vessels. This, itself, can be a function of chemicals released from activation of the coagulation pathway (e.g., bradykinin) or from other activated cells (e.g., macrophages/lymphocytes) releasing cytokines. The reader will be introduced to the mechanism(s) by which other molecules (chemokines), produced following cellular activation, also serve as potent chemoattractants recruiting different cells to the inflammatory site, and how bystander activation of the complement system can produce mediators (C5a) with similar function.

Effective localized inflammatory reactions depend also on the ability of recruited cells to migrate into the tissues. Accordingly, the reader must understand how cytokines, in particular, serve to regulate the expression and avidity of the receptor:counter-receptor interactions occurring between cells and blood vessel endothelium, which are intimately involved in controlling this extravasation of cells into tissues. The clinical disorders occurring as a result of interference with these pathways will be described.

Clinical Immunology, by Reginald Gorczynski and Jacqueline Stanley. 2001 Landes Bioscience

INFLAMMATION

General Features

Inflammation is a term used to describe the events that either occur locally, following trauma or infection and leading to redness, heat, edema and pain, or occur systemically (generally following release of chemical mediators from this local reaction). With some local infections, accumulation of pus is also observed. In localized inflammation, heat and redness reflect increased blood flow (vasodilatation) and red blood cell extravasation; **edema** is caused by the leakage of fluid from the circulation into tissues (increased vascular permeability); pain is the result of stimulation of nerve endings by **bradykinin** (see below); pus is the accumulation of dead phagocytes and bacteria along with byproducts of tissue destruction.

Tissue damage, microbial infections, or toxic agents are classical inducers of inflammation (Fig. 10.1). These stimuli activate:

  i. the complement system
 ii. mast cell degranulation
iii. the blood coagulation contact system, leading indirectly to production of bradykinin
 iv. macrophages

The integrated effect of these processes (Fig. 10.2) produce biological changes culminating in the diapedesis of leukocytes at the site of infection (Fig. 10.1). These biological changes include:

  i. secretion of chemokines and cytokines
 ii. generation of inflammatory mediators
iii. altered expression and/or enhanced affinity of adhesion molecules
 iv. increased vascular permeability
  v. localized degradation of the basement membrane
 vi. extravasation of neutrophils, monocytes and lymphocytes from the circulation

Inflammatory changes normally initiate the processes that eliminate the source of infection and restore the integrity of damaged tissue. Many of the responses observed in inflammatory states represent the functioning of both nonimmune and innate immune processes. However, some components of the adaptive immune system may serve both to initiate and perpetuate the inflammatory process.

Vasodilatation, Increased Vascular Permeability and Edema

Classical inducers of inflammation (see above) give rise to an increase in blood flow at the site of inflammation. Increased blood flow is caused by vasodilatation,

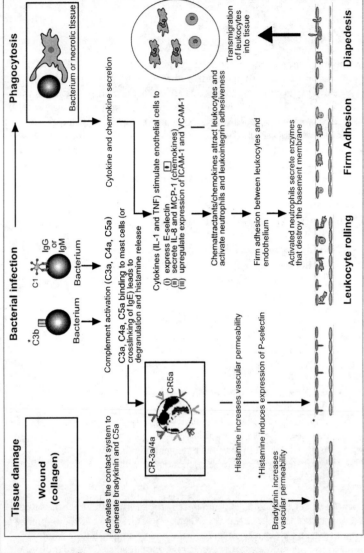

Fig. 10.1. Various stimuli initiate inflammation processes leading to diapedesis of leukocytes. Tissue damage, and microbial infections are common inducers of inflammation. These stimuli lead to activation of the coagulation system, mast cell degranulation, complement activation, and macrophage activation with cytokine release. Cytokines activate vascular endothelial cells to express adhesion molecules, and secrete chemokines. Integration of these processes results in diapedesis of circulating leukocytes into the site of infection.

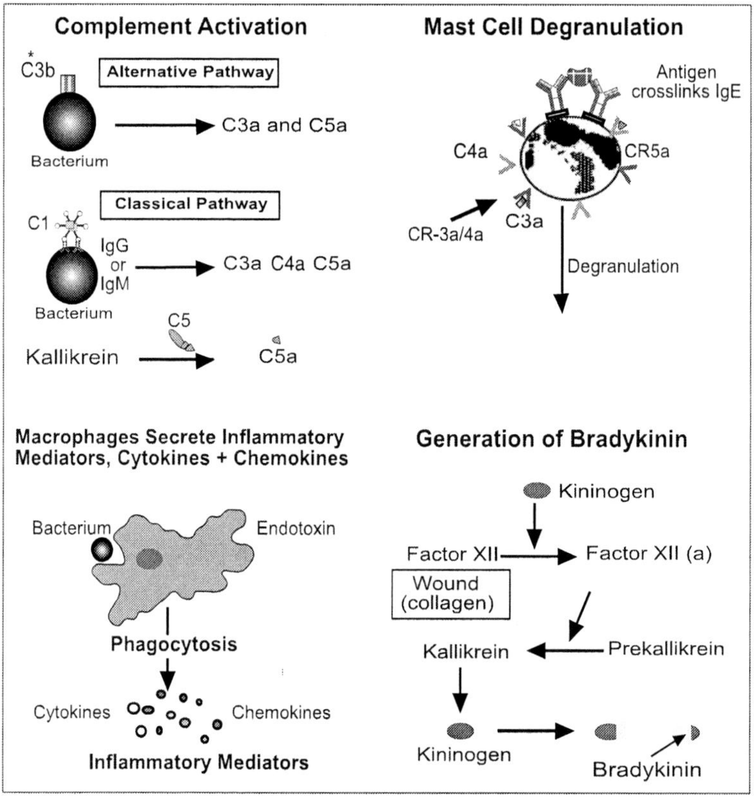

Inflammation

Complement Activation

Alternative Pathway

C3b, Bacterium → C3a and C5a

Classical Pathway

C1, IgG or IgM, Bacterium → C3a C4a C5a

Kallikrein —C5→ C5a

Mast Cell Degranulation

Antigen crosslinks IgE

C4a, CR5a

CR-3a/4a, C3a

Degranulation

Macrophages Secrete Inflammatory Mediators, Cytokines + Chemokines

Bacterium, Endotoxin → Phagocytosis → Cytokines, Chemokines (Inflammatory Mediators)

Generation of Bradykinin

Kininogen

Factor XII → Factor XII (a)

Wound (collagen)

Kallikrein ← Prekallikrein

Kininogen → Bradykinin

Fig. 10.2. Early events in the inflammatory response. Complement may be activated by the alternative or the classical pathway, leading to the production of proteolytic fragments that induce the degranulation of mast cells with histamine release. Histamine is a vasodilator and increases vascular permeability. Tissue damage activates the coagulation pathway, with the subsequent production of bradykinin, a potent vasodilator. Phagocytosis of microbes or other antigens activates macrophages with associated increases in cytokines and chemokines.

which occurs in response to mast cell derived histamine and leukotriene B4. Bradykinin, a product of the activated kinin system, is a contributing factor to the vasodilatation seen.

Mast cells

Mast cell *activation* or *degranulation* results in exocytosis of intracellular granules liberating **histamine** and other inflammatory mediators following the binding of various molecules to their cognate receptors (Fig. 10.3). Histamine causes vasodilatation of precapillary arterioles resulting in increased blood flow to capillary beds. This, coupled with histamine induced contraction of the endothelial

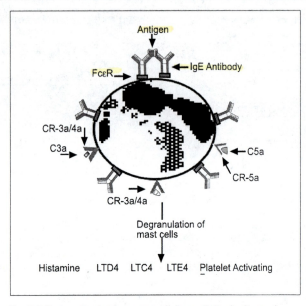

Fig. 10.3. Various signals trigger mast cell degranulation leading to the secretion of histamine and other inflammatory mediators. Antigen crosslinking of IgE bound to mast cells via the FcεR stimulates mast cell degranulation, as does binding of complement fragments C3a, C4a, and C5a to their receptors on the mast cell. In addition to histamine release, mast cell degranulation leads to the production of leukotrienes C4, D4, and E4 (LTC4, LTD4, and LTE4).

cells in the capillary beds and postcapillary venules, produces an increase in vascular permeability and associated edema.

Activation of complement by either the alternative or classical pathways of complement (Chapter 5) generates the anaphylatoxins C3a and C5a (Figs. 10.1, 10.2). Interaction of these **anaphylatoxins** with their cognate receptors on mast cells causes mast cell degranulation and release of histamine and other inflammatory mediators (Fig.10.3). In addition, **kallikrein** (see next section) mediated hydrolysis of C5 generates the C5a fragment (see below).

Mast cells express FcεR (Fig. 10.3). These receptors bind IgE antibodies via the Fc region, thus arming the cell for activation following re-exposure to the antigen recognized by that IgE. Antigen binding to the Fab region of the IgE molecule crosslinks the FcεR, which triggers exocytosis of intracellular mast cell granules and release of histamine and other inflammatory mediators.

Contact system: Source of bradykinin

Tissue damage, regardless of the initiating agent, triggers activation of the coagulation pathway contact system. The contact system is composed of four proteins

Inflammation

(**Factor XII,** Factor XI, **prekallikrein**, and high molecular weight kininogen). Collagen exposed in damaged tissue serves as a target for Factor XII binding and activation to an enzymatically active state. Platelet membranes also serve as a target for Factor XII. Activated Factor XII converts prekallikrein to an enzymatically active form, kallikrein (Fig. 10.4). Kallikrein enzymatically cleaves kininogen to release the nonapeptide molecule, bradykinin. Bradykinin is a potent vasodilator and increases vascular permeability (Fig. 10.5). Kallikrein also cleaves the complement component C5 to generate C5a, an anaphylatoxin that binds receptors on basophils and mast cells inducing degranulation and histamine release.

RECRUITMENT OF NEUTROPHILS AND MONOCYTES TO THE SITE OF INFLAMMATION

General features
Macrophages and neutrophils (phagocytes) mediate the clearance of necrotic tissue and/or invading organisms present at inflammatory sites. Although tissue macrophages are present in most tissues, neutrophils are circulating blood cells and generally represent the first leukocyte actively recruited to an inflammatory

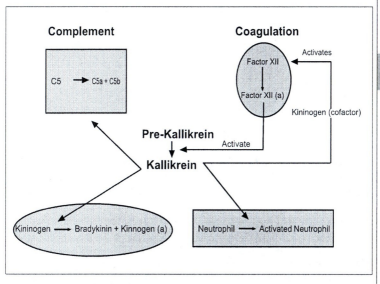

Fig. 10.4. Interrelationship of the coagulation system and complement. The complement and coagulation pathways are intimately linked via the plasma protein kallikrein, the enzymatic form of the zymogen, prekallikrein. The conversion of prekallikrein to kallikrein follows the enzymatic action of activated Factor XII, the initiator of the contact pathway of intrinsic coagulation. Substrates for kallikrein include the complement component C5, as well as kininogen, a protein that serves as a cofactor in the activation of Factor XII. Additionally, kallikrein, in the presence of calcium and magnesium, aggregates and activates neutrophils.

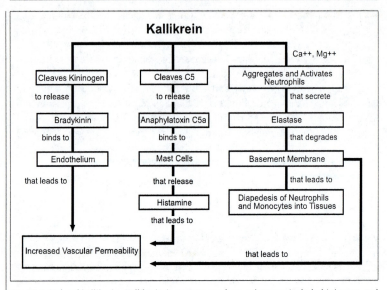

Fig. 10.5. Role of kallikrein. Kallikrein is a protease whose substrates include kininogen and complement component C5. Proteolytic hydrolysis of kininogen by kallikrein produces bradykinin, which mediates vasodilatation and increased vascular permeability. Kallikrein also cleaves the complement component C5 into fragments C5a and C5b. C5a, an anaphylatoxin, binds to basophils and mast cells inducing degranulation and histamine release. Histamine alters vascular permeability. C5b is an initiating component in the formation of the MAC on susceptible cells.

site. Circulating monocytes (immature macrophages) are also recruited to sites of inflammation, where in the presence of the appropriate microenvironmental stimuli they mature to macrophages.

Recruitment of neutrophils and monocytes into inflamed tissues occurs sequentially. Although the general processes are similar to those described for non-inflammatory states, there are differences. The steps leading to diapedesis are:

   i. leukocyte rolling on activated endothelium
  ii. expression of cytokine induced counter-molecules on the endothelium
 iii. enhancement of the adhesiveness of integrins present on leukocytes
  iv. firm adherence of leukocytes to vascular endothelium
   v. squeezing in-between the endothelial cells
  vi. degradation of the basement membrane
 vii. migration of leukocytes into inflamed tissue

Leukocyte rolling and firm adherence between leukocytes and the endothelium is mediated by two classes of adhesive molecules, the **selectins** and **integrins**, respectively (Fig. 10.6). Selectin/ligand interactions induce leukocyte rolling;

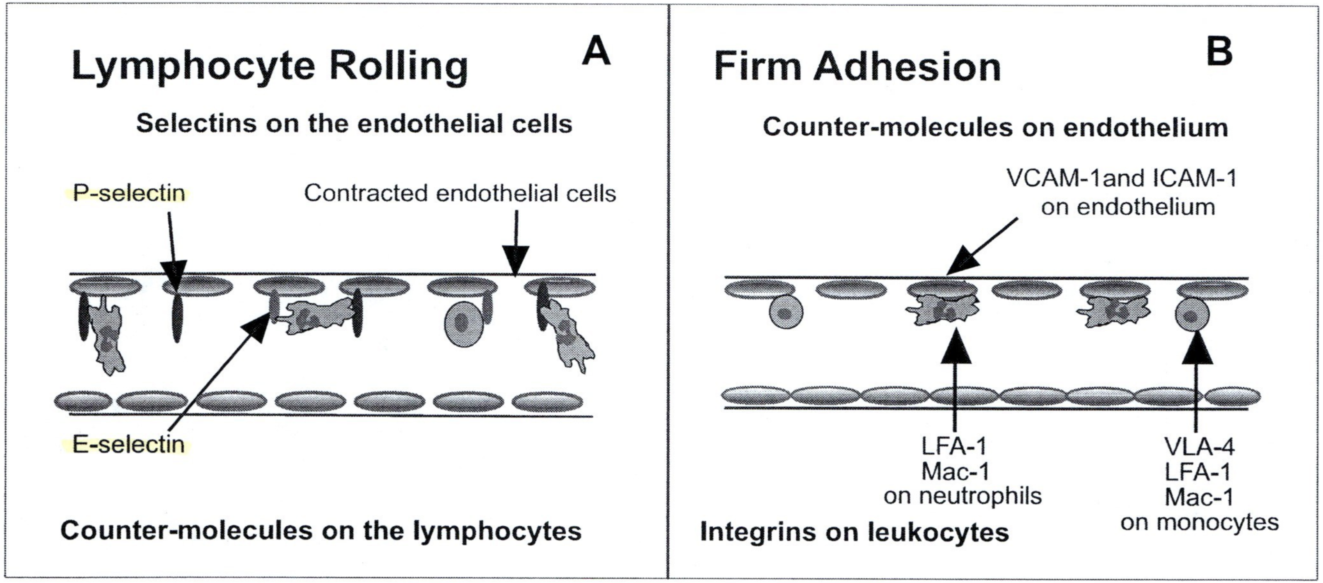

Inflammation

Lymphocyte Rolling — A

Selectins on the endothelial cells

P-selectin
E-selectin
Contracted endothelial cells

Counter-molecules on the lymphocytes

Firm Adhesion — B

Counter-molecules on endothelium

VCAM-1 and ICAM-1 on endothelium

LFA-1
Mac-1
on neutrophils

VLA-4
LFA-1
Mac-1
on monocytes

Integrins on leukocytes

Fig. 10.6. A). P-selectin and E-selectin are induced on endothelial cells during inflammatory responses. During an inflammatory response, P-selectin and E-selectin are sequentially expressed on activated endothelium. P-selectin rapidly translocates to the plasma membrane from cytoplasmic stores, in the presence of mast cell derived histamine. E-selectin expression is induced by cytokines derived from activated macrophages (e.g., TNF, IL-1) and requires de novo protein synthesis. P-selectin, and E-selectin on the activated vascular endothelium interact with their cognate carbohydrate ligands on leukocytes, leading to leukocyte rolling on endothelium. B). Integrins exist in different activation states, depending on the local microenvironment. Leukocyte integrins in a high affinity state interact with counter molecules on the activated endothelium, leading to firm adhesion of the leukocyte with the endothelium.

integrin activation followed by high affinity integrin/ligand interaction stimulates firm adherence of leukocytes to the vascular endothelium and migration into tissues.

Leukocyte rolling: Selectins

Selectins are monomeric proteins that bind carbohydrate molecules, producing transient and weak adhesion between two cells (Fig. 10.6, Table 10.1). Selectin family members include **L-selectin, E-selectin**, and **P-selectin**. L-selectin is constitutively expressed on naive lymphocytes, monocytes, and neutrophils, and regulates cell trafficking during *noninflammatory states*. In contrast to L-selectin, the P-selectins and E selectins are **not** expressed on circulating cells but instead on postcapillary venules *during inflammatory states*. The preferential expression of P and E selectins on postcapillary venules correlates with the greater migration of leukocytes into inflammatory sites. The ligands for the selectins are complex carbohydrate molecules present on glycoproteins. For P-selectin, the (cell associated) counter-receptor is an O-linked, sialylated carbohydrate. These cell surface carbohydrate molecules are expressed only on discrete populations of circulating cells, thus causing tissue specific migration. Each selectin interacts with distinct carbohydrate ligands.

During an inflammatory response, P-selectin and E-selectin are sequentially expressed on activated endothelium. P-selectin is rapidly translocated to the plasma membrane from cytoplasmic stores, in the presence of mast cell derived histamine. In contrast, E-selectin expression is induced by cytokines derived from activated macrophages (e.g., TNF, IL-1) and requires de novo protein synthesis. In brief, P-selectin, and E-selectin on the activated vascular endothelium interact with their cognate carbohydrate ligands on leukocytes. These interactions lead to leukocyte rolling on the endothelium (Fig. 10.6). Leukocyte rolling prolongs the duration of time to which leukocytes are exposed to chemoattractants and activators secreted into this inflammatory microenvironment.

Firm adhesion and stable conjugates: Integrins on leukocytes

Integrins are heterodimeric proteins, consisting of noncovalently associated alpha and beta polypeptides, that exist in different activation states depending on the stimulatory signals in the local environment. Integrin activation reflects a transition from a nonadhesive, constitutive, low affinity state to a transient high affinity state. High affinity state integrins mediate strong adhesion between activated endothelium and leukocytes, a prerequisite for migration of leukocytes into inflamed tissues.

Integrins are classed into *families* based on the **beta chain** that they express (Table 10.1). Thus, integrins that have a β2 polypeptide belong to the **β2 integrin family**; integrins that have a β1 polypeptide belong to the β1 **integrin family**, and integrins that have a β7 polypeptide belong to the **β7 integrin family**. The counter molecules for these integrins are expressed on endothelium in a tissue specific manner, thus determining the tissues into which leukocytes will migrate (Fig. 10.7). Some of the counter-receptors for the integrins are constitutively expressed on

Inflammation

Table 10.1. Interactions of adhesion molecules and their counter-molecules

Adhesion Molecule	Expression	Counter-Molecule	Expression
Selectins			
L-selectin	naïve lymphocytes, monocyte, neutrophils	GlyCAM-1, CD34 MAdCAM-1	peripheral lymph node HEV, endothelium** mucosal lymph node HEV, Peyer's patches HEV
P-selectin	histamine activated endothelium	PSGL-1 PSGL-1 like	monocytes and neutrophils activated or memory lymphocytes
E-selectin	cytokine activated endothelium	E-selectin ligand (ESL) ESL (CLA in skin)	monocytes and neutrophils activated or memory lymphocytes
Integrins			
β^1Integrins			
VLA-4 ($\alpha^4\beta^1$)	monocytes activated or memory lymphocytes	VCAM-1	cytokine activated endothelium
β^2 Integrins			
LFA-1 ($\alpha^L\beta^2$)	lymphocytes, monocytes, and neutrophils	ICAM-1 ICAM-2	cytokine activated endothelium endothelium, constitutive
Mac-1 ($\alpha^M\beta^2$)	monocytes and macrophages	ICAM-1	cytokine activated endothelium
β^7 Integrins			
LPAM ($\alpha^4\beta^7$)	mainly activated or memory T cells	MAdCAM-1 VCAM-1	mucosal lymph node HEV, Peyer's patches HEV cytokine activated endothelium

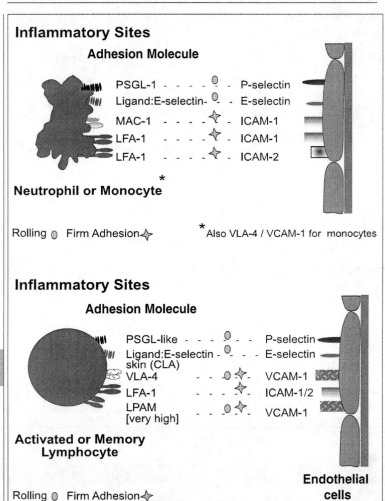

Fig. 10.7. Adhesion molecules and their counter-molecules. Adhesion molecules and their counter-molecules mediate interaction of leukocytes with endothelial cells during inflammation. Selectins mediate leukocyte rolling on inflamed endothelium; integrins mediate firm adhesion between leukocytes and the inflamed endothelium.

endothelium, while others are induced by cytokines/chemokines generated during inflammation (Table 10.1).

High affinity interaction between these integrins and their counter-receptors is contingent upon activating signals from molecules (chemokines and cytokines) in the local milieu. These molecules alter the adhesive properties (and/or enhance expression) of integrins.

Role of cytokines and chemokines

Cytokines and chemokines play a major role in inflammatory responses (Figs. 10.1, 10.2). Activated macrophages secrete a host of inflammatory mediators, both cytokines (e.g., TNF, IL-1) and chemokines (e.g., IL-8, MCP-1, MIP-1 etc.). Mast cells have been shown to secrete cytokines, but the stimulus for their secretion remains unknown. The inflammatory cytokines, **TNF** and **IL-1** have pleiotropic activity, serving to stimulate endothelial cells to express the adhesive molecules E-selectin and VCAM-1, as well as to secrete the chemokines **IL-8** and **MCP-1**. IL-8 induces increased adhesiveness of the β2 integrins, LFA-1 and Mac-1, and shedding of L-selectin. The consequence of L-selectin shedding is unclear at this time.

Chemokines also have profound chemoattractant activity for different cells, and indeed this was the function by which chemokines were first characterized. **MCP-1** and **RANTES** are chemotactic for both monocytes and lymphocytes, but not for neutrophils, whose primary chemoattractant is IL-8. In the early phase of the inflammatory response C5a (complement fragment) and PAF (produced by mast cells and activated endothelial cells) also serve as potent chemoattractants and activators of neutrophils.

Macrophage derived cytokines and chemokines initiate and propagate the inflammatory response. The actions of inflammatory cytokines are not restricted only to the local milieu. TNF and IL-1 can act systemically, producing a vasodilatation, which contributes to the production of low blood pressure in "shock", a corollary of systemic inflammation. Both of these cytokines also act on the hypothalamus to induce fever. IL-6 acts on hepatic cells to release a number of acute phase proteins such as C-reactive protein that serves as an opsonin for enhanced phagocytosis of bacteria. Macrophage activity is further enhanced by T cell derived cytokines (TNF, IFNγ) when adaptive immune responses are mobilized (see below).

Basement membrane transmigration

The subendothelial basement membrane is normally a barrier to the entry of leukocytes into tissues. However, under inflammatory conditions, localized enzymatic degradation of the basement membrane by activated cells permits leukocyte entry into tissues. Several classes of enzymes, proteases, heparanases, and sulfatases have been implicated in this destruction, based on their ability to degrade subendothelial extracellular matrix in vitro. More recently, the endopeptidase gelatinase B, a member of the family of zinc binding **matrix metalloproteinases,** has been shown to degrade Type IV collagen in reconstituted membranes.

Gelatinase B is secreted as a zymogen, **progelatinase B,** which is activated following limited proteolysis with elastase, or other endopeptidases. Inhibitors of gelatinase B, or of elastase, inhibit leukocyte transmigration across the reconstituted membranes. Although naive lymphocytes that traffic to serve an immunosurveillance role can produce low levels of the enzymes that degrade the basement membrane in noninflammatory states, the numbers of leukocytes reaching **sites of inflammation,** together with their state of activation, both contribute to the increased enzymatic digestion of the basement membrane which increases the flow of cells into inflamed tissues.

The existence of this redundant "battery" of enzymes secreted by monocytes, platelets, neutrophils, and endothelial cells, all contributing to the degradation of the subendothelial basement membrane, reflects the crucial role of leukocyte migration to sites of inflammation in host defense.

ADAPTIVE IMMUNE RESPONSES IN INFLAMMATION

General features
Adaptive immunity refers to immunological responses in which T cells, B cells, or their effectors play a role. The first (primary) exposure to an antigen in secondary lymphoid tissues leads to the differentiation of CD4+ T cells and B cells into effector cells. While most of the T cells and B cells will die following resolution of infection, some will become memory cells and recirculate in immunosurveillance. In the presence of the antigen that triggered the initial differentiation (secondary immune response) of these cells, lymphocytes can be activated at the site of infection (Fig. 10.8).

Recruitment of Th cells to the site of inflammation
During inflammation the process of lymphocyte rolling, adhesion, and **diapedesis** of T cells occurs in a multistep fashion as described above—see "Recruitment of Neutrophils and Monocytes to the Site of Inflammation". Differences in the recruitment of activated T cells, versus that of monocytes and neutrophils to the site of inflammation, can be explained in terms of the adhesion molecules, or their counter-molecules, used in the formation of a stable leukocyte/endothelial cell conjugate (Table 10.1). In particular, activated and memory lymphocytes express high concentrations of the integrins, LPAM and VLA-4. The model in which *only selectins* mediate rolling has been challenged by reports that rolling followed low affinity interactions between VLA-4 or LPAM on VCAM-1. This rolling step is rapidly followed by firm adhesion.

Transmigration of lymphocytes
Recent in vitro studies have shown that a family of matrix metalloproteinases (MMP) proteolytically degrade Type IV collagen to generate channels in the subendothelial basement membrane thus facilitating lymphocyte transmigration into tissues. T cells secrete **MMP-2** and **MMP-9,** also known as progelatinases A and B, respectively. Both enzymes are secreted in an inactive form and require

proteolytic cleavage for activation. During inflammation, secretion of progelatinase A is induced, while that of progelatinase B is enhanced both by a vasoactive intestinal peptide, as well as by the interaction of VLA-4 on activated or memory lymphocytes with the endothelial counter-molecule, VCAM-1. In vitro studies have shown that the conversion of progelatinases to their active form is mediated by elastase, as well as by other MMP family members secreted by macrophages and other inflammatory cells.

Role of Type 1 cytokines at inflammatory sites

The phenotype of Th cells generated in response to antigen determines the course of inflammation. Th1 cells secrete Type 1 cytokines (IL-2, IFNγ, and TNF) which enhance inflammatory responses (Fig. 10.8). IFNγ is a potent activator of macrophages, leading to enhanced phagocytosis and associated increases in inflammatory mediator/cytokine secretion. A role for CD40 (on macrophages) and CD40L (on T cells) interaction in the activation of macrophages has been postulated because (i) IFNγ induces expression of CD40 on monocytes (ii) activated T cells express CD40L, and (iii) activation of macrophages with soluble CD40L has been observed.

Role of Type 2 cytokines at inflammatory sites

The Type 2 cytokines IL-4 and IL-10 dampen development of Th1 responses. Indeed the reciprocal regulation of Th1/Th2 development by IL-4 (IL-10) and IFNγ serves an important regulatory influence on inflammatory reactions. Interestingly, TGFβ, another cytokine secreted predominantly by Th2 cells, serves to decrease activation both of Th1 cells and probably also other cells (e.g., macrophages) contributing to the inflammatory cascade. Other control mechanisms include the elimination of microbes, tissue healing, and shedding of adhesion molecules that competitively inhibit leukocyte binding to counter-molecules on the endothelium.

ROLE OF INNATE AND ADAPTIVE IMMUNITY IN INFLAMMATION

In general the innate immune system initiates inflammation when complement is activated, mast cells degranulate and tissue macrophages are activated. Tissue damage recruits nonimmune systems such as the coagulation system, producing bradykinin, a potent vasodilator. When the stimulus is an antigen to which CD4+ T cells have been previously sensitized, trafficking memory cells are activated in tissues to secrete cytokines (e.g., IFNγ) that enhance inflammation by inducing the differentiation of monocytes to macrophages, and by activating mature macrophages (Fig. 10.8). Activated macrophages, as well as activated mast cells and neutrophils, secrete cytokines and inflammatory mediators.

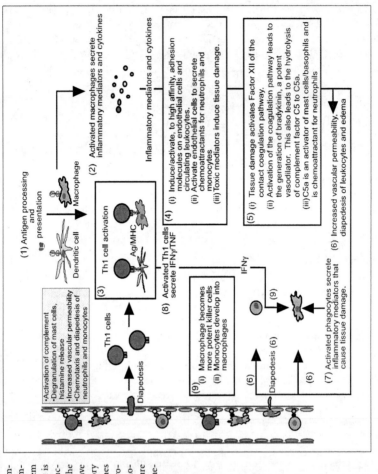

Fig. 10.8. Inflammation is initiated by innate immune processes and enhanced by adaptive immunity. In general the innate immune system initiates the inflammation when complement is activated, mast cells degranulate and tissue macrophages are activated (see Fig. 10.2). When the stimulus is an antigen to which CD4+ T cells have been previously sensitized, trafficking memory cells are activated in tissues to secrete cytokines (e.g., IFNγ) that enhance the inflammatory processes by inducing the differentiation of monocytes to macrophages, and by activating mature macrophages. Other sources of inflammatory mediators include the activated mast cell.

CLINICAL RELEVANCE

Leukocyte adhesion deficiency, Type I
Leukocyte adhesion deficiency (LAD) is an autosomal recessive disorder caused by a deficiency in CD18. CD18 is the **β2 integrin chain** of LFA-1 and Mac-1. LFA-1 is present on lymphocytes, monocytes and neutrophils; Mac-1 is present on monocytes and neutrophils. Consequently, transmigration of these cells to sites of inflammation, or of naive lymphocytes to secondary lymphoid tissues, does not occur. Since leukocyte and lymphocyte transmigration is crucial for immune responses, individuals with this deficiency have multiple infections, with the frequent occurrence of localized pustular infections.

Unlike other immunodeficiency disorders (Ig deficiency, **chronic granulomatous disease**, etc.) which also lead to an increased incidence of bacterial infections, this disorder has normal numbers of healthy leukocytes and lymphocytes. In LAD, the cause of the problem is the inability of those cells in vivo to extravasate into sites of infection. The diagnosis becomes essentially one of exclusion, with confirmation made by documenting (by immunofluorescence) the absence of the relevant cell surface integrins. Patients are treated by repeated systemic antibiotic infusion although, in severe cases, bone marrow transplant is an option.

Systemic inflammatory response syndrome (SIRS)
A number of factors tend to dampen inflammatory responses to prevent pathophysiogical destruction of normal tissue. Occasionally however, this does not occur and a so-called systemic inflammatory response syndrome (SIRS) develops. Mortality in patients with SIRS (and commonly multi-organ failure) is often as high as 50%. The defective regulation in SIRS is now becoming clear. It seems that activated neutrophils, invading tissue in inflammatory responses, generally die by apoptosis over a period of 12-24 hrs. In SIRS, apoptotic death is, itself, inhibited. One of the mechanisms by which this occurs seems to be an IL-1 triggered induction of anti-apoptotic mediators in the affected neutrophils. Selective inhibition of these anti-apoptotic stimuli may offer hope of improved treatment of SIRS.

SUMMARY

Inflammation encompasses a number of interrelated events that occur following infection, tissue damage, or exposure to toxic agents, leading to local redness, heat, edema and pain. These stimuli activate tissue macrophages, the complement system, the blood coagulation contact system, and mast cell degranulation. Cytokine and chemokine secretion by activated tissue macrophages is also a primary event in inflammation, inducing other cells also to secrete molecules that are chemotactic for neutrophils and monocytes. The combined effects of an adhesive endothelium, chemotactically derived leukocytes, and enhanced vascular permeability, along with the enzymatic degradation of the subendothelial basement membrane, fulfill the requirements for subsequent migration (diapedesis) of neutrophils and monocytes into tissues. Neutrophils are rapidly activated and secrete a plethora of inflammatory mediators. In contrast, monocytes must undergo differentiation to macrophages before they can secrete cytokines and inflammatory mediators.

In the presence of antigen, the inflammatory response includes activated memory CD4+ T cells and the cytokines they release. Type 1 cytokines sustain the inflammatory response by further stimulating macrophages. Type 2 cytokines dampen Type 1 cytokine secretion, and hence the inflammatory response. The actions of inflammatory cytokines are not restricted to the local milieu; TNF and IL-1 act on the hypothalamus to induce fever; IL-6 acts on hepatic cells to release acute phase proteins such as C-reactive protein, which serves as an opsonin for enhanced phagocytosis of bacteria. Because leukocyte transmigration into tissues is crucial for immune responses, individuals deficient in expression of adhesion molecules, and defective leukocyte extravasation to sites of infection, suffer increased localized infections as seen in the disorder, leukocyte adhesion deficiency (LAD).

CLINICAL CASES AND DISCUSSION

Clinical Case #19
DE is a 50-year-old male with severe arthritis in multiple joints of unknown etiology. He has failed all conventional anti-inflammatory therapies, and is interested in being considered for more experimental approaches. What treatment(s) would you suggest? Explain why the treatment(s) might work?

Discussion Case #19
Background
In the absence of repeated stress/chronic trauma, leading to joint inflammation and the arthritis referred to as osteoarthritis, most other arthritides are considered autoimmune disorders, recognizable by immune attack directed at, and associated with inflammation and tissue destruction in, the joints. It has been known for a long time that a number of immune cells (T cells/B cells) and inflammatory cytokines accumulate in the joint fluid in association with this inflammation. We now believe that these cytokines are intimately involved in the disease process, including the recruitment of lymphoid cells to the inflamed joint.

Normal lymphocyte recirculation through lymphoid/nonlymphoid tissues occurs in a nonrandom fashion, under the control of the expression of a number of receptors/counter-receptors expressed on the lymphocyte/target tissue respectively. Under noninflammatory conditions, T cells migrate into peripheral lymph nodes under the control of L-selectin, binding to specialized endothelial target counter-receptors, glyCAM-1 and CD34 (Table 10.1). Integrins (LFA-1, binding to the target molecule ICAM-1 and ICAM-2 on the endothelial) may also be important. Migration of naive lymphocytes into the mucosal tissue, in contrast, depends on L-selectin binding to MAdCAM-1.

Following development of an inflammatory response the expression of a number of these adhesion molecules changes dramatically. VCAM-1, E-selectin and P-selectin, are all up-regulated on the inflamed vascular endothelium following cytokine stimulation. L-selectin expression on T cells is decreased, while on activated lymphocytes VLA-4 (a counter-molecule for VCAM-1) and LFA-1 expression is dramatically increased. VLA-4:VCAM-1 interactions are crucial for transmigration through the endothelium.

Tests
DE will already have undergone those tests that might help determine his disease (according to the criteria of the American Rheumatological Association, ARA). You have been unable to clarify whether this is an example of rheumatoid arthritis, psoriatic arthritis, mixed connective tissue disease, etc. Most of the other tests you might perform serve only to confirm the status of the disease (active or quiescent). Amongst these, for instance, one could measure release of so-called acute phase reactants (C-reactive protein, CRP), or the erythrocyte sedimentation rate (ESR; this is elevated following increased production of the acute phase protein fibrinogen). These biochemical tests could be used in conjunction with physical exam (e.g., joint effusions indicate inflammation and altered permeability of basement membranes in the joint capsule). Since many of these alterations occur following local/systemic cytokine production, one could envisage a situation where we may eventually use such measures (of cytokines) as more useful (definitive) tests both to confirm diagnoses and to aid therapy (below).

Experimental Treatments
Note that this discussion concentrates on novel approaches only. The reader must be aware that there are conventional, generally quite successful, treatment methodologies available to most individuals, which usually involve some combination of so-called anti-inflammatory drug therapies. However, there is a subset of persons who "fail" conventional treatments. This has focused attention on other therapeutic modalities, which, if successful (and less toxic than conventional therapy), may even replace conventional treatment for most patients.

Based on experimental studies, novel approaches to inflammatory diseases have been suggested, many of which use antibody directed therapy. As example, because the expression of adhesion molecules on the inflamed endothelium is upregulated by the presence of distinct cytokines (e.g., TNF) administration of anti-TNF antibodies might decrease the expression of the adhesion molecules. Alternatively, pilot studies have begun using antibodies to the adhesion molecules themselves. Because the LFA-1:ICAM-1, and VLA-4:VCAM-1 interactions are crucial for lymphocyte migration at sites of inflammation, antibodies to these have been amongst the first under consideration.

ICAM-1 is a cytokine inducible molecule and so is not normally expressed on peripheral tissue endothelial cells in noninflammatory states, except on HEV endothelium. Both HEV and normal peripheral tissue endothelial cells constitutively express ICAM-2. Because LFA-1/ICAM-2 interactions are relevant in the recruitment of trafficking lymphocytes to peripheral tissues during noninflammatory conditions, the anti-ICAM-1 antibody therapy should not, in principle, interfere with the normal trafficking of lymphocytes to either the lymph nodes or to peripheral tissues. Data to date suggest that use of such anti-LFA-1:ICAM-1 combinations, may prove of value, particularly when used in conjunction with anti-cytokine antibodies (e.g., TNF).

Clinical Case #20
You are asked to consult on a 4-year old boy who has had recurrent outbreaks of severe pustular bacterial infections on his arms and legs in the last 15 months. All cleared with antibiotic treatment. Routine blood tests reveal a normal white cell count with a normal differential, and normal levels of serum Ig. Complement activity is within the normal range. Both parents are well. What might be going on? What additional tests might you order?

Discussion Case #20
Background
The reader should recognize that he/she is being "pointed" towards the innate defense mechanisms here. This child has a normal white cell differential, implying normal lymphocyte numbers (and, with the other information, we can thus assume normal B/T-cell numbers) as well as normal numbers of neutrophils. The data do not fit the picture of a case where absolute numbers of immunologically important cells are altered. We might therefore now begin to wonder whether it is cell function, not numbers, that are altered. In particular, we should be thinking of possible phagocytic cell defects.

In chronic granulomatous disease, there is a defect in NADPH oxidase enzyme pathways, and patients can certainly present with increased susceptibility to bacterial infections. However, in this patient, the lack of systemic (blood borne) disease suggests this is unlikely to be simply a defect in the functional activity of cells important in defense. Patients with chronic granulomatous disease generally present with frequent inflammatory granulomas and abscesses (Chapter 15), and this child is not developing repeated lung and sinus infections, nor is he developing abscesses.

The caregivers have noticed an increased susceptibility to localized skin outbreaks, as though getting immune cells (e.g., macrophages/neutrophils) to compromised tissues is the major problem. Lymphoid (and other) cells of the immune system migrate within the body using discrete receptors:coreceptor interactions. Molecules expressed on their surface (and the surface of target cells/tissue) thus regulate whether cells "flow" in the circulation, or become arrested at certain sites for subsequent migration into tissues. The adherence of cells to, and their transmigration through, endothelium into tissues depends on the expression of adhesion molecules on the surface of migrating cells and the cytokine activated endothelium, e.g., LFA-1 on lymphocytes with ICAM-1 on the endothelium.

Defective genes for these so-called *adhesion* molecules will result in the cells being unable to adhere/undergo transmigration, even in the face of cytokines that normally induce increased expression of those adhesion molecules. One of the first such defects, leukocyte adhesion deficiency disease (LAD) is, in fact, characterized by repeated bouts of localized pustular bacterial infections as the infecting organisms proliferate locally, without neutrophil access to the infected site and with the tissue macrophages themselves not capable of completely sterilizing the infection. All of these pathophysiological changes thus occur in the face of an apparently normal immune system, yet this subtle defect in adhesion molecule expression *is in fact the cause* of the problem.

Tests
To test for chronic granulomatous disorder, a nitroblue tetrazolium test (NBT) would be ordered. The dye used to test for this defect changes color when it is reduced by activated NADPH oxidase enzyme. The reduced dye turns blue on the test slide (hence the name NBT).

The simplest definitive way to test for leukocyte adhesion deficiency disease is to perform immunofluorescence studies on cytokine stimulated peripheral blood cells of the patient, using antibodies to LFA-1 and ICAM-1. Lymphocytes express LFA-1; many activated cells express ICAM-1. Decreased or absent expression of these molecules, along with the clinical picture, would confirm the diagnosis. It is theoretically possible that a more subtle defect may exist, in which cell surface expression is apparently normal, but the molecules do not serve their normal adhesive function. This could be tested by direct measurement of adhesive function (using radiolabeled cells, adhering in culture to endothelial monolayers, and quantitating the radioactivity (cells) adherent to the monolayer after washing).

Treatment
Long-term treatment for this disease is with antibiotics. As our technologies improve one could envisage a future in which bone marrow transplantation (already an option in severe cases) and/or gene therapy might become the norm.

TEST YOURSELF

Multiple Choice Questions
1. Mast cell derived histamine induces vasodilatation. Which of the following inflammatory mediators induce degranulation of mast cells and histamine release?
    a. Crosslinking of IgE bound to mast cell FcεR
    b. Binding of complement fragment C3a
    c. Binding of complement fragment C5a
    d. All of the above
    e. Only a and c
2. Activation of the contact system leading to coagulation during tissue damage leads to the generation of bradykinin. Bradykinin is a fragment derived from which one of the following.

a. Factor XII
b. Factor XI
c. High molecular weight kininogen
d. Prekallikrein
3. Selectin/ligand interaction mediates leukocyte rolling on inflamed endothelium. Which of the following selectins are induced on endothelial cells during the inflammatory response?
   a. P-selectin
   b. E-selectin
   c. L-selectin
   d. All of the above
   e. Only a and b
4. Which one of the following molecules is chemotactic for neutrophils and induces enhanced adhesiveness of Mac-1 and LFA-1?
   a. IL-2
   b. IL-4
   c. IL-6
   d. IL-8
   e. IL-10
5. Which of the following T-cell/endothelium interactions may have a dual role in the steps leading to T-cell diapedesis?
   a. LFA-1/ICAM-1
   b. LFA-1/ICAM-2
   c. VLA-4/VCAM-1
   d. LPAM/VCAM-1
   e. Both c and d

Answers: 1d ; 2c ; 3e ; 4d ; 5e

Short Answer Questions
1. In general terms, what is the cause of (a) redness and heat (b) edema at inflammatory sites?
2. What class of molecules induces leukocyte (a) rolling (b) firm adhesion on endothelium?
3. Explain why leukocytes preferentially emigrate from the postcapillary venules into inflamed tissue.
4. Activated neutrophils secrete elastase and progelatinase B. What is the proposed role of these enzymes in the emigration of cells into sites of inflammation?
5. How does interferon gamma contribute to the inflammatory response?

Immunological Responses to Microbes

Objectives	211
Immunity to Microbes	212
General Features	212
Host Defenses to Extracellular Bacteria	212
Resistance to Immunity: Extracellular Bacteria	217
Host Defenses to Viruses	217
Resistance to Immunity: HIV	222
Host Defenses to Intracellular Bacteria	225
Resistance to Immunity: Intracellular Bacteria	226
Host Defenses to Fungi	227
Resistance to Immunity: Fungi	229
Summary	230
Clinical Cases and Discussion	232
Test Yourself	236

Objectives

The following chapter explores the mechanism(s) by which the immune system defends the host from pathogenic organisms. In addition to the dichotomy already discussed (Chapter 2) between the so-called innate (primitive) immune system and acquired immune defenses, the heterogeneity of mechanisms apparent in the acquired immune system is enormous. However, some order to this is readily apparent when we consider immunity to virus, bacteria (intra- or extracellular bacteria) and fungi.

Generally efficient eradication of an organism occurs before the immune system is overwhelmed by further proliferation of the infectious agent. Thus, antiviral immunity depends upon recognition of a virally infected cell before production of further infectious virus. Both of the effector cells involved (NK cells and CD8+ killer cells/CTL) recognize cell surface changes (different for each effector cell) which reflect invasion by virus. In contrast, phagocytes most effectively eradicate extracellular bacterial organisms, particularly when marked for recognition by the host immune system. These "tags" (opsonins) facilitate recognition by macrophages, and so the organism is destroyed.

Intracellular bacteria (including those responsible for tuberculosis, *Mycobacterium tuberculosis*) and fungi are eliminated by promoting the natural lytic machinery in the infected cell. CD4+ T-cell recognition of cell surface changes, reflective of infection (this time by intracellular bacteria), results in secretion of molecules (cytokines) which enhance destruction of the intracellular organisms.

During evolution a continual coadaptation of both host and infectious agent has occurred in an attempt to circumvent the hurdles each developed to thwart

Clinical Immunology, by Reginald Gorczynski and Jacqueline Stanley. 2001 Landes Bioscience

the survival of the other. Viruses have developed mechanisms to prevent generation of killer CTL, while some bacteria surround themselves with "carbohydrate coats" to deflect recognition by other host cells. One particular virus (human immunodeficiency virus (HIV), responsible for acquired immunodeficiency syndrome (AIDS)) has a particularly effective mechanism of evading host immunity, infecting and destroying the very cells responsible for protection.

IMMUNITY TO MICROBES

GENERAL FEATURES

Microbes invade the body by penetrating the normally protective physical and chemical defenses. Having breached these barriers, microbes now face the onslaught of the innate and adaptive immune systems, comprised of tissues, cells, and soluble mediators. Different subsets of the immune system are recruited during immune responses, depending on the organism and its mode of infection. As an example, viruses infect cells and either integrate into the host cell DNA (latent virus) or subvert the host cell's synthetic machinery to make new virus. Viruses generally remain sequestered in the cell until they bud from the cell membrane and/or "burst" the host cell, now infecting new populations of cells. Intracellular bacteria also infect cells, but many thrive within macrophages having evolved mechanisms to evade the proteolytic degradation that normally occurs in the phagolysosome. Extracellular bacteria are not sequestered, but many have become pathogenic because they have a polysaccharide capsule that hinders phagocytosis. Other extracellular bacteria secrete toxins that "poison" various aspects of normal cell/tissue physiology (e.g., altering the function of enzymes which regulate ion flow across cell membranes, leading ultimately to altered ion secretion and (in the intestine) diarrhea; altering the state of activation of lymphocytes, leading to massive proliferation followed by cell death (apoptosis), etc.). The immune system has evolved ways to counteract many of the protective mechanisms of microbes, which reflect the different components of the immune system mobilized in response to infection with these different organisms.

HOST DEFENSES TO EXTRACELLULAR BACTERIA

General features
Extracellular bacteria thrive within the host environment, but are not sequestered within cells. They are generally vulnerable to soluble mediators of the immune system and phagocytosis. Extracellular bacteria may enter the body by various routes. As an example, **Borrelia burgdorferi**, the causative agent of **Lyme's disease**, is transmitted to humans by ticks and enters the bloodstream directly. In contrast, **Staphylococcus aureus**, the (frequent) causative agent of localized skin infections (**boils, furuncles** etc.) is found on the skin of most individuals, but

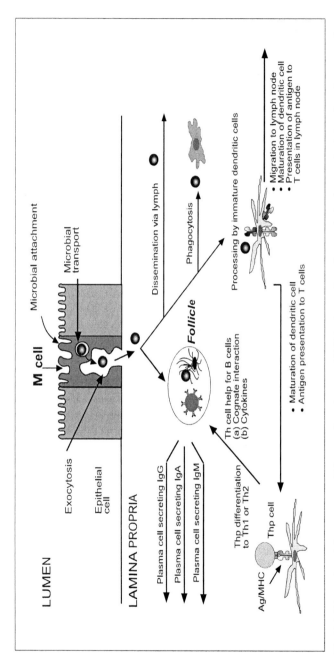

Fig. 11.1. Primary host defenses to extracellular organisms that enter MALT in the gut. Bacteria enter the lamina propria via M cells and encounter host defense mechanisms. Bacteria may be: (i) phagocytosed and destroyed by resident macrophages, (ii) disseminated via lymph to the mesenteric lymph nodes; (iii) processed by immature dendritic cells with antigens displayed with class II MHC for recognition by T cells in the lamina propria or the mesenteric lymph nodes; (iv) bound to B-cell membrane immunoglobulin in local follicles, or regional draining lymph nodes, initiating B-cell differentiation.

only becomes pathogenic when intact skin barriers are broken, and a significant bacterial load enters the body. Some extracellular bacteria adhere to mucus membranes of the neopharynx, respiratory, genitourinary, or gastrointestinal tracts as a preliminary step to tissue invasion (Fig. 11.1). When ***Neissseria gonorrhea***, the causative agent of **gonorrhea**, encounters mucus membranes it adheres to the epithelium and propagates (e.g., vagina). Immunity involves complement mediated osmotic lysis because this organism has evolved mechanisms to resist both direct and opsonin mediated phagocytosis. ***Streptococcus pneumoniae***, a common cause of bacterial pneumonia, is airborne and invades the respiratory tract. For primary immune responses, the site of entry determines the secondary tissue where the initial immune response will occur.

Physical and chemical barriers

Extracellular bacteria must penetrate the host's physical barriers such as intact skin or mucosal surfaces. Bacteria that adhere to intact skin are cast off along with the regular shedding of dead skin. Bacteria present in mucosal secretions encounter **bactericidal** (bacterial killing) or **bacteriostatic** (bacterial growth inhibiting) proteins. As one example, mucosal surfaces contain **lactoferrin**, a protein that binds iron, reducing the amount available to bacteria so that they are unable to grow. Mucosal secretions also contain **lysozyme**, a protein that weakens the cell wall of some bacteria by cleaving specific bonds in the peptidoglycan layer (cell wall). While the mucus layer is protective, it is not as impervious a barrier as intact skin. Once physical barriers have been breached, bacteria gain access to interstitial fluid, blood, or lymph. To survive within this environment, they must thwart the subsequent attack by the immune system.

Phagocytes, phagocytosis, and cytokines

Phagocytosis is the primary mechanism by which extracellular bacteria are eliminated (Fig. 11.2). The process of phagocytosis is enhanced by molecules generated following the activation of B cells, T cells, and complement. Nonspecific recognition of bacteria by phagocytes, leading to phagocytosis, represents an early phase of host defense. The deposition of molecules termed **opsonins** enhances recognition of bacteria via receptors that are specific for the opsonin, a process referred to as opsonin mediated phagocytosis.

The term opsonin does not refer to a single protein, but refers to any host protein that binds to bacteria and is recognized in a specific manner leading to phagocytosis. Opsonins are generally proteolytically derived complement proteins, or IgG antibodies. Opsonin mediated phagocytosis therefore occurs only after the complement system has been activated or after B cells differentiate into plasma cells secreting IgG antibodies.

Opsonins facilitate recognition of bacteria but do not alter the process by which the organism is destroyed. This process depends upon fusion of lysosomes with the endocytic vesicle containing the bacteria, and the release of bactericidal and bacteriostatic products into the phagocytic vacuole. Oxygen-dependent mechanisms are also recruited following activation of NADPH oxidase and nitric oxide

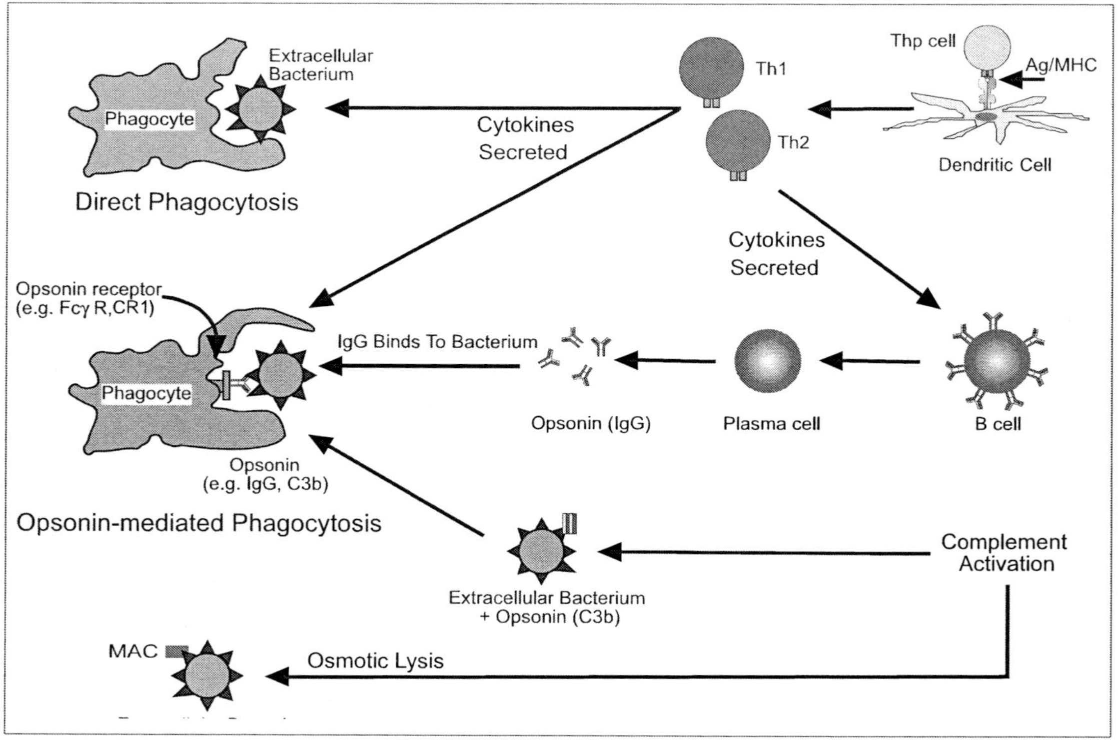

Immunological Responses to Microbes

Fig. 11.2. Role of immune cells and complement in host defense to extracellular bacteria. Phagocytosis, the primary means by which extracellular bacteria are eliminated, is enhanced by molecules generated following the activation of B cells, T cells, and complement. Nonspecific recognition of bacteria by phagocytes is termed direct phagocytosis, while phagocytosis that follows binding of opsonin is termed opsonin mediated phagocytosis.

synthase, which leads to the production of bactericidal products including reactive oxygen intermediates, nitric oxide and other reactive nitrogen intermediates formed when the reactive oxygen intermediates react with nitric oxide. Activated macrophages secrete cytokines. Some cytokines enhance the inflammatory response, while others influence the course of naive CD4+ T-cell differentiation with respect to phenotype, Th1 or Th2. The production of many bactericidal factors by the host cell is, in turn, enhanced in the presence of CD4+ T-cell derived cytokines (e.g., interferon gamma (IFNγ) and tumor necrosis factor (TNF)).

Complement

Complement refers to the complex system of proteins found in normal blood serum and interstitial fluid (Chapter 5). The role of complement in the elimination of bacteria is 2-fold: (i) proteolytically derived complement fragments serve as opsonins; (ii) the generation of a membrane attack complex, and its insertion into the bacterial cell surface, causes destruction of the bacterium by osmotic lysis.

Complement activation can proceed via the *alternative pathway* or the *classical pathway*. The former is activated when spontaneously derived C3b is deposited on bacteria, leading to the production of more C3b and other complement proteins that play a role in host defense. The deposition of C3b onto the bacterial surface facilitates opsonin mediated phagocytosis. Bacteria that are not destroyed in this manner may undergo osmotic lysis following the insertion into the bacterial membrane of a complement-derived molecular complex, the so-called membrane attack complex. Complement activation by the classical pathway requires antibodies. Therefore, activation via this pathway occurs only after recruitment of adaptive immunity. The final role of complement in bacterial host defense is the same regardless of whether activation was mediated by the alternative or the classical pathway (Chapter 5).

Antibodies

Antibodies contribute to the destruction of extracellular bacteria by activating the classical pathway of complement and by serving as opsonins for opsonin mediated phagocytosis. IgM and IgG antibody isotypes activate the classical pathway of complement. IgM is more effective at activating complement than IgG because of its pentameric structure (Chapter 5). Antibodies also play a protective role in host defense by binding to and neutralizing toxins secreted by some bacteria. B-cell responses to T-dependent antigens require T-cell help delivered in the form of cytokines and cognate interaction.

CD4+ T cells and cytokines

CD4+ T-cell derived cytokines augment the bactericidal activities of the phagocytes. Cytokines that enhance killing by phagocytes are Type 1 cytokines, IFNγ and TNF, which activate the intracellular cascades (producing reactive oxygen/nitrogen products) important for killing phagocytosed organisms. Naive CD4+ T cells (Thp) are activated in secondary lymphoid tissues when they bind bacterial peptide/class II MHC complexes displayed on the surface of antigen presenting cells. Appropriate costimulatory molecules are also required (Chapter 9). The

Immunological Responses to Microbes

cytokine pattern present in the local microenvironment influences whether Thp cells differentiate into Th cells secreting Type 1 cytokines or Type 2 cytokines. T-cell derived cytokines are required for B-cell activation leading to isotype switching and differentiation to antibody secreting plasma cells.

Resistance to Immunity: Extracellular Bacteria

Streptococcus pneumoniae

Streptococcus pneumoniae is one of the common causative agents of bacterial pneumonia. Infections begin with inhalation of respiratory secretions containing the pneumococci. Generally these bacteria are cleared by the physical and chemical defense mechanisms of the respiratory tract as described above. Organisms that breach these defenses are protected from phagocytosis by the presence of a polysaccharide capsule until B cells are activated and IgG opsonins are produced.

B-cell activation occurs in response to mIg crosslinking by the polysaccharide capsule. B cells undergo differentiation to antibody secreting plasma cells. While most of the antibodies generated are IgM, some isotype switching to IgG also occurs. Polysaccharides are not processed for presentation with class II MHC on the surface of antigen presenting cells. Therefore, CD4+ T cells are not activated in response to this antigen, and so pneumococcal polysaccharide is referred to as a T-independent antigen. The lack of T-cell activation accounts for the relative lack of class switching in response to infection by this organism. The little IgG produced presumably reflects low (endogenous) levels of some cytokines believed to be important for class switching. There may also be some cytokine production from γδ TCR+ T cells, which do not depend upon conventional class I/II MHC restricted presentation of antigen for stimulation of cytokine production (Chapter 9).

A lack of opsonins can lead to multiplication of this bacterium resulting in bacteremia. Immune responses to T-independent antigens do not generate memory cells, and so each infection is potentially life threatening. That is, innate responses are inadequate in the absence of IgG antibodies that serve as opsonins, and activation of B cells leading to IgG production requires several days.

Host Defenses to Viruses

General features

Viruses are a heterogeneous group of infectious agents composed mainly of nucleic acid surrounded by a protein coat. Following entry into the cell the virus makes use of the host cell's synthetic "machinery" to manufacture the proteins and nucleic acids required for its replication. These components are then assembled and released as viral particles. Viruses cause diseases ranging from acute infections (e.g., polio) to chronic infections that are relatively benign (e.g., herpes), as well as life-threatening chronic infections (e.g., HIV). The development of sterile immunity to viruses is a challenge immunologically, because viruses are sequestered within cells and replicate rapidly, potentially producing mutations rapidly. When these mutations occur at the antigenic epitope, previously active immune effector cells may no longer recognize the altered virus producing immunological resistance. Some viruses have evolved mechanisms that sabotage immune responses, synthesizing products that subvert the host immune system. As an example, the virus causing mononucleosis (Epstein-Barr Virus, EBV) encodes a (viral) IL-10-like molecule which inhibits the development of effective antiviral cytotoxic T cells needed to kill virally infected cells (Figs. 9.5 and 9.7).

In general, elimination of a viral infection requires the *destruction* of virally infected cells by osmotic lysis as a result of natural killer (NK) or cytotoxic T-cell (CTL) activation, before the production of newly infective viral particles. Immune cells active in these processes must "see" something unique to the surface of virally infected cells, not present on noninfected cells. An effector system that awaits cell release of newly synthesized virus before initiating destruction (e.g., antibody) would be ineffective, since infectious viral particles replicate exponentially in infected cells. Activation of anti-viral recognition processes requires cytokines secreted by antigen presenting cells, or Type 1 cytokine producing CD4+ T cell (Figs. 11.3, 11.4). During the initial phase of infectivity and when the viral particles bud from the cell, the particles can be targeted by antibodies or phagocytes.

Phagocytes, phagocytosis and cytokines

Immune responses to viruses vary according to the site where the virus is detected and whether the infection is primary or secondary. When viruses are found within blood, lymph, or interstitial fluid, they may be phagocytosed. Viruses are found only transiently in fluids during the initial infectivity stage, and when they are released from infected cells. Therefore, phagocytosis is not a primary mechanism for the eradication of viral infections.

Natural killer cells and osmotic cell lysis

Natural killer cells (NK cells) express an "NK receptor", which recognizes viral proteins that remain embedded within the cell membrane following viral entry into the cell or viral budding from the cell. NK cells have a rather broad specificity and so the NK receptor recognizes a variety of targets. NK cells can also interact, via the FcγR, with virally infected cells to which IgG antibodies have bound.

Natural killer cells destroy virally infected cells following recognition of, and conjugate formation with, the virally infected cell. There follows a polarized release of granules containing perforin, a protein that induces osmotic lysis of the target by forming pores in the membrane. Although perforin induces osmotic lysis of the infected cell, it does not harm the natural killer cell (Fig. 2.9).

Natural killer cells are most effective during the early phase of infection because virally infected cells secrete interferon α/β, cytokines that enhance the expression of class I MHC. NK cells also express a receptor, the so-called killer inhibitory receptor (KIR), whose ligand is class I MHC. This prevents NK cell killing of ubiquitous class I MHC expressing host cells. Increased expression of class I MHC following IFNα/β signaling by virally infected cells "shuts off" NK mediated activity, limiting the time over which NK cells provide effective viral immunity.

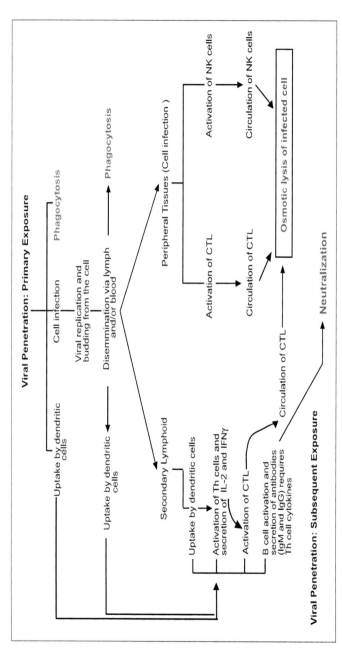

Fig. 11.3. Concept map depicting the immune response to viral infection. Viral infections activate numerous components of the immune system. The key response involves destruction of the infected cell. Phagocytosis and neutralization by antibodies are mechanisms that come into play when the viral particle is in the fluid phase, rather than sequestered within a cell.

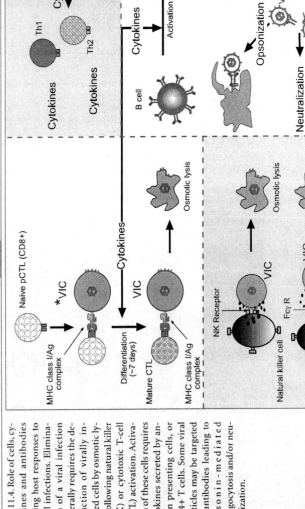

Fig. 11.4. Role of cells, cytokines and antibodies during host responses to viral infections. Elimination of a viral infection generally requires the destruction of virally infected cells by osmotic lysis following natural killer (NK) or cytotoxic T-cell (CTL) activation. Activation of these cells requires cytokines secreted by antigen presenting cells, or CD4+ T cells. Some viral particles may be targeted by antibodies leading to opsonin-mediated phagocytosis and/or neutralization.

CD4+ T cells and cytokines

Activation of CD4+ T cells leading to cytokine secretion follows recognition of viral peptides/class II MHC, along with costimulator molecules, expressed on the surface of dendritic cells. Because dendritic cells detect viral particles in interstitial fluid, blood or lymph, antigen presentation occurs only during the initial infectivity stage or when viral particles are released from the cells. For effective viral immunity CD4+ T cells must differentiate to the Th1 subset secreting IL-2 because this cytokine is required for differentiation of naive CD8+ T cells to CTL that kill virally infected cells (Fig. 9.7).

B cells and antibody production

B cells are not key players in viral immunity. B cells are activated and differentiate to antibody secreting cells when mIg binds to virus, in the presence of appropriate CD4+ T-cell help. Circulating IgG antibodies can neutralize free virus by binding to the site of cell attachment and promoting phagocytosis (Fig. 2.4).

CD8+ T cells and osmotic cell lysis

Virus sequestered within cells is effectively protected from the immune system, leaving destruction of the infected cell as the only recourse. Infected cells are veritable "viral factories", which are destroyed by NK cells (see above) and by CD8+ cytotoxic T cells (CTL). Like NK cells, CTLs deliver their lethal hit following conjugate formation with the infected cell and release of granules containing perforin. Naive CD8+ T cells, also known as precytotoxic T cells (pCTL), must differentiate to mature CTLs before they become lytic effectors. This differentiation process requires interleukin-2 (IL-2). For the most part, the CD4+ T cell (Th1) is the source of the IL-2 required for differentiation of the pCTL (Fig. 9.7).

Comparison of CTL and NK cell responses to viral infections

NK cells and CTLs deliver the lethal hit to the infected cell in the same manner. IL-12, a macrophage/dendritic cell derived cytokine, promotes differentiation of Type 1 cytokine producing cells, thus providing IL-2 for CD8+ T-cell expansion. IL-12 provides a proliferative and stimulatory signal to NK cells. Major differences in the induction of anti-viral activity in NK cells and CTLs include:

i Following initial contact with an infected cell, NK cells can deliver the lethal hit without further differentiation. In contrast, CD8+ pCTL cells must differentiate to CTLs before performing their biological function. This process requires both antigen contact (an infected cell) as well as the presence of IL-2. IL-2 also enhances NK cell cytotoxicity, but its presence is not absolutely required for cytotoxicity.

ii NK cell recognition of infected cells is mediated by a broad specificity NK receptor. In addition, the FcγR on the NK cell interacts with infected cells via IgG antibodies bound to viral proteins present in the cell membrane. In contrast, pCTLs (and CTLs) recognize infected cells by virtue of the class I MHC/viral peptide expressed on the cell surface.

iii NK cell cytotoxicity is inhibited by excessive class I MHC expression on the target cell. Interaction of the killer inhibitory receptor (KIR) on the NK cell with MHC class I on the target cell delivers this inhibitory signal to the NK cell. In contrast, up-regulation of class I MHC expression on the infected cell *enhances* CTL cytotoxicity, probably because this increases the number of viral peptides displayed on the cell surface.

RESISTANCE TO IMMUNITY: HIV

General features
The **human immunodeficiency virus (HIV)** is the causative agent of the **acquired immunodeficiency syndrome (AIDS)**. HIV disables the immune system by destroying the CD4+ T cells directly, or indirectly. Because CD4+ T cells secrete cytokines that are required for virtually all aspects of immunity, this destruction predisposes individuals to opportunistic infections and some malignancies. Destruction of CD4+ T cells is partially mediated by the same normal host defenses that destroy virally infected cells.

Transmission of HIV
HIV is transmitted between humans in several ways:
i   sexual intercourse,
ii exposure to contaminated blood or body fluids;
iii perinatally.

HIV targets the CD4 molecule present on the surface of a subset of T cells, dendritic cells, and macrophages. Binding to a second coreceptor, such as those for the CC chemokine family (**RANTES; MIP-1α, MIP-1β**), namely **CCR5**, may be a requirement for target cell entry for macrophage (M-) tropic strains of HIV (Fig. 11.5). T-tropic strains of HIV seem to use primarily **CXCR4**, the receptor for the CXC chemokine, **SDF-1 (stromal cell-derived factor 1)**.

Seroconversion
Entry of HIV into bodily fluids (rather than directly into a cell) provides a small "window" in which HIV specific B cells can be activated, providing that adequate T-cell help is available. As a result neutralizing and opsonizing antibodies are generated. When these antibodies are detected in serum, the individual is said to be seropositive with respect to HIV. As noted above, the effectiveness of antibodies is limited to free viral particles, and not to those viral particles sequestered within a cell. In consequence there is little evidence that seropositivity is a useful marker for protective anti-viral immunity.

Productive infection of CD4+ T cells
Replication in T cells occurs optimally in activated T cells. CD4+ T cells stimulated with viral peptide/class II MHC, and appropriate costimulatory molecules, become activated. In one model of CD4+ T-cell infectivity, an infected antigen presenting cell releases viral particles into the microenvironment where the T cell

Immunological Responses to Microbes

is being activated (Fig. 11.5). This "ensures" productive infection of the CD4+ T cell.

Syncytia formation and cell destruction

Following infection, cell conjugates form, resulting in **syncyctia formation**. This occurs when CD4 molecules, present on the T-cell surface, interact with residual viral proteins embedded within the infected cell membrane leading to the fusion and functional destruction of the two cells. Syncytia formation may contribute to the decrease in uninfected CD4+ T cells observed during HIV infection.

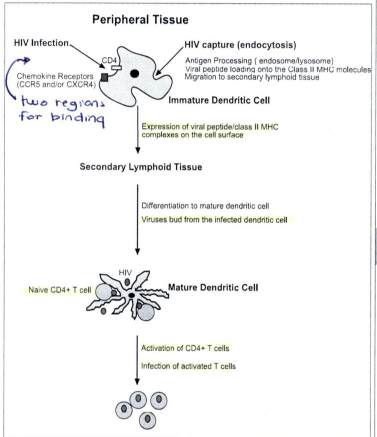

Fig. 11.5. Model for HIV infection of dendritic cells and CD4+ T cells. HIV targets the CD4 molecule on the surface of a subset of T cells, dendritic cells, and macrophages. However, binding to a coreceptor such as the chemokine receptor, CCR5, for macrophage tropic strains of HIV, may be a requirement for cell entry. T cells must be activated to be productively infected by HIV.

Disease progression

CD4+ T cells are the main target of HIV infection, regardless of their antigenic specificity. This produces a decline in the CD4+ T-cell numbers and a non-antigen specific immunosuppression. Similar diseases strike this population, as are seen in other nonspecifically immunosuppressed individuals (transplant patients; individuals receiving cancer chemotherapy; the elderly, etc.). The decline in CD4+ T-cell numbers is a useful marker of disease progression. Some six months after the initial infection, the viral load reaches a steady state, which is maintained for varying periods of time depending on as yet unidentified factors, that vary between individuals. For the average individual this steady state will be sustained for eight to ten years. While some individuals die within a year of infection, others survive for more than 15 years. With recent improvements in polypharmaceutical treatments with antiviral agents, life expectancy following initial infection with HIV has been considerably increased. The potential for co-opting immune mechanisms into this defense offers the hope of eventual cure of this disease.

HOST DEFENSES TO INTRACELLULAR BACTERIA

General features

Intracellular bacteria live inside host cells. Although any cell may be infected, the macrophage phagolysosome serves as a favorite niche, in contrast to viruses that are normally found in the cytosol. Sequestration in cells protects the organisms from the (humoral) immune system, and again cellular immunity is the primary effector mechanism. Key cells in immunity to intracellular bacteria are cytokine activated macrophages, where cytokines are derived from activated natural killer cells and CD4+ T cells (Fig. 11.6). While most intracellular bacteria enter the host through mucosal tissues, some can enter the circulation directly via bites from an intermediate vector (animal/insect).

Food borne/oral-fecal intracellular bacteria

Food-borne intracellular bacteria are generally removed from the intestine by peristalsis. However, some bacteria escape this fate by binding to M cells (Fig. 11.7). M cells are interspersed between epithelial cells, in distinct regions devoid of a protective mucus covering. Bacteria pass through M cells in vesicles from which they are released into the lamina propria and phagocytosed by tissue macrophages where they are either destroyed or establish infection. A similar fate awaits bacteria in mesenteric lymph nodes if they leave the lamina propria via efferent lymphatics. Bacteria that have evolved mechanisms to resist degradation in the macrophage use this niche to proliferate because they are concealed from humoral effectors of immunosurveillance. Not all the intracellular bacteria, however, use the macrophage as a habitat (e.g., *Shigella sp*).

Airborne intracellular bacteria

Airborne intracellular bacteria are generally trapped by the mucus coated, ciliated epithelium and removed by coughing. Some bacteria are phagocytosed by alveolar macrophages and destroyed. Bacteria escaping these fates bind to epithelial

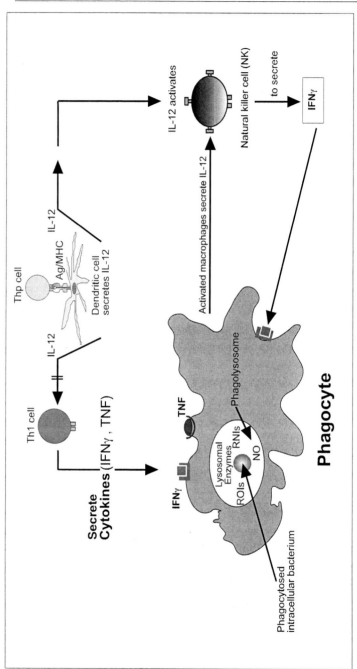

Fig. 11.6. Cells and cytokines in host responses to infection with intracellular bacteria. Key cells in immunity to intracellular bacteria are cytokine activated macrophages. The cytokines involved are derived from activated natural killer cells and CD4+ T cells.

cells and enter the lung by transcytosis through the epithelial cells. Alternatively, bacteria may enter the lung inside macrophages (a "trojan horse") as the macrophages enter tissue spaces. Macrophages squeeze between alveolar cells and penetrate the alveolar basement membrane (diapedesis) following their localized enzymatic degradation by macrophage derived proteins. Bacteria that have evolved mechanisms to resist degradation in the macrophage proliferate, effectively secluded from antibodies and complement. As an example, phagocytosed *Mycobacterium tuberculosis* organisms prevent phagosome/lysosome fusion and replicate within the phagosome.

Resistance to Immunity: Intracellular Bacteria

Mycobacterium tuberculosis
Tuberculosis is a disease resulting from infection with the intracellular bacterium, ***Mycobacterium tuberculosis***. Infection occurs primarily via the respiratory route and is transmitted from person to person. More than 1.5 billion people are infected world-wide with this organism. Many remain healthy if the cellular immune system keeps the infection in check. However, bacteria frequently persist in the lungs and are reactivated when the individual becomes immunocompromised, as occurs for instance in an aged and/or chronically debilitated population. Because most infected individuals do not develop overt symptomatology, a skin test is used to confirm exposure. This consists of an intradermal challenge with purified protein derivative (PPD) from *Mycobacterium tuberculosis*. Previously infected individuals develop a cutaneous reaction, a consequence of reactivation of memory CD4+ T cells at the site of challenge. This cutaneous reaction (redness, edematous, cellular infiltration) is referred to in general as a **delayed-type-hypersensitivity (DTH)** reaction, and in this particular case as a **Mantoux reaction**. Ten million new cases of tuberculosis arise yearly, and more than two million people die each year from infection. In many third world countries, where tuberculosis is rampant, immunization with *Bacillus Calmette-Guerin* (BCG), an attenuated strain of *Mycobacteria bovis*, provides some protection from *Mycobacterium tuberculosis*. There is a pressing need to develop more effective and safer vaccines for this disease.

Host defense
Key cells in immunity to *Mycobacterium tuberculosis* are cytokine (IFNγ, TNF) activated macrophages. IL-12 produced by activated macrophages is a potent activator of IFNγ production by NK cells. Macrophages also secrete TNF. The significance of TNF in *Mycobacterium tuberculosis* infections was shown during studies with mice in which the gene for TNF was disabled. These animals showed significant impairment in their ability to resist challenge with the organism. IFNγ has a dual role in host defense to this intracellular organism. First, IFNγ enhances the production of reactive oxygen intermediates, nitric oxide, and reactive nitrogen intermediates. Secondly, ongoing production of IFNγ by CD4+ Th1 cells in host defense to infection with *Mycobacterium tuberculosis* is contingent on the pres-

ence of this cytokine (NK cell derived initially) during the differentiation of naive CD4+ T cells (Fig. 9.4).

Some *Mycobacterium tuberculosis* organisms may survive in alveolar macrophages because components of their cell wall prevent the fusion of lysosomes with the phagosomes. As a result lysosomal enzymes cannot destroy the microbe. The enhanced virulence of *Mycobacterium tuberculosis*, in comparison with other organisms that also prevent phagolysosome fusion, may reflect the additional effect of scavenging reactive oxygen species, as has been shown for *Mycobacterium leprae*.

A notable feature of the immune response to *Mycobacterium tuberculosis* is the formation of granulomas. A granuloma is an aggregation of macrophages surrounded by CD4+ T lymphocytes secreting Type 1 cytokines, particularly IFNγ. When the cells are arranged in this formation, cytokines secreted by activated T cells are available to large numbers of infected macrophages. In healthy individuals, the intracellular organisms are destroyed, or contained, with a residue of bacteria surviving in a quiescent state, and no observable clinical symptoms. Disruption of this homeostasis in previously infected individuals results in disease. Individuals at risk for overt disease are those with CD4+ T-cell defects, or those in whom differentiation of naive CD4+ Thp cells results in a polarization to Th2 cells secreting Type 2 cytokines rather than Type-1 cytokines.

Shigella dysenteriae

Shigelle dysenteriae, the causative agent of Shigella dysentery, infects epithelial cells in the intestinal lumen. *Shigella dysenteriae* produces a toxin, Shiga toxin, believed to be associated with damage to the colonic vasculature thus causing bloody diarrhea. *Shigella dysenteriae* variants that do not produce the toxins remain pathogenic but are less virulent. Shigella organisms that escape expulsion from the gastrointestinal tract by peristalsis, bind to M cells and are endocytosed within these cells. However, unlike most organisms, *Shigella dysenteriae* lyses the endosomal wall and escapes into the M cell cytoplasm where they replicate (Fig. 11.7). From there, many of these organisms spread laterally to infect adjacent epithelial cells. *Shigella dysenteriae* that do not infect the adjacent epithelial cells pass through the M cell, into the lamina propria, where they are phagocytosed by macrophages, which are induced to undergo apoptosis.

HOST DEFENSES TO FUNGI

General features

Fungal infections are often called **mycoses**. Fungal infections generally pose a serious threat only to immunocompromised individuals, including AIDs patients, as well as those receiving immunosuppressive drugs, or chemotherapy (for malignancy).

Fungi that are part of the normal flora, or that are wide spread in the environment, are termed "opportunistic" fungi because they are relatively harmless to healthy hosts. **Candida albicans** and various species of ***Aspergillus***, a mold, are common **opportunistic** fungi.

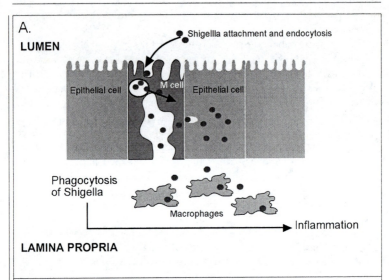

Fig. 11.7. Invasion by Shigella causes death of epithelial cells and apoptosis of macrophages. *Shigella sp.* bind to M cells and are endocytosed within these cells. They lyse the endosomal wall and escape into the M cell cytoplasm where replication occurs. Many of the organisms then spread laterally to infect adjacent epithelial cells. Organisms not infecting adjacent epithelial cells pass through the M cell, into the lamina propria, where they are phagocytosed by macrophages, which are stimulated to undergo apoptosis.

Fungi that are not part of the normal flora, or widespread in the environment, can cause infection following human contact with contaminated soil, or animals, and even other humans. Fungi transmitted from human to human generally cause superficial infections such as ringworm and athlete's foot. Systemic infections and serious disease result from infection with airborne fungi such as the dimorphic *Cryptococcus neoformans*. This is found primarily in its mold form in soils contaminated with pigeon droppings. Clinical infection is believed to be initiated with inhalation of the yeast form.

Cryptococcus neoformans is a common infection in AIDS patients. The presence of a polysaccharide capsule surrounding the organism protects it from phagocytosis. Opsonin mediated phagocytosis occurs when IgG antibodies are secreted following B-cell differentiation to antibody secreting plasma cells. B-cell activation leading to isotype switching requires cytokines. Low endogenous levels of cytokines probably serve to promote sufficient IgG production for opsonization of the organism. Following sequestration in macrophages, other CD4 derived cytokines (e.g., IFNγ) are required for optimal activation of intracellular killing mechanisms. Patients with reduced CD4+ T-cell counts have impaired killing of this organism.

RESISTANCE TO IMMUNITY: FUNGI

Candida albicans
Opportunistic fungi are a normal part of the human flora and produce disease only when the individual is immunosuppressed. *Candida albicans* is a yeast found primarily in mucosal tissues such as the oral cavity and female genital tract, colonizing these regions by binding to glycoproteins present in the secretions of mucus membranes, or on the epithelial cell surface. *Candida albicans* may invade the underlying basement membrane by forming budding protrusions termed "hyphae". Conditions (e.g., chemotherapy) leading to the loss of epithelial cells allows *Candida albicans* to bind to the glycoproteins in the basement membrane and invade the tissues below the basement membrane by forming hyphae.

In immunosuppressed hosts, oral infection with *Candida albicans* manifests as white plaques (thrush) weakly adherent to the mucosal surface. Vaginal infection manifests as a thick discharge and itching of the vulva. Vaginitis is more common during states of pregnancy, diabetes, or when using oral contraceptives (localized steroid-induced immunosuppression). Both yeast infections are referred to as *candidiasis*.

Phagocytosis is the main mechanism by which *Candida albicans* are destroyed. Individuals with neutrophil defects have serious infections with these fungi. Phagocytosis is more efficient in the presence of opsonins, IgG or complement fragments, and hence immunity to *Candida albicans* requires the activation of both B cells and CD4+ T cells. Secreted IgG may act as an opsonin. IgM or IgG activate the classical pathway of complement leading to production of complement proteins that serve as opsonins (Chapter 5).

When the hyphae are too large for phagocytosis, activated neutrophils can still destroy them by secretion of an array of proteolytic molecules into the local microenvironment. Attachment of neutrophils to the hyphae ensures that the fungi are within "range" of these metabolites.

In addition to their role in B-cell activation, cytokines secreted by activated CD4+ T cells play a significant role in immunity to Candida species. IFNγ augments the production of reactive oxygen intermediates, nitric oxide, and reactive nitrogen intermediates by phagocytes. The role of CD4+ cytokines is underscored by the fact that individuals who lack T cells with antigen specific T-cell receptors recognizing Candida peptide/class II MHC have recurrent candidiasis. This disorder is termed **chronic mucocutaneous candidiasis** and results from a so-called "hole" in the T-cell repertoire.

SUMMARY

Microbes penetrate the normally protective physical and chemical defenses. Having breached host barriers, they face the onslaught of both the innate and adaptive immune systems. Different components of the immune system are recruited during immune responses, depending on the organism and its mode of infectivity (Fig. 11.8). Viruses infect and replicate within cells. Intracellular bacteria also infect cells, often thriving within macrophages because they have evolved mechanisms to evade the proteolytic degradation that occurs in the phagocytic vacuole. Extracellular bacteria are not sequestered, and many have become pathogenic because they have a polysaccharide capsule that hinders phagocytosis.

Extracellular bacteria thrive within the host environment, but are not sequestered within any cell. These microbes are vulnerable to soluble mediators of the immune system. Phagocytosis is the primary vehicle by which extracellular bacteria are eliminated. The process of phagocytosis is greatly enhanced by molecules generated following the activation of B cells, T cells, and complement. The deposition of molecules termed opsonins allows phagocytes to bind bacteria via receptors that are specific for the opsonin. Activated macrophages also secrete cytokines, some of which enhance the inflammatory response, while others influence the course of naive CD4+ T-cell differentiation. Antibodies contribute to the destruction of extracellular bacteria by activating the classical pathway of complement, and by serving as opsonins for opsonin mediated phagocytosis. Antibodies may also play a protective role in host defense by binding to, and hence neutralizing, toxins secreted by some bacteria.

Immune responses to viruses vary according to the site where the virus is detected and whether the infection is primary or secondary. When viruses are found within blood, lymph, or interstitial fluid, they may be phagocytosed. However viruses are found only transiently in fluids during the initial infection and when they are released from infected cells. Thus while phagocytosis of viral particles does occur, this is not a primary mechanism for the eradication of viral infections. Viruses are sequestered within cells, protected from the immune system. Destruction of the infected cell, a veritable "viral factory", is mediated by NK cells, and by

Immunological Responses to Microbes

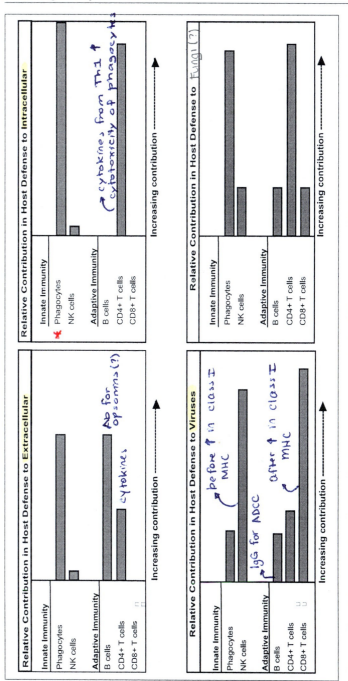

Fig. 11.8. The relative contribution of various cells in immune responses to microbes. Different components of the immune systems are recruited during immune responses, depending on the organism and its mode of infectivity.

CTL. Both release lytic granules following conjugate formation with the infected cell.

Intracellular bacteria live inside host cells. Although any cell may be infected, the macrophage phagolysosome serves as a favorite niche, unlike viruses that are normally found in the cytosol. Once again sequestration inside cells protects the organism from humoral immunity, and so cellular immunity becomes the primary mechanism for controlling infection. Key cells in immunity to intracellular bacteria are cytokine activated macrophages, with the cytokines derived from activated natural killer cells and CD4+ T cells. Food-borne intracellular bacteria are generally removed from the intestine by peristalsis. Some bacteria escape this fate by binding to M cells, interspersed between epithelial cells in regions devoid of a protective mucus covering. Bacteria pass through M cells inside vesicles from which they are released into the lamina propria and phagocytosed by tissue macrophages where they are either destroyed or establish infection.

Fungal infections generally pose a serious threat only to immunocompromised individuals. Phagocytosis is the principal mechanism by which some fungi (e.g., *Candida albicans*) are destroyed, and individuals with a defect in neutrophil function sustain serious infections. Phagocytosis is again more efficient in the presence of opsonins, IgG or complement fragments, and so immunity to *Candida albicans* requires the activation of both B cells and CD4+ T cells. Secreted IgG and IgM may function as opsonin, or activate the classical pathway of complement leading to the generation of complement-derived opsonins. In addition to their role in B-cell activation, cytokines secreted by activated CD4+ T cells enhance the ability of phagocytes to destroy the phagocytosed organisms. The role of CD4+ cytokines is underscored by the fact that individuals who lack T cells with antigen specific T-cell receptors recognizing candida peptide/class II MHC have recurrent candidiasis. This disorder is termed chronic mucocutaneous candidiasis and results from a "hole" in the T-cell repertoire.

CLINICAL CASES AND DISCUSSION

Clinical Case #21
FH, a 36-year-old male heterosexual, is brought to your urban hospital with recurrent fevers (he has been seen here repeatedly over the last several weeks). He is a known iv drug user, and a resident of a local men's shelter. Three weeks ago you obtained permission for an HIV test, and the results, available only 4 days ago, indicate sero-negativity. He has no cough or weight loss, denies using drugs for a week, but has a temperature of 40ºC, has general myalgias (muscle aches/pains), and feels "weak". What tests might you order and why?

Discussion Case #21
Background
The indigent represent a population at significant risk for a number of acute and chronic infectious diseases, both because of increased risk of exposure (close

contact with other infected individuals) and because this population often shows subtle signs of immunocompromise, again frequently reflective of lifestyle. Tuberculosis (TB), of widespread concern globally, is a particularly acute problem in this group. Because of poor medication compliance, control of diagnosed infections can become a separate but equally difficult problem, and has led to the emergence of drug resistant organisms over the last 10 years, with concern that TB might become an even bigger scourge (globally) than it already is.

This gentleman fits a population for whom TB is a major concern. He also falls within a category at clear risk for HIV infection, namely iv drug use. While he denies homosexual intercourse, you should be aware that unprotected intercourse is itself a major risk factor, with a significant frequency of infected females, particularly in sex workers in inner city environments. You are told that, at a recent visit to the ER, HIV testing revealed sero-negativity. You need to be alert to the possibility of false negative results here, particularly if he is recently infected and has not developed antibodies. Perhaps he is chronically unable to produce anti-HIV antibody; or maybe the test itself was a technical failure, and was falsely negative. Other tests, looking directly for evidence of replicating virus in the blood with PCR based technology, are available clinically. Finally, the iv drug use brings to mind another, not uncommon infectious disorder, with high incidence in this population, namely hepatitis (particularly Hep B and C).

We are given some other information (other than the negative HIV serology) that can help here. He denies a cough or recent iv drug use, and has multiple (albeit vague) symptoms of recent viral infection (the myalgias, weakness and fever). While testing for all of the above disorders is appropriate, acute presentation of a chronic disorder may best fit this picture. You need to ask about his sexual lifestyle (protected vs unprotected intercourse), and consider checking on contacts.

Tests

Conventional blood work (looking for evidence for anemia (multiple causes), low white cell counts) is important. Perhaps he is at risk of infection because of an acquired disorder (e.g., leukemia) not related to lifestyle but which has depleted either lymphocytes (viral/fungal immunity) or neutrophils/macrophages (bacterial immunity). You could retest for HIV sero-conversion (sero-conversion itself can take up to 6 weeks post infection), but given the previous (recent) negative result, you are justified in asking for a quantitative virus test. In addition, serology for Hep B/C should be drawn along with liver biochemistry (these viruses infect hepatic cells). A chest X-ray should be performed to look for active infection and/or previously resolved infection (old granulomas representing healed TB). In addition, a Mantoux test should be ordered (it is important to use a control antigen to which everyone has been exposed, e.g., Candida antigen, so that any failure to react in the Mantoux test is not misinterpreted because of a general lack of immune responsiveness).

Treatment
He admits to multiple sexual partners and to unprotected intercourse with all. Despite the negative HIV serology, high titers of virus are detected in his blood. He becomes sero-positive over the next 3 weeks. He has a normal white cell and CD4 count, and is sero-negative for Hep B/C. He has a negative Mantoux but positive Candida test (suggesting no exposure to TB). *This is the picture of recent HIV infection.* Contact tracing is important, as is counseling on the need for changes in lifestyle (no shared needles, use of condoms, etc.). Discussion of longer-term care in relation to use of combinations of multiple anti-viral agents should also be begun, along with planning for frequent (and long-term) follow-up.

Clinical Case #22
You see this young boy for the first time at 3 years of age. Mom says he was well for the first 9 months of his life, but thereafter developed multiple bacterial infections of the upper respiratory tract (bronchi, nasal passages, otitis) and skin infections. All were treated successfully with antibiotics. His mother had had 3 brothers who died at an early age (before 3 years), in an era where antibiotics were not readily available, but has four healthy sisters, one of whom has a healthy son and daughter and two of the others each have one healthy daughter. This patient seems a bright and active child, and he has gained weight, grown, and developed normally. He has another ear infection (this will be his fifth infection in the first 6 months of the year). What are your thoughts, what tests might you order, and what therapy is appropriate?

Discussion Case #22
Background
The picture of recurrent bacterial infections is suspicious for defects somewhere in the process of production of immunoglobulin for host defense, or in the auxiliary cells/factors which contribute to that defense. Note that he was well in the first months of life. This is not unexpected, because passive transfer of maternal Ig (across the placenta; in colostrum) is protective. Despite the (greater) likelihood of exposure to viral infections over the first 3 years of life, and indeed common exposure to fungi (e.g., Candida is present in all warm moist areas of the skin surface, including the axillae and groin) no-one has been concerned at any suggestion of increased susceptibility to viral and /or fungal infections in this young boy. Thus you expect to find no evidence for defects in the T cell (or NK) arm of the immune response.

Amongst the pathways for eradication of bacterial infections, not only is Ig important (both IgM, IgG and IgA), but also complement and other phagocytic cells (macrophages, neutrophils). Defects in the complement pathway can have multiple presentations (Chapter 5), but a significant susceptibility to *N. gonnorhea* is a classical presentation of defects in production of a membrane attack complex (for destruction of this extracellular organism). A number of defects in metabolic pathways lead to ineffective development of the intracellular mechanisms needed to kill intracellular pathogens (e.g., NADPH oxidase deficiency etc., Chapter 2). Most of these defects leading to immunodeficiency disease are autosomal recessive however, and in this family background we are told only of affected males, with unaffected females. This pattern is characteristic of an X-linked recessive trait, which eliminates a number of other immunoglobulin deficiency states (Chapter 15). Note we cannot yet tell if his mother's sisters necessarily carry a defective gene because none of them has had an affected male child.

Tests

Serum immunoglobulin levels should be investigated. The results show 60 mg/dl IgG (normal 600-1500 mg/dl); no IgA (normal 50-125 mg/dl), and only 30 mg/dl IgM (normal 75-150 mg/dl). All are in keeping with a profound agammaglobulinemia (hypogamaglobulinemia). You need to perform a "differential" count on the white cells, to ensure there is no obvious developmental defect in cells responsible for control of infection. Laboratory studies at the time showed a white blood cell count of 6200/µl (normal). The differential revealed 50% neutrophils (normal), 37% lymphocytes (normal), 12% monocytes (elevated) and 1% eosinophils (normal).

Further flow cytometry (FACS) scan of the cells can provide additional information here. In this case it showed that (i) 83% of the lymphocytes bound an antibody to CD3, a T-cell marker (normal), (ii) 57% helper (CD4+) T cells reacted with an anti-CD4 antibody and (iii) 26% cytotoxic T cells reacted with an anti-CD8 antibody (both values within normal limits). Nevertheless, none of the peripheral blood lymphocytes were stained by antibody to the B-cell marker CD19 (normal 12%-20%). This failure to develop mature cells in the B-cell lineage is characteristic of X-linked agammaglobulinemia (Chapters 8 and 15).

Finally, you might consider a simple test for T-cell function. Since polyclonal proliferation and production of cytokines (e.g., IL-2) takes place after stimulation with certain mitogens (Chapter 1), a useful test would be to stimulate cells with certain mitogens (e.g., phytohemagglutinin) and measure proliferation and IL-2 production (this was done and it was normal). At this stage you would be interested in investigating evidence for the "carrier" state in unaffected females in this family. The gene involved in this defect (Bruton's tyrosine kinase gene, *Btk*) can be detected by testing for the presence of a mutant btk gene. Because in all somatic cells in females one of the two X chromosomes is inactivated, the normal phenotype in this patient's mother clearly indicates that all her B cells have the normal X chromosome active. Genetic marker analysis of the X chromosomes in the patient's 4 aunts (looking for identity or distinction from his mother) will enable you to predict whether any are carriers or not.

Treatment

Monthly intramuscular injections of gamma globulin are begun, along with treatment of the current otitis. The aim should be to maintain a serum IgG level in the 200 mg/dl range. Note that individuals with immunodeficiency disease should not be given live viral vaccines. There are cases where male infants with X-linked agammaglobulinemia have been given live (albeit attenuated so that the virus does not replicate in nerve cells) oral polio vaccine and subsequently developed paralytic poliomyelitis. Presumably the recipients were unable to make (the normally) protective IgG and IgA antibodies following mucosal immunization, which would neutralize the poliovirus and prevent the infection from spreading. In the gut of normal healthy individuals, following immunization with the attenuated virus, as infected cells die the infection is terminated. Delivery of the same vaccine to male infants with X-linked agammaglobulinemia can lead to persistent infection, excretion of poliovirus in the gut, and in some cases a reversion of the virus to reacquire an ability to enter nerve cells (neurotropism). Dissemination of these viral revertants through the bloodstream and infection of neurons in the spinal cord can cause paralytic poliomyelitis.

TEST YOURSELF

Multiple Choice Questions
1. Immunological responses to extracellular bacteria in the lamina propria could include activation of all the following EXCEPT
   a. CD8+ T cells
   b. CD4+ T cells
   c. Dendritic cells
   d. Macrophages
   e. B cells
2. *Shigella sp.* induce apoptosis in which of the following cells?
   a. M cells
   b. Epithelial cells
   c. Macrophages
   d. Only a and b
   e. All of the above
3. Which of the following does not play a role in host defense to *Mycobacterium tuberculosis*?
   a. reactive oxygen intermediates
   b. interferon gamma
   c. tumor necrosis factor
   d. lysosomal enzymes
   e. nitric oxide
4. Natural killer cells secrete IFNγ in response to stimulation by which of the following cytokines?
   a. IL-2
   b. IL-12
   c. IL-1
   d. IL-10
   e. TNF
5. Which cell's activity is inhibited in the presence of high concentrations of class I MHC?
   a. Natural killer cells
   b. CD4+ T cells
   c. CD8+ T cells
   d. Macrophages

e. Dendritic cells

Answers: 1a; 2c; 3d; 4b; 5a

Short Answer Questions
1. Explain why CD4+ T cells are required for host defenses to microbes irrespective of whether they are extracellular bacteria, intracellular bacteria, viruses or fungi.
2. How do microbes in the lumen reach the lymphoid cells in the lamina propria?
3. Compare and contrast destruction of virally infected cells by natural killer cells and CTL.
4. List the major host defense mechanisms for each of the following: extracellular bacteria, viruses, intracellular bacteria, and fungi.
5. Explain why phagocytosed *Mycobacterium tuberculosis* are difficult to eradicate.

Section II

Clinical Immunology in Practice

In Section II of this text we endeavor to address a discussion of the diseases which the clinical immunologist finds most familiar. While this section provides an integration of the knowledge the reader will have acquired from the previous chapters, we hope that any of these chapters can nevertheless themselves be read in isolation, with appropriate referral to the more relevant basic immunobiological chapters as the reader feels appropriate. There is one other important difference from the Section I chapters that the reader will see immediately, and that concerns our discussion of the clinical cases in this section. In the Section I chapters we have used these cases to highlight important points made in the text of each chapter, emphasizing for the reader the relevance to the clinician of individual facts noted therein. However, in the cases in Section II we use a different format. A patient problem is presented, and the clinician is invited to "work through" this case by answering a series of questions, with a broader discussion of their relevance to the problem at hand. We feel this is a more realistic approach to evaluation of a "real-life" patient. Nevertheless, we acknowledge that in real clinical practice patients do not "present" with a label "autoimmune disease", "hypersensitivity" etc. Therefore, the reader must be aware that even our broader discussion of these cases makes no attempt to consider exhaustively a "differential diagnosis" of disorders that may, in clinical practice, present in the same fashion as the cases we discuss. This would include a discussion of metabolic, infectious, congenital disorders etc., and both time and space constraints dictate that we make at least this (artificial) restriction to the discussion presented. We hope, nevertheless, that the reader finds these case discussions useful, and that educators find a class discussion of the problems a rewarding experience for both students and instructors.

Immunization

Objectives	240
Immunization	241
Passive Immunization	242
Active Immunization or "Vaccination"	244
Forms of Vaccines	247
Vaccine Efficacy and Safety	254
Successful Application of Vaccine Technology	255
Limited Use Vaccines and Experimental Vaccines	256
Uses of Vaccines (For Other than Control of Infection)	257
Summary	258
Clinical Cases and Discussion	259
Test Yourself	264

OBJECTIVES

Protection from the ravages of infectious diseases represents a major success story for clinical immunology. Different concepts are involved in vaccination versus post exposure prophylaxis, and different regimes are used to vaccinate for different diseases. Safety limitations have forced us to consider molecular technologies, including so-called "naked DNA", rather than whole organisms for vaccination. Lack of understanding of the immunobiology of the response to pathogens leaves us without vaccines for scourges like *Mycobacterium tuberculosis*, malaria, schistosomiasis, filariasis, etc. It is sobering to realize that the most effective of vaccines is useless unless it can be delivered to the population at risk with appropriate speed and cost.

There is some hope that current vaccination practices will be expanded to include immunization for *post exposure infection* in such diseases as hepatitis and HIV. What does the future hold in terms of further exploration into the concomitant use of cytokines and other nonspecific therapies in improving immunization strategies? Clinical trials are beginning in areas such as cancer immunotherapy, where vaccination may become useful for increasing resistance to tumor growth. Similar approaches may come into development in other areas, including protection from autoimmune disorders (using e.g., anti-idiotype vaccination), though this field is still in its infancy.

Clinical Immunology, by Reginald Gorczynski and Jacqueline Stanley. 2001 Landes Bioscience

IMMUNIZATION

General features

Immunization represents a deliberate attempt to protect an individual from disease. In **passive immunization,** the patient receives antibodies generated in another individual (or animal). In **active immunization** the patient receives the antigen which stimulates the generation of an immune response, (antibody or cell mediated), by the patient. Passive and/or active immunization can be administered simultaneously or independently.

Active immunization is often referred to as **vaccination,** following its discovery by Jenner 200 years ago who observed protection against smallpox following vaccination with the cowpox virus (*vaccinia*). Understanding of the immune processes involved awaited formulation of theories of clonal selection and development, which explained how prior antigen exposure selected for an expanded pool of memory cells capable of responding faster, and with greater magnitude, on rechallenge with the inciting antigenic stimulus. Antigens used in vaccines must be safe to administer, produce the appropriate type of immunity (antibody vs cell-mediated) for the disease in question, and be inexpensive for the target population. There are many infectious diseases of global significance for which these criteria remain unmet. Table 12.1 lists the antigen formulations in current clinical use.

Understanding the type of immunity needed for protection from the organism(s) in question imposes constraints on the antigen used (Chapter 11). Antibacterial immunity generally involves opsonization and/or phagocytosis, needing immunoglobulin and complement. Cell-mediated immunity is more important for intracellular bacteria (*Mycobacterium tuberculosis*). Where anti-toxins (which bind avidly to target, and are not displaced by IgG) are used for passive protection from toxin-producing bacteria (tetanus) the antitoxin must be present

Table 12.1. Immunization schedule(s) for currently used vaccines

Disease	Vaccine	Immunization Schedule
Tetanus	Toxoid	Given together (DPT) at 2, 4 and 6 months
Diphtheria	Toxoid	
Pertussis ("whooping cough")	Killed (whole organisms)	Booster with tetanus (Td) and diphtheria every 10 years
Polio	Live or Attenuated	Given at 2, 4 and (5-15) months
Measles	Attenuated Virus	
Mumps	Attenuated Virus	Given together at 12-18 months of age (MMR)
Rubella	Attenuated Virus	

early after exposure. Antifungal immunity depends on cell-mediated immune reactivity (and T-cell cytokine-mediated macrophage activation) and IgE production, depending on the stage of the life cycle of the organism, while antiviral immunity depends upon both CD8+ CTL and preformed neutralizing antibody.

Passive Immunization

Natural

Passive immunization can be natural or artificial (Fig. 12.1). Natural passive immunization occurs in the fetus when maternal IgG antibodies (antiviral, antibacterial) cross the placenta, or in the neonate during breast feeding because IgG and IgA are present in colostrum. This protects the neonate from enteric pathogens (*E.Coli, coxsackie* etc.) which may otherwise cause a life-threatening disease, necrotizing enterocolitis. The colostrum contains other protective factors for microbial infection, including lysozyme, lactoferrin, interferons, and leukocytes.

Artificial

Artificial passive immunization refers to deliberate administration of immunoreactive serum, or concentrated immunoglobulin (gamma globulin) isolated from pooled human plasma/serum of individuals that have recently recovered from disease, or from volunteers who have been intentionally immunized. Recipients are generally immunocompromised individuals (e.g., varicella immune globulin given to immunodeficient individuals exposed to chicken pox virus), or immunocompetent individuals who need protection from disease during the time before active immunization could be effective (postexposure prophylaxis from infectious disease). Examples of the latter include use of hepatitis immune globulin given to nonimmune health care workers following accidental needle sticks.

Most immune globulin preparations used for passive immunization are of the IgG isotype. Some preparations are only adequate for intramuscular injection (IgIM), whereas other preparations may be used intravenously (IgIV). The IgIM form contains high molecular weight aggregates that may activate complement if given intravenously. Even pooled *normal human serum* contains sufficient antibody for protection from common infectious disease (presumably because the donor pool is continually rechallenged with the pathogens of interest). This is used for routine passive protection of hypogammaglobulinemic patients (doses of the order of 100-400 mg IgG given monthly). All passively delivered sera must be pathogen free (tested for HIV, hepatitis B and C virus, etc.-see below).

Protection from a number of diseases, including hepatitis A, hepatitis B, rabies, tetanus, and measles can be mediated by passive immunization, in situations where exposure (to infection) has already occurred (in a nonimmunized individual) before active immunity develops. Immune preparations are also available for snakebites, Rh incompatibility, diphtheria, and botulism. In ideal cases, antibody fractions derived from animals would only be used when human globulin preparations are unavailable. Infusion of heterologous antibodies can cause serum sickness, and a second injection of the same animal serum may cause

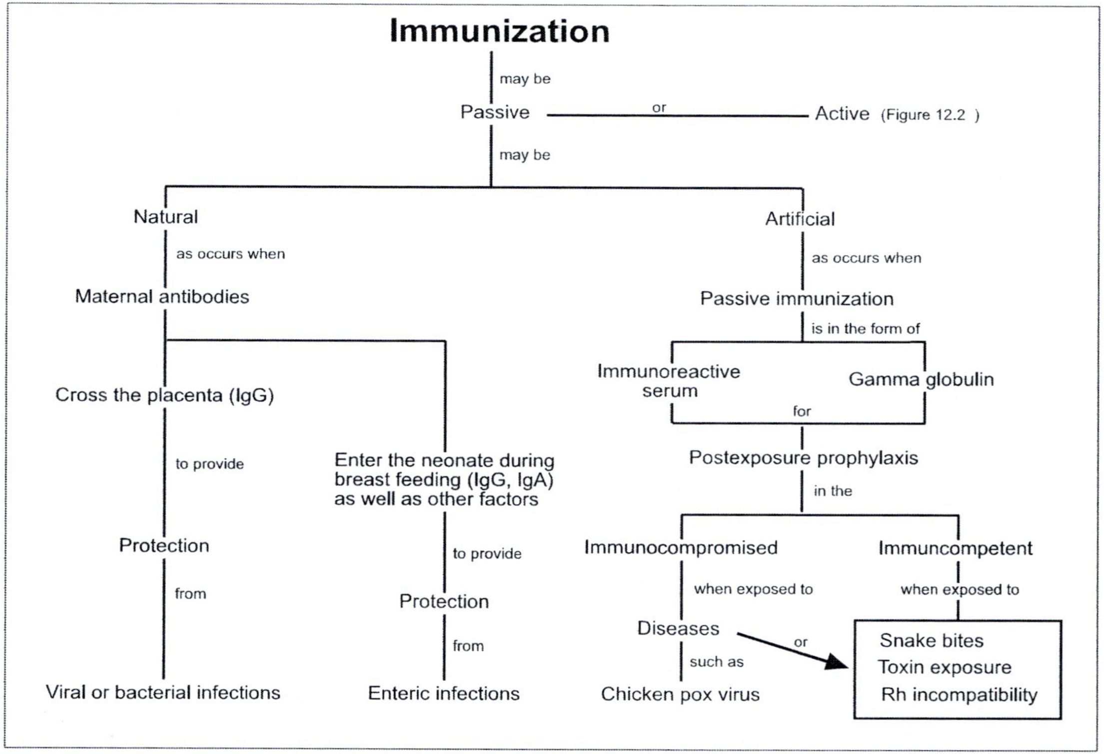

Immunization

Immunization

- **Passive** (may be)
  - **Natural** — as occurs when
    - Maternal antibodies
      - Cross the placenta (IgG) — to provide Protection from Viral or bacterial infections
      - Enter the neonate during breast feeding (IgG, IgA) as well as other factors — to provide Protection from Enteric infections
  - **Artificial** — as occurs when
    - Passive immunization
      - Immunoreactive serum, or
      - Gamma globulin — is in the form of
    - for Postexposure prophylaxis in the
      - **Immunocompromised** — when exposed to Diseases such as Chicken pox virus
      - or
      - **Immunocompetent** — when exposed to:
        - Snake bites
        - Toxin exposure
        - Rh incompatibility
- **Active** (Figure 12.2) (may be)

Fig. 12.1. **Passive immunization**. Passive immunization can be natural or artificial. A natural process is when maternal IgG antibodies (antiviral, antibacterial) cross the placenta, or when the neonate breast feeds receiving IgG and IgA from colostrum. Artificial passive immunization reflects the administration of immunoreactive serum or concentrated immunoglobulin (gamma globulin).

anaphylaxis (Chapter 13). One of the major current goals in this field of medicine is to replace polyclonal heteroantibodies used for passive protection with humanized monoclonal antibodies of the appropriate specificity (Chapter 4).

ACTIVE IMMUNIZATION OR "VACCINATION"

General features

Vaccination, may be unintentional, occurring when someone is inadvertently exposed to a pathogen, or intentional, when the individual is exposed to a safe form of the pathogen in the hope of inducing sterile immunity to the pathogen (Fig. 12.2). Vaccines may be: (i) live natural organisms; (ii) attenuated microbes; (iii) killed microbes; (iv) purified proteins prepared from the pathogen; (v) recombinant proteins made using molecular biological techniques; and (vi) "naked DNA" preparations (Fig. 12.2 and Table 12.2). In some cases, e.g., tetanus or diphtheria bacteria, a detoxified form of the bacterial toxin is used as an antigen. Vaccines can be administered by different routes (Fig. 12.3). The usual site of injection is the arm using either intramuscular or subcutaneous modes of injection; less commonly, intradermal injection occurs. When mucosal immunity is the goal, vaccines are given orally, or intranasally. For DNA vaccines current practice is to deliver the DNA directly by "gene gun" into muscle tissue.

The age for optimal vaccination is important. *In utero* the mother provides protection, but by 3-6 months post birth, the majority of the serum IgG is fetal in origin and has reached 50% of adult levels. Cell mediated immune potential is poorly developed at birth and is reflected in the sensitivity to, amongst other infections, those caused by *Toxoplasma, Herpes simplex virus, Listeria monocytogenes*, and *Mycobacterium tuberculosis*. Despite this sensitivity, immunization too early may be blocked by maternal IgG, or may even risk tolerization to vaccine antigen (Chapter 7-tolerance). Before 12-18 months of age the poor response to T dependent antigens sometimes results in the risk of tolerance induction outweighing any benefit of immunization. Theoretically the inclusion of multiple antigens in a vaccine runs the risk of immune interference at the "antigen handling" stage, though there is little evidence for this in practice, and multiple antigens are given routinely (e.g., measles/mumps and rubella, the MMR vaccine).

Adjuvants and nonspecific immunostimulation

Vaccination preparations often include an **adjuvant** that enhances the immune response (Fig. 12.4). Different adjuvants mediate their effects in different ways. Most are believed to increase immunogenicity by prolonging the period of antigen presentation (providing a "depot" effect for concentrating antigen locally at the site of injection), and/or by stimulating the antigen-presenting cell (APC) itself by promoting local cytokine production (e.g., of IL-12, a cofactor in antigen presentation). The most commonly used adjuvants in human vaccines are inorganic salts, based on aluminum hydroxide (alum) or calcium phosphate. Both act primarily to produce a depot effect. So-called immune stimulating complexes (ISCOMs) have recently been introduced to produce similar effects, this time by

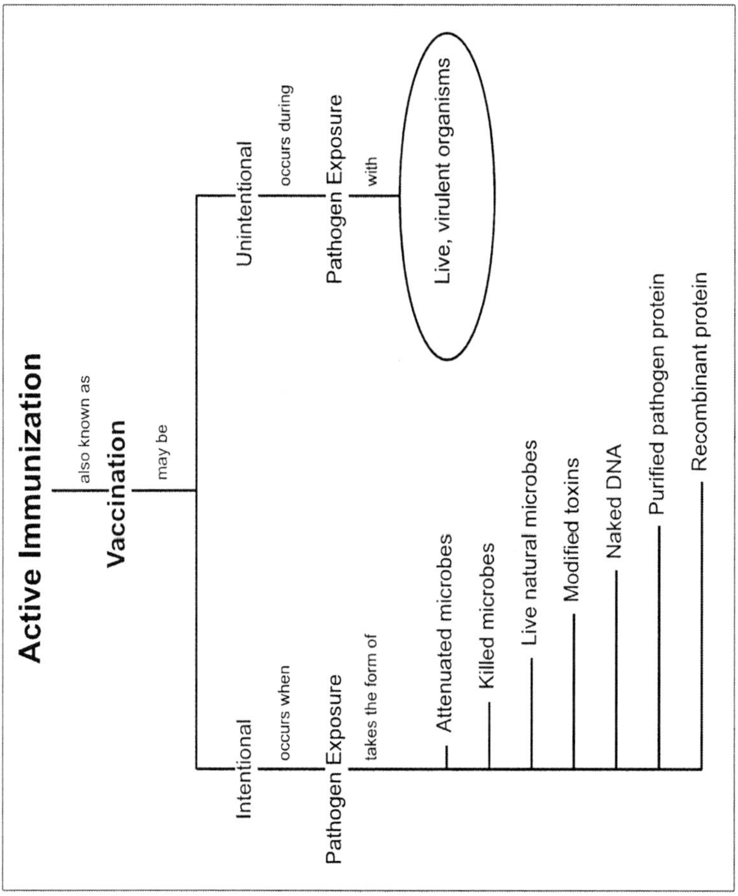

Active Immunization

- also known as **Vaccination**
- may be:
  - **Intentional**
    - occurs when Pathogen Exposure takes the form of
      - Attenuated microbes
      - Killed microbes
      - Live natural microbes
      - Modified toxins
      - Naked DNA
      - Purified pathogen protein
      - Recombinant protein
  - **Unintentional**
    - occurs during Pathogen Exposure with (Live, virulent organisms)

Fig. 12.2. Active immunization. Active immunization is referred to as vaccination. Vaccination may be unintentional, following inadvertent exposure to a pathogen, or intentional, when the pathogen is delivered under controlled conditions in the hope of developing sterile immunity. Various vaccine forms have different risks and efficacy.

Table 12.2. Different forms of vaccines

Form of Vaccine	Mode of Administration	Vaccine	Comments
Live, Virulent	Intramuscular	*Vaccinia*	Smallpox vaccination; rarely used (WHO data suggests disease eradicated)
	Natural infection (buttock)	*Leishmania*	"Controlled" development of sterile immunity; safety a concern
Live, Attenuated	Oral	Sabin polio virus	Small risk, but less effective than live natural virus
	Intramuscular	*Mycobacterium tuberculosis* (BCG)	In rare cases attenuated organisms revert to wild type
	Intramuscular	Measles, Mumps, Rubella	
Inactivated / Killed	Intramuscular	Salk polio virus	Safer, but less effective than live or attenuated organisms.
	Intramuscular	Rabies virus,	
	Intramuscular	Influenza virus (moderately effective)	May be used in the immunocompromised
	Intramuscular	Cholera bacteria (only moderate effectiveness)	
	Intramuscular	*Bordetella pertussis*	Note—Pertussis bacterial vaccine has significant toxicity
Inactivated Toxin and Toxoids	Intramuscular	Bacterial vaccines for tetanus and diphtheria	Most successful vaccines yet tested
	Intramuscular	Carrier molecule for vaccination with malaria organism	Useful as carriers because of highly effective T cell memory development following prior immunization with toxin!
Recombinant Vaccines	Intramuscular	Antigen peptide e.g. hepatitis B (HBs) e.g., Salmonella proteins	Fewer side effects than other vaccines. Advantage of ability to manipulate (add/subtract) epitopes of importance
DNA Vaccines	Gene gun into the dermis, IM, SC, ID, IV, and IN	Plasmid containing genes encoding pathogen protein	In experimental animals gives rise to both B and T cell immunity, without evidence for tolerance induction (a worry, given an unlimited antigen supply); trials to start soon for influenza (other viruses).

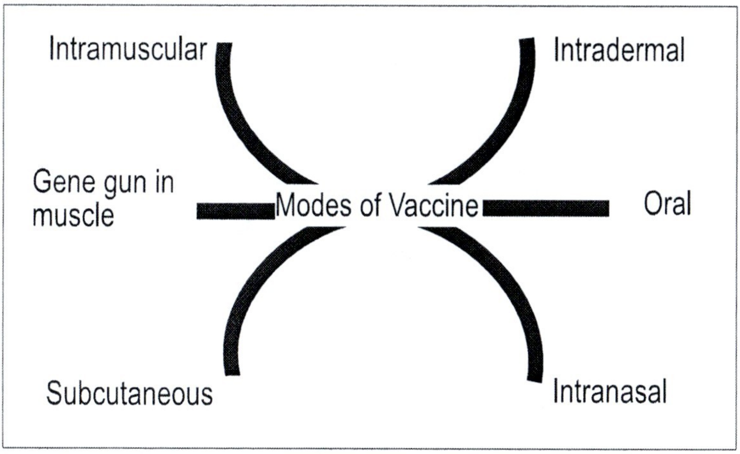

```
                Intramuscular              Intradermal


       Gene gun in
       muscle          ← Modes of Vaccine →    Oral



                Subcutaneous               Intranasal
```

Fig. 12.3. Various modes of vaccine administration. Vaccination may use: (i) live organisms; (ii) attenuated microbes; (iii) killed microbes; (iv) purified proteins prepared from the pathogen; (v) recombinant proteins made using molecular biological techniques; and (vi) naked DNA preparations.

incorporating the antigen within a liposomal particle that is presented to APC. Less commonly used are products of bacterial cells (e.g., *Bordetella pertussis*, used in combination with tetanus and diphtheria toxoids) which act to stimulate local cytokine production. In the future recombinant cytokine delivery systems might be improved/manipulated such that these can be incorporated into clinical vaccines. Similar thoughts apply to the use of other agents (e.g., cytokine inhibitors) that might improve immunity nonspecifically as is the case in other inflammatory states (e.g., **IL-1 receptor antagonist**). Auxiliary agents that block access of the organism to the site where pathology can develop are also under consideration (e.g., CD4 and/or chemokine receptor blockade to prevent infection by HIV-see Chapter 11).

FORMS OF VACCINES

Live natural virulent vaccination

Maximum protection is best achieved using live organisms as antigen, though there are obvious risks. Despite this, and in the absence of any safer alternative, in the Middle East parents often expose the buttocks of their children to sandfly holes, ensuring infection with cutaneous *Leishmania species* (an organism carried by sandfly vectors). Infection is self-limited and provides long-lived sterile immunity (without the risk of scarring on visible body areas, as occurs following natural infection).

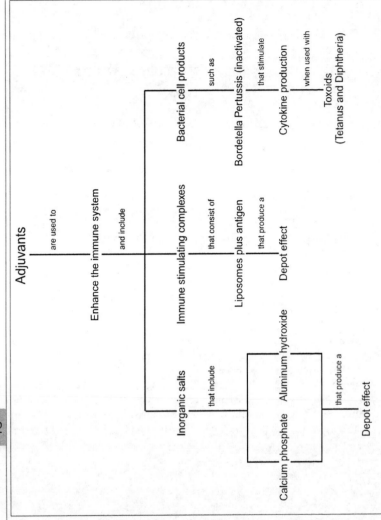

Fig. 12.4. Adjuvants used in vaccines. Adjuvants enhance the immune response when administered as components of a vaccine. Most common in human vaccines are inorganic salts (based on aluminum hydroxide (alum) or calcium phosphate). Both act primarily to produce a depot effect. Immune stimulating complexes (ISCOMs) have been introduced to produce essentially the same effect, by incorporating the antigen within a liposomal particle that is presented to APC. Less commonly used adjuvants are products of bacterial cells e.g., *Bordetella pertussis*, (used with tetanus and diphtheria toxoids), which act to stimulate local cytokine production.

Attenuated vaccines

Generating attenuated organisms

Attenuated organisms are avirulent but maintain the antigenic epitopes of virulent strains. This is frequently achieved by modifying the culture conditions in which the organisms grow, as was the case for the first successful application of this technology, by Calmette and Guerin. They passaged a bovine strain of *Mycobacterium tuberculosis* in culture to produce the less virulent *Bacillus Calmette Guerin* (BCG), which provides some protection against human tuberculosis. Greater success was achieved for virally induced disorders, where live attenuated viral vaccines decreased the incidence of measles, mumps, rubella and poliomyelitis well over 100-fold.

Attenuated organisms and reversion to wild type

Attenuated organisms harbor the risk of reversion to virulence (e.g., for types 2 and 3 poliomyelitis virus). In Sweden this led to the withdrawal of the live attenuated polio vaccine from routine use. Molecular biological investigations help us understand these cases. An attenuated form is produced in culture after accumulation of mutations at random which, while preserving antigenicity, decrease virulence. For the type 1 polio vaccine (which has never reverted), over 50 mutations exist in the attenuated form, while for types 2/3 only *two* important mutations occurred to produce the attenuated forms-thus their reversion rates were much higher. Using molecular tools to introduce multiple mutations (site-directed mutagenesis) live attenuated vaccines may be produced in the future which have low risks of reversion.

Attenuated viruses commonly used

Two live attenuated viral vaccines commonly used in North America/Europe are the Sabin polio vaccine and a measles vaccine. Because the natural route of polio infection is the gastrointestinal tract, the Sabin vaccine is generally administered orally to protect individuals against a disease that causes paralysis and death. Children receive Sabin poliovirus vaccine at two, four, and six months of age, with a booster dose administered just before school entry. Measles vaccine is also a live attenuated virus, which protects individuals from an infectious disease that may be accompanied by pneumonia or encephalitis. Children are generally vaccinated at twelve months, with a booster injection given just before school entry.

Inactivated (killed) organisms

Inactivated or killed viruses and bacteria are also used in vaccines. They are generally safer, but less effective. The Salk polio vaccine, used in Scandinavia following problems with the attenuated Sabin vaccine, is an inactivated poliovirus vaccine for intramuscular injection. Less effective than the Sabin vaccine, it is safer and can be used in immunocompromised individuals. Rabies virus vaccine is also reasonably efficacious. Killed organisms in cholera (bacteria) and influenza (virus) vaccines are only moderately effective for vaccine purposes. Even killed pertussis vaccine is toxic with measurable risk of damage to the central nervous system, though the incidence of risk from vaccination does not exceed that from infection. Considerable effort is underway to develop a safer useful recombinant pertussis vaccine.

Inactivated toxins and toxoids as vaccines

The most successful bacterial vaccines (for tetanus and diphtheria) use the inactivated exotoxins, in the case of tetanus, given in an alum precipitate. Their efficacy is evident from the decline in reported cases of diphtheria following introduction of this vaccine in the United Kingdom (from 70,000 cases annually in 1935 to less than 1,000 by 1950). Now tetanus toxoid is used as a "carrier" molecule for trial vaccination with other peptides (e.g., of malaria organisms etc.) which are otherwise nonimmunogenic. The tetanus toxoid provides carrier determinants recognized by memory T cells (most individuals have high levels of T-cell memory to tetanus toxin following vaccination) while the novel hapten antigen linked to it stimulates B cells for antibody production.

Recombinant vaccines

Advantages of recombinant vaccines

Recombinant DNA technology has now been used to generate purified viral peptides with fewer side effects in vaccines because they do not have the culture medium impurities associated with growing organisms. Viruses grown in chicken embryo cells caused significant problems in individuals with unsuspected allergies to egg protein. The use of DNA recombinant proteins also avoids isolation of infectious organisms from the blood plasma of humans, as was the case for the first hepatitis B vaccines developed, where there was a risk of overt infection with contaminating live virulent hepatitis B virus. The gene encoding the surface antigen (HBs) of hepatitis virus has now been cloned into a vector and used to transfect yeast cells for expression and production of the protein material used in vaccination. Use of such cloning strategies allows manipulation of the recombinant protein, such that epitopes may be added/deleted to improve immunogenicity or directly immunize distinct arms of the immune system i.e., to the development of delayed type hypersensitivity (DTH) responses (Chapter 13), or antibody production (Chapter 8).

Potential vectors

Future interest surrounds the use of vectors to carry the gene encoding the relevant antigen into the host, where it can be expressed, immunizing the host in vivo. Vaccinia was predicted to be a suitable viral vector. However, given the high level of immunity to the parent vaccinia virus vector following routine immunization against smallpox, it was decided that the virus would be eliminated before sufficient time elapsed for the expressed product, encoded by the vector, to immunize the host. With smallpox essentially eradicated globally and the subsequent decline in routine smallpox vaccination, this concern over the use of vaccinia virus vectors may diminish.

Immunization

Given the high global incidence of diarrhea, a vector system capable of immunizing within the gastrointestinal tract is desirable. Attenuated *Salmonella* (bacterial) vectors may prove useful. In addition, there already exist a number of mutant strains of *Salmonella* that are eliminated before they cause significant disease, a key issue when considering any vector for vaccination purposes. Furthermore, because other phagocytic cells eventually take up the attenuated bacteria, some degree of systemic immunity should develop following this immunization route.

DNA vaccines

DNA vaccines have many potential advantages: (i) there is no risk of infection; (ii) the protein is produced in native form without the risk of denaturation during purification; and (iii) DNA is very stable, which may be advantageous in developing countries.

DNA as an immunizing agent

In DNA vaccines, plasmids containing genes encoding proteins of pathogenic origin serve as the vehicle for producing expressed protein in an individual (Fig. 12.5). Plasmids for DNA vaccines are engineered so that they cannot replicate in eukaryotic cells, and they cannot integrate into the host chromosomal DNA. These plasmids contain a strong viral promoter, and a polyadenylation/transcriptional termination sequence so that the protein of interest is made successfully. DNA vaccines are particularly effective in the induction of viral immunity.

Administering DNA vaccines

Delivery is via intramuscular, subcutaneous, intradermal, intranasal, or intravaginal routes. Early studies used intramuscular injection of DNA, but in an alternative approach, the plasmid is coated onto gold beads and propelled directly into the dermis and epidermis using a "gene gun". Langerhans cells present in the skin

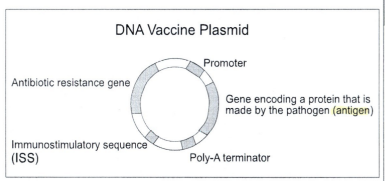

Fig. 12.5. DNA vaccine plasmid. The DNA vaccine plasmids contain a strong viral promoter, the cDNA for the pathogen-encoded protein, and a polyadenylation/transcriptional termination sequence so that the protein of interest is made in the cell. An additional noncoding immunostimulatory sequence (ISS) stimulates the innate immune system.

are directly transfected; there is transient gene expression using host protein-synthesizing machinery; and these Langerhan cells serve as antigen presenting cells.

Immune response to DNA vaccines
DNA vaccination has been shown to lead to the production of antibodies, the generation of Th cytokines, and the activation of CTL responses. Generation of antibodies and cytokine production implies that the protein encoded by the plasmid DNA has been expressed, secreted from the cell, and taken up by antigen presenting cells for presentation to CD4+ T cells. To generate antigen specific CTLs, the protein expressed by the plasmid is presented either directly on the muscle cell in the context of class I MHC, or again after expression, release and representation in association with class I MHC on another cell. Th1 cytokines must also be available. Immune responses with gene gun delivery are not as predictable as with intramuscular injections because the response does not preferentially bias the differentiation of CD4+ T cells to Th1 cells.

Areas of concern of DNA vaccines
Three main areas of concern have been identified by regulatory agencies: (i) random integration of the plasmid into host chromosomes or homologous recombination; (ii) tolerance induction; and (iii) autoimmunity. Integration of plasmids into host DNA does not occur readily. Nevertheless the theoretical concern remains that it will occur and disrupt a gene vital for normal cell homeostasis (potentially leading to transformation to cancer cells). Repeated injection of some antigens induces tolerance rather than protection, though in experimental studies this effect seems to be species and model dependent. Finally, there is concern that immune responses to foreign DNA may induce anti-DNA antibodies in humans. In animal models to date this has not been a problem.

Anti-idiotype vaccines for use when the antigen is unavailable/unidentified
Frequently glycolipids and/or carbohydrate antigens are most effective at inducing protective T cell (e.g., CD1-restricted T cells for *Mycobacterial* immunity-Chapters 3/9) or antibody immunity (to encapsulated bacteria) respectively. Here recombinant DNA technology is not useful for cloning such antigens. An alternative approach can be used in such circumstances, based on the premise that immunoregulation in the immune system uses networks of interacting idiotypes and anti-idiotypes on cells with complementary receptors (Chapters 4/8). If we could identify the anti-idiotype complementary to an immunoglobulin recognizing a given carbohydrate epitope, this could serve as an "antigen image" and be used as antigen. This concept has been tested successfully in experimental animals.

Widespread clinical use has not yet developed. Other instances of applications of anti-idiotype vaccines exist, particularly in cancer therapy (Chapter 16) using immunization against chronic lymphocytic lymphomas, (CLL). An advantage of using anti-idiotype immunization for immunity to lipids/carbohydrates is that protein immunization, like this, produces memory cells, whereas this is not normally the case for immunity to lipids/carbohydrates.

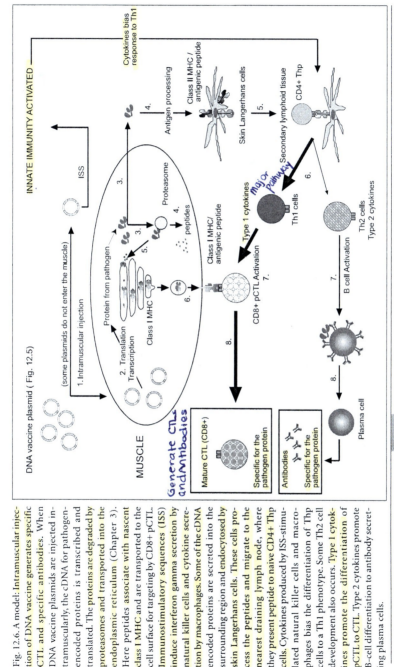

Fig. 12.6. A model: Intramuscular injection of DNA vaccine generates specific CTL and specific antibodies. When DNA vaccine plasmids are injected intramuscularly, the cDNA for pathogen-encoded proteins is transcribed and translated. The proteins are degraded by proteasomes and transported into the endoplasmic reticulum (Chapter 3). Here peptides associate with nascent class I MHC and are transported to the cell surface for targeting by CD8+ pCTL. Immunostimulatory sequences (ISS) induce interferon gamma secretion by natural killer cells and cytokine secretion by macrophages. Some of the cDNA encoded proteins are secreted into the surrounding region and endocytosed by skin Langerhans cells. These cells process the peptides and migrate to the nearest draining lymph node, where they present peptide to naive CD4+ Thp cells. Cytokines produced by ISS-stimulated natural killer cells and macrophages bias the differentiation of Thp cells to a Th1 phenotype. Some Th2 cell development also occurs. Type 1 cytokines promote the differentiation of pCTL to CTL. Type 2 cytokines promote B-cell differentiation to antibody secreting plasma cells.

Vaccine Efficacy and Safety

Vaccine efficacy requires stimulation of the appropriate arm of the immune system

After identifying the relevant antigen(s), development of an appropriate vaccine depends upon: (i) understanding the mechanism(s) of protection against a particular microorganism; and (ii) ensuring that the vaccine induces that form of protective immunity (Clinical case #18). Thus, for extracellular organisms (*Streptococcus pneumoniae*) and toxins, antibody mediated immunity is crucial (producing phagocytosis and destruction of the organism, or neutralization of the toxin, respectively). For intracellular organisms such as *Mycobacterium tuberculosis*, cell-mediated immunity is important (leading to cytokine release from immune T cells stimulated by antigen, activation of infected macrophages and intracellular destruction of the organism). When the important immune mechanisms remain unclarified (e.g., for a number of tropical diseases of global importance, including malaria) development of an effective vaccine is more difficult.

Vaccine efficacy is altered by the inclusion of adjuvants and mode of storage

Often significant storage time occurs in transfer from the manufacturer to the clinic, which compromises the value of vaccines dependent upon cold storage (e.g., live vaccines) for efficacy. In addition, macromolecules differ in their inherent immunogenicity (carbohydrates are notoriously poorly immunogenic), which often necessitates the use of adjuvants to improve immunogenicity. A major advance in vaccine development would come from development of potent and safe adjuvants for routine clinical use in man that could differentially stimulate antibody or cell-mediated immunity.

Vaccine efficacy depends on the form of the vaccine

Killed vaccines, or components thereof, used to avoid the safety issues associated with live vaccines, may be less effective by virtue of decreased antigen dose and/or altered sites of immunization, leading to development of different types of immunity. Peptide vaccines produce MHC-restricted T-cell recognition, and there is a theoretical risk that certain individuals may lack the necessary T-cell receptor in the T-cell recognition repertoire to develop immunity, or express MHC genes unable to present certain epitopes to responder T lymphocytes (Chapters 3/9). This may explain why some 5% of the population are unresponsive to recombinant hepatitis B vaccine. Because most proteins used in recombinant vaccines are large, and responsiveness reflects the ability of peptides (10–20 amino acids long) to "fit" in the groove of an MHC molecule, this normally poses insignificant problems for population immunization.

When the killed vaccine material produces T-independent immunity (e.g., polysaccharides used for immunization against extracellular bacteria) the material is coupled to a standard protein carrier (tetanus toxoid), or to protein derived from the immunizing organism as a carrier. Thus the membrane protein of

Haemophilus influenzae is used in such a vaccine and has decreased the incidence of meningitis caused by *Haemophilus* in the pediatric population.

Vaccine efficacy is linked to cost

While immunization using recombinant hepatitis B vaccine costs less than $100 per person, this is still unaffordable for over 90% of those individuals at risk (especially in underdeveloped countries). Furthermore, as noted by the World Health Organization, the major global diseases are parasitic infestations. There is little basic science research on these diseases, and even less into vaccine development because they do not affect countries with developed Research and Development expertise.

Hazards that decrease vaccine efficacy

In an increasingly litigious society vaccine safety is an overriding concern. Most individuals accept minor discomfort (local pain, swelling, and even a mild fever, for a few days), but remember that vaccines are normally given to otherwise apparently healthy people, so the level of acceptance of side-effects is low. For attenuated vaccines a concern is reversion to wild type organisms, as well as the possibility that an attenuated vaccine may cause significant disease in immunocompromised individuals (e.g., disseminated varicella infection has been seen in leukemia patients exposed to varicella vaccine for immunization against chicken pox).

During the swine flu epidemic in 1976 there was a rush to vaccinate the population most at risk (particularly the elderly). Significant neurological complications (e.g., **Guillain-Barre** disease) were seen in a number of individuals, related to cross-reactive immunity induced against antigens found within the central nervous system. There is a risk of hypersensitivity reactions to bystander materials in the vaccine (egg antigens) in allergic patients; even the preservatives used in vaccines (neomycin/merthiolate) can cause allergic reactions. Killed vaccines pose significant risk, beyond that attributable to failing to kill the organisms in question (responsible for past accidents with polio vaccine). Contamination with animal viruses during the preparation process has been documented for polio virus vaccines, and was a concern in the preparation of hepatitis B antigen for immunization from the blood of carriers (risk of contamination with e.g., HIV, hepatitis C etc.). For pertussis vaccine, a major problem has been contamination with endotoxin (the vaccine itself is a bacterial product). Moving to recombinant vaccine development alleviates many of these concerns.

SUCCESSFUL APPLICATION OF VACCINE TECHNOLOGY

Vaccination has the ability to **eradicate** certain diseases as shown by the phenomenal success in achieving control/eradication of smallpox by universal worldwide vaccination. Polio, measles, mumps and rubella have been "earmarked" for eradication by the early 21st century, using current technology. The major limitation to success seems to be socio-political (and economic) rather than scientific/

immunologic. Current vaccination protocols for the following diseases, while holding hope for improvement in the state of world health, do not suggest likely eradication of the organisms concerned:

1. Side effects from pertussis vaccination (see earlier) have decreased the willingness of the public to "take up" vaccination, although the risk (individual) of vaccination is much less than that of virulent infection.
2. Eradication of hepatitis B in endemic areas depends upon breaking the carrier state. In carriers, virus is integrated into the host genome without causing clinical disease in the host, but providing a reservoir for continued infection of other individuals (e.g., by blood transfer; mother to infant transmission). Few strategies have been tested for efficacy in this area.
3. Some current vaccines are known to be suboptimal (e.g., BCG vaccine and even the pertussis vaccine). Infectious organisms for which there is a known animal host will not be eradicated by a strategy directed only to man (e.g., parasitic organisms where a significant portion of the life cycle takes place in animal hosts).

Medicine occasionally falls victim to its own success. As we improve our ability to immunize populations and the "reservoir" of infection shrinks, we have seen more cases of infection in elderly (moderately immunocompromised) populations, often with significantly more severe symptomatology.

LIMITED USE VACCINES AND EXPERIMENTAL VACCINES

Immunization of select groups

For a variety of reasons a number of vaccines are routinely offered only to selected groups. BCG and hepatitis B vaccine currently fit this category in the developed world, although in North America, there is a move to consider universal vaccination for hepatitis B (risk:benefit advantage). For diseases with significant geographical restriction (yellow fever), and/or for which the risk of exposure is low (rabies) cost and risk/benefit considerations limit vaccination to at-risk groups (travelers or animal handlers, respectively). In some instances where universal immunization might be useful there is a supply:demand problem. Developing a suitable influenza vaccine involves an ongoing annual commitment of time, energy and resources, because each influenza outbreak is caused by a different strain (with variability in the **haemagglutinin** and **neuraminidase** antigens). Thus, in general, these vaccines are often given only to groups (the elderly) at greatest risk of significant disease following infection.

Trial vaccines

Trial vaccines in development

In parasitic diseases, where the parasite produces a chronic infection, development of an effective vaccine may be quite difficult ("nature" has presumably also failed over a long period of time). Often this is understandable in terms of the biology of the infecting organism(s). Rapid antigenic variability can occur in some organisms after infection, following development of host immune responses. In cattle, *trypanosoma* cycle through expression of multiple coat proteins after infection, as the infected host makes repeated antibody responses to newly emerging variants in an attempt to eradicate the parasite. **Plasmodium falciparum** (causing malaria in man) similarly undergoes antigenic variation within a single infected host. Understanding the life cycle of the parasite in the infected host is also important, as exemplified by malaria which has both a liver and a red cell infectious stage of development (as well as growth in the mosquito vector). Trial vaccines for malaria are directed at a number of these stages, including: (i) inducing antibodies to gametocytes to block transmission of sexual forms to the vector when it feeds on infected humans, (ii) producing antibodies to the sporozoites, the first stage in the blood following biting by infected mosquitoes, (iii) developing cell mediated immunity to sporozoite infected liver cells, blocking development of the parasite in infected humans and (iv) producing merozoite specific antibodies to block transmission from ruptured infected liver cells to erythrocytes, the last stage of the cycle in humans.

Limitations of trial vaccines
One concern is the possibility that antibody might make the infection worse, facilitating parasite entry into host cells, e.g., via an Fc receptor in the case of antibody coated organisms. This was observed in one experimental malaria vaccine. In other instances it seems the immune response to the parasite is, under normal circumstances, a contributor to immunopathology, so vaccination runs the risk of worsening this problem. **Trypanosoma cruzi** (the cause of **Chagas** disease) is associated with myocardial injury from autoreactive antibodies (produced following an immune response to trypanosmal antigens in vivo).

Diseases for which no vaccine is available
Human immunodeficiency virus (HIV), while under intense investigation, still has no clinically proven suitable vaccine. Understanding the nature of natural immunity (e.g., in HIV resistant sex workers) suggests that a vaccine stimulating $CD8^+$ T-cell immunity may be important (Chapter 9). The immune reactions stimulated by a vaccine suitable for preexposure prophylaxis might be quite different from those needed for postexposure vaccination in individuals with existing disease symptoms. There is a pressing need to develop a superior vaccine for tuberculosis, given the poor (and variable) efficacy of BCG vaccine. There are no effective vaccines for organisms such as *chlamydia* (a prominent cause of blindness globally, and of reproductive failure in developed countries); *candida/ pneumocystis* (opportunistic pathogens in immunocompromised individuals); or for any of a number of parasitic disorders of underdeveloped countries, including *malaria, trypanosomiasis, leishmaniasis, schistosomiasis* and others.

USES OF VACCINES (FOR OTHER THAN CONTROL OF INFECTION)

Cancer immunotherapy

Immunizing with "cancer vaccines", often in the form of antigen presenting cells (dendritic cells) pulsed in culture with a putative cancer antigen, has come to the fore as a technique to improve therapy of established cancers (Chapter 16). A number of relatively melanoma-specific antigens, the so-called **MAGE-1 to –3** antigens, have been used in phase I and II clinical trials with some success (measured by disease control). MAGE-3 has been used in immunotherapy because it induces CTL that are HLA-A1 restricted (i.e., CTL whose T-cell receptors recognize a MAGE-3 peptide fragment displayed on the cell surface with the class I MHC molecule, HLA-A1). This is important because basic immunobiological studies suggested that CTL are important for immunity to established melanoma.

Widespread use of hepatitis B vaccine (and the development of a hepatitis C vaccine) would likely have significant impact on the incidence of hepatocarcinoma. In Asia, where hepatitis B is endemic, preliminary data suggests that introduction of HepB vaccine has already been associated with a decreased incidence of chronic cirrhosis and hepatocarcinoma.

Antifertility vaccines

Both the conception and implantation stages of pregnancy are amenable to interruption by antibodies binding hormones intimately involved in the normal ordered development of the fertilization process. One targeted hormone has been human chorionic gonadotropin (hCG), responsible for maintaining an active corpus luteum. In the absence of the necessary hormonal environment to promote further growth and development of the normal placental:fetal environment, development of anti-hCG antibodies should induce spontaneous fetal loss. Vaccines were developed using the β-chain of human hCG coupled to tetanus toxoid, and were found to interrupt, transiently, fertility in a human population, with no significant adverse effects. Widespread trials have not been performed, and the efficacy of this form of contraception in comparison with others is undocumented.

SUMMARY

Immunization is generally used to protect individuals from infectious disease. In **passive immunization,** the patient receives antibodies generated in another individual (or animal), while in **active immunization (or vaccination)** the patient receives the antigen that stimulates the immunity. Vaccination strategies often use additional nonspecific stimuli, or **adjuvants,** to "boost" the immune response to the delivered antigen.

Key issues in using vaccination in clinical practice concern cost, efficacy, and safety. Vaccines are normally given to otherwise perfectly healthy individuals who, while perceived to be at some theoretical and quantifiable risk of disease, may nonetheless, during their lifetime, never encounter the pathogen for which the vaccine offers protection. Development of a suitable vaccine implies knowledge of the host immune mechanisms responsible for protection from disease under conditions of active infection.

Vaccination uses either live/attenuated organisms or killed organisms (or even material derived from them). There has been a general drift away from the use of attenuated infectious agents (because of a risk of reversion) towards a search, where feasible, for immunogenic products (toxins) of the infectious agent (e.g., in the case of *tetanus, diphtheria*), and even for proteins derived by recombinant DNA technology (hepatitis B surface antigen). Sometimes the relevant antigen may not be protein in nature (e.g., carbohydrates for extracellular bacteria), and in these situations the antigen may be coupled to an immunogenic carrier (e.g., tetanus toxoid) for immunization or an anti-idiotype vaccine may be used.

There are many success stories in the history of vaccination, including the recent eradication of smallpox as a major world health problem. However there are a number of diseases for which vaccines are currently unavailable, or are of poor efficacy (e.g., tuberculosis). Many of these represent parasitic diseases of the underdeveloped world, and our understanding of the basic biology of the infectious cycle is often so limited that a rationale approach to vaccine design is impossible. Application of the concepts of vaccination which were developed for protection from infectious disease have now been extended to other areas of clinical medicine, including tumor immunotherapy (Chapter 16) and the regulation of fertility.

CLINICAL CASES AND DISCUSSION

Clinical Case #23
A young woman comes to your Emergency Department in the late stages of labor. She delivers a healthy baby girl after a further one hour of uneventful labor. She is a known prostitute and iv drug user. She admits to being HIV positive but is under no current treatment. She has none of the stigmata of AIDS (no documented lymphadenopathy; no reports of cervical infection; no skin lesions or respiratory problems; her white count is normal). What is your course of action?

Questions and Discussion: Case #23
1. List the six likely key features we need to bear in mind in discussing this case.
Pregnant female
Prostitute
IV drug user
HIV positive
Healthy baby
Normal white blood cell count

2. Of immediate concern is the risk of blood group incompatibility between the mother and the fetus. Which incompatibility are we considering?
Immediate risks relate to possible blood (rhesus) incompatibility between mother/infant. A rhesus negative mother, carrying a rhesus (Rh) positive child, can become immunized to Rh antigen during bleeding during the pregnancy or

following delivery. Transfer of anti-Rh Igs across the placenta can cause fetal loss (hydrops) in subsequent pregnancies with Rh positive children. This is avoided by passive delivery of anti-Rh antibody (RhoGam) to all Rh negative mothers at birth, or to all mothers if, as here, Rh status is unknown. Your first step is to give RhoGam to the mother.

3. The mother's lifestyle puts her at risk for several infectious diseases in addition to HIV. Explain.

This lifestyle (sex worker; iv drug abuse) clearly puts her at risk for HIV, hepatitis B and C, and a number of (more conventional) infections, including chlamydia, syphilis, gonorrhea and other sexually transmitted diseases. Serology should be sent to test for viral infections (acute/chronic infection with hepatitis B, C and HIV are critical). Rapid testing is important, because this has an impact on the treatment given to the child (see below). Begin a work-up for other infectious disorders (cultures of blood, urogenital tract, and sputum). Remember infection with HIV, and her lifestyle, lead to increased risk of tuberculosis.

4. HIV transmission to the fetus is worrying. What is the optimal strategy for preventing perinatal transmission of HIV? Is there any benefit to postpartum treatment, in the absence of antepartum and intrapartum therapy?

We have two patients to consider, and you are the patient advocate for one of them (the baby). Over the past 10 years effort has gone into clinical trials to understand how best to prevent perinatal transmission of HIV. Currently a three-part regimen of zidovidine (AZT) given antepartum, intrapartum, and to the newborn is believed the optimum strategy. However, we couldn't give this drug antepartum or even during labor. Is only postpartum use efficacious?

A recent study by the Pediatric AIDS Clinical Trials Group in the USA investigated this issue. Even when given only postpartum, AZT reduced transmission rates from some 30% (with no treatment) to a mean of 9% when begun during the first 48 hours of life. Time is crucial, since starting AZT therapy at three days of life was associated with a mean transmission rate of 18%.

5. What technique identifies HIV virus in the blood and confirms transmission? Explain the technique in general terms.

In the study cited in #4, investigators used a polymerase chain reaction (PCR) to identify the virus and confirm transmission. In PCR technology DNA nucleotide sequences complementary to "ends" of the virus genome are used to amplify (over one million-fold) viral DNA in the blood. This is readily detected by a radiolabeled antiviral (DNA) probe, or even by direct visualization in an agarose gel. AZT therapy should therefore be promptly initiated in this child, with follow-up of HIV virus titers by PCR.

6. Postexposure prophylaxis with AZT for treatment after accidental needle sticks has been well documented. How does AZT work when given immediately following exposure, and what is the duration of the therapy?

Data for postexposure prophylaxis with AZT in neonates are similar to data from trials using postexposure treatment after accidental needle sticks (in health care workers). A Center for Disease Control (CDC) case-control study reported

Immunization 261

an 80% reduction in transmission. Both trials imply that the drug exerted its potent protective effect by causing rapid decline in the titers of infectious particles, thus avoiding productive infection in the host. Accordingly, it was felt that long-term treatment would not be necessary, and generally only a 4-week postexposure treatment is offered to needle stick victims.

7. According to USA Public Health guidelines, what should be the duration of prophylaxis for this baby? Should an HIV mother breast-feed her child?

There is some dispute in cases of *blocking perinatal transmission* as to how long AZT should be given. This depends to some degree on whether the infant will be breastfed or not. In underdeveloped countries, the advantages of breast feeding to avoid an increased risk of other diseases must be taken into consideration before advocating artificial feeding. In more developed countries one might prefer to avoid further transmission risk. Recent USA Public Health guidelines suggest continued prophylaxis of the baby for only 6 weeks.

8. What additional postexposure prophylaxis should you consider for this baby?

There are other possible infectious exposures for this infant. There is no postexposure treatment for HepC, but hepatitis B immune globulin is available. Make plans to monitor evidence for HepB, C and to give HepB vaccine when the child reaches a suitable age (12-18 months). Simpler (but no less immediately life-threatening) infections with other (bacterial) organisms should be assessed and treated as necessary.

9. Assuming that the mother has an acute bacterial infection, how would you treat it?

We now begin to develop a treatment plan suitable for this mother. Acute infections with bacterial pathogens are treated symptomatically (with antibiotics as needed).

10. Assuming that the mother has been exposed to hepatitis B virus, how would you determine the acuteness of the HepB exposure?

There are few treatment options open for acute viral infections, though this is an area of intense study. Some idea of the acuteness of HepB exposure is obtained by measuring viral antigens and IgM (or IgG) antibodies to them (See Case #15). HepBe antigen (a core antigen) reflects an acutely infectious episode, while anti-HepBe antibody is often transiently present as the infection clears. HepBs (surface antigen) is present in cases of both acute and chronic (carrier state) infection, while IgG anti-HepBs antibody reflects a (sterile) immune state; IgG anti-HepBc (another core antigen) reflects both past (chronic) and acute exposure, but *not a state of sterile immunity*. Acute exposure (e.g., in health care workers by needle stick) could be treated with Hep B immune globulin.

11. What treatment options are available for HepB during viral relapse, as opposed to acute exposure?

Some clinical trials with interferon-alpha have proven successful in both HepB and C during viral relapse. Ribavirin is another antiviral agent under investigation for treatment of hepatitis.

12. The mother is HIV positive, how would you treat?

Survival following seroconversion (for HIV infection) has increased substantially over the last 5-10 years. Current guidelines suggest induction therapy with a triple drug regimen that includes two independent antiviral nucleoside analogues, zidovudine (AZT) and lamivudine, along with an HIV protease inhibitor (e.g., indinavir). Once the HIV viral titer has dropped below 500 copies/ml of blood the optimum maintenance therapy remains controversial. There is no evidence that regimens including only two drugs are as effective as triple therapy.

13. HIV positive patients have an increased incidence of diseases that are normally handled by cell mediated (T-cell) immunity. Name one disease and how you would treat?

The incidence of tuberculosis has increased significantly in underprivileged groups in North America (and in the global population) over the last few years, and is particularly high in the HIV positive population. PPD conversion/positivity, without clinical disease, could be treated by single drug prophylaxis (isoniazide), though the risk of drug-related hepatotoxicity might be a concern. With clinically active disease, particularly where compliance with out-patient therapy is problematic, a policy of supervised treatment, has successfully curbed a rising infection rate amongst this population.

14. How would you counsel this mother?

Finally there are a number of public health issues that need to be considered. We have touched on some of these, including protection of the local population from such transmissible disorders as tuberculosis by supervised treatment. However the mother should be counseled in safe-sex practices, and arrangements need to be made for appropriate long-term care and follow-up of both mother and infant.

Clinical Case #24

A known poisonous snake has bitten a keeper (T.J.) from the local zoo. In the hospital he is sweating profusely, has profound hypotension (low blood pressure), some petechiae (small vessel hemorrhages) in the arms, and is very tachycardic with a pulse of 160 (normal healthy male 60-85). The Center for Disease Control (CDC) was contacted and they sent anti-snake venom immediately. They recommended infusion of 8 vials sequentially. After the first 5 vials were administered T.J. felt noticeably improved, the tachycardia had resolved, and he asked to go home. Over the following day, his joints began to ache, he developed a fever, and he again became hypotensive. What is happening and how do you proceed?

Questions and Discussion: Case #24

1. List the six likely key features we need to bear in mind in discussing this case.

The initial physiological changes reflect an effect of snake toxin. Consider also the following:

  Male zoo keeper with recurrent symptoms
  Snake bite (known poisonous)
  Profound hypotension

Some petechiae in the arms
Very tachycardic
Heterologous antibody

2. The early improvement showed that the antisnake venom was effective. How does this treatment work?

T.J. sustained a life-threatening exposure to a snake toxin (unknown etiology). The signs and symptoms alerted you to the danger and, appropriately, you ordered the only curative treatment, namely one that neutralized the toxin, rather than just treating its effects. The improvement in symptoms occurred as antibody neutralized the toxin.

3. This is an example of serum-mediated, passive, artificial immunoprophylaxis. Under what conditions should this type of therapy be administered? Give specific examples.

This form of protection is given for accidental exposures to infectious agents (e.g., HepB immune globulin-see Case #23; anti-tetanus immune globulin; anti-varicella immune globulin, etc.) as well as after exposure to many toxins, of which snake venom exposure is a classic example. The antibody binds the toxin avidly so neutralizing its toxin activity. Speed in administration of the anti-venom is crucial.

4. Serum-mediated, passive immunoprophylaxis occurs both naturally and artificially. When do we receive the natural form? What serum components mediate protection in each case?

A natural form of passive antibody prophylaxis occurs during life in utero (transfer of IgG across the placenta) and when breast feeding (IgG and leukocytes in the colostrum, along with other antimicrobial factors such as lactoferrin, lysozyme etc.).

5. Recurrence of symptoms could mean that the anti-venom stopped working, which seems unlikely. More plausible is that another reaction is confusing the picture. Remember that the snake anti-venom currently in use is a heterologous antibody, made in horses. Why might this induce complications?

Although the horse antibodies are neutralizing the toxin, these antibodies are foreign to the host, and serve as antigens. An immune response is triggered and antibodies, IgM and IgG, are generated.

6. What is the consequence of this excess of antigen and antibodies?

Type III hypersensitivity reactions, characterized by production of IgM and IgG antibodies to soluble antigens (the heterologous horse serum proteins) with subsequent formation of an excess of immune complexes, occurs (Chapter 13). The large numbers of circulating immune complexes overwhelm the normal clearing mechanisms of the reticuloendothelial system and complexes are deposited in the capillary walls where they stimulate complement activation.

7. How does excessive complement activation manifest?

Anaphylatoxins (e.g., C5a) are produced following complement activation. Anaphylatoxins bind to mast cells/basophils causing the release of vasoactive amines, hypotension and increased vascular permeability. C5a is also chemotactic for neutrophils, and activated neutrophils secrete multiple inflammatory mediators. These further damage the endothelium, and the exposed subendothelium is a stimulus for activation of the intrinsic coagulation pathway, producing kallikrein and bradykinin (a potent vasodilator). Inflammatory mediators (e.g., IL-1) are also responsible for the fever.

8. *Excessive numbers of immune complexes occur in a number of other diseases and are associated with this same form of hypersensitivity reaction (following immune complex formation). Name three autoimmune diseases caused by immune complexes deposition in different sites (Chapters 13/14).*

In systemic lupus erythematosus (SLE), complexes are mainly deposited in the kidney glomeruli to cause glomerulonephritis; in rheumatoid arthritis, complexes are deposited in the joints; and in farmer's lung, they are deposited in the lung.

9. *Is there any historical precedent for the reactions described in this individual?*

Serum sickness (following heterologous antibody infusion) was much more common in years past and was seen in patients who received passive treatment with horse serum containing anti-diphtheria toxin antibodies (as therapy for diphtheria). These patients often developed fever, edematous rashes, enlarged lymph nodes and swollen joints about one to two weeks after treatment. If the cause was not realized, then a second injection of the horse serum led to anaphylaxis and death.

10. *How would you treat the zoo keeper who is still being infused with anti-snake venom?*

The infusion should be stopped, at least temporarily, while we plan how to deal with the problem. Most of the symptoms are amenable to therapy, with high dose steroids and antihistamine therapy being prominent amongst these. Short-term therapy with steroids has few risks. There are significant risks associated with stopping infusion of anti-venom (namely recurrence of toxin-mediated disease!).

If the symptoms stabilize, the risk:benefit would be in favor of restarting the anti-venom with close monitoring and ongoing prophylaxis with steroids (for the symptoms associated with hypersensitivity reactions). The precipitating feature here was the use of a heterologous antibody containing multiple proteins to which the individual could, and did, make an immune response. This could be avoided in the future by using humanized monoclonal forms of antivenom for protection. Research is underway to realize this goal!

TEST YOURSELF

Multiple Choice Questions
1. An 8-year-old boy was bitten by an angry playmate near her house two hours ago, breaking the skin. All the child's immunizations are up to date. However, the other child's family is currently being investigated for possible HepB infection. Appropriate treatment after the wound care (and antibiotics) would be
   a. tetanus immunization
   b. demand blood test from the playmate for Hep B serology
   c. begin course of HepB vaccine

d. administer anti-HepB immunoglobulin and start a course of HepB vaccine injections
2. Johnny is 10 years old and you find he was NOT vaccinated as an infant. Which of the following is the recommended schedule of immunizations?
   a. Td, Polio and MMR at first visit
   b. DPT, Polio and MMR at first visit
   c. DPT, Polio, MMR and HIB (Haemophilus influenza B) at first visit
   d. Td, MMR and HepB at first visit
3. A heroin addict, in her last month of pregnancy is diagnosed with a right lower lobe pneumonia. Response leads to the formation of IgG antibodies. The fetus would be protected when born due to
   a. active artificial immunity
   b. active natural immunity
   c. passive natural immunity
   d. passive artificial immunity
   e. no protection of the fetus would occur
4. A cancer patient needs immunoprophylaxis against possible HepB exposure. You decide on antibody prophylaxis followed by active HepB immunization. All the following are correct EXCEPT
   a. This represents an example of "natural" passive immunization.
   b. IgM (high molecular weight aggregate) must be given by IM injection to avoid complement activation.
   c. HepB immune globulin is ineffective after acute exposure.
   d. HepB vaccine immunization must use a different site from administration of HepB immune globulin.
   e. Anti-Hep titers should be monitored after vaccination to check efficacy of immunization.
5. Mr. and Mrs. Webb come to visit you for their annual check-up. They are both in their early 70s. Which of the following would you NOT recommend as a routine immunization for them?
   a. pneumococcal vaccine
   b. tetanus
   c. measles/mumps/rubella
   d. influenza

Answers: 1d; 2a; 3c; 4a; 5c

Short Answer Questions
1. What is an adjuvant and what role do adjuvants play in immunization?
2. How do DNA vaccines generate both a B-cell and a T-cell (both CD4 and CD8) response?
3. What is vaccination? What is the mode of antigen delivery for mucosal immunity?
4. Attenuated organisms are normally used for immunization. Explain why, giving examples.
5. List the advantages and disadvantages of DNA vaccines.

Hypersensitivity Reactions

Objectives	266
Hypersensitivity Reactions	267
General Features	267
Type I: Immediate Hypersensitivity Reactions	267
Type II: Antibody-mediated Hypersensitivity Reactions	272
Type III: Immune-complex Mediated Hypersensitivity	276
Type IV: Cell-mediated Hypersensitivity	278
Summary	282
Clinical Cases and Discussion	283
Test Yourself	287

OBJECTIVES

Hypersensitivity reactions are primarily discussed under a terminology (Types I-IV reactions) which classifies them according to the nature of the immune mechanisms involved, ranging from IgE mediated to T-cell derived. It is important to understand and differentiate the sensitization stage from the effector phase of the response (which is associated with observed clinical pathology). This immune pathology ranges from immediately life-threatening (associated with so-called anaphylaxis reactions) to more chronic disorders, such as those resulting in granulomatous formation, again a function of the immune response elicited and the inflammation or other physiological process which ensue.

The reader will find him/her self well-armed to understand the discussion that follows from the readings in the previous chapters. Brief re-review of this material may be helpful at key points in the text, particularly when we consider the multiple mediators and inflammatory mechanism(s) triggered by immunoglobulin with/without associated complement activation. Reactions as diverse as thrombosis, associated with a (hyperacutely) rejected foreign kidney graft, to the itchy skin we associate with contact ivy exposure, have an easily understood, immunological basis which lies within the domain of hypersensitivity reactions. The rationale for trying to understand this mechanism of disease is that it makes immediate sense of the treatment protocols that are adopted to treat the disease itself. While the reader may previously have struggled with understanding, in isolation, the clinical and pathophysiological manifestations of diseases such as Farmer's lung or tuberculosis, we hope that by considering them as hypersensitivity reactions, the host response to the disease and our treatment of it becomes more understandable.

HYPERSENSITIVITY REACTIONS

GENERAL FEATURES

Hypersensitivity reactions are exaggerated immune responses of detriment to the host. They are classified according to the system devised by Gell and Coombs, categorizing the immune mechanisms involved in the response (Figs. 13.1, 13.2). There are four types of hypersensitivity reactions:

Type I	immediate hypersensitivity
Type II	antibody-mediated hypersensitivity
Type III	immune complex-mediated hypersensitivity
Type IV	cell-mediated hypersensitivity

Regardless of the immune mechanisms involved, hypersensitivity reactions can be divided into two phases, a sensitization phase and a detrimental effector phase.

TYPE I: IMMEDIATE HYPERSENSITIVITY REACTIONS

Sensitization phase
The sensitization phase of Type I immediate hypersensitivity reactions occurs when antigen exposure induces IgE production with IgE binding to FcεR on mast cells and basophils (Fig. 13.3). IgE antibodies, rather than other isotypes, are produced depending on the CD4+ T-cell derived cytokines present in the B-cell microenvironment during its activation (Chapters 8 and 9). T-cell clones, specific for defined allergens and isolated from atopic individuals, are predominantly a Th2 phenotype associated with production of the cytokines IL-4 and IL-10, rather than IL-2 and IFNγ. The presence of IL-4/IL-10 during T-dependent B-cell activation induces isotype switching to IgE. IgE antibodies bind to high affinity Fcε receptors present on mast cells and basophils, "awaiting" re-exposure to the initiating antigen.

Effector phase
Tissue damage is caused by inflammatory mediators, (histamine, prostaglandins, leukotrienes, and platelet activating factor) released from mast cells and basophils following antigen binding to cell bound IgE. These substances induce increased vascular permeability, vasodilatation, and smooth muscle contraction, either locally or systemically, depending on the site of antigen exposure. Contact allergens generally produce localized skin responses, but systemic exposure can often produce immediate life-threatening pathology (Fig. 13.3). Because pre-existing antibodies are obligatory for immediate hypersensitivity reactions, primary exposure to an antigen cannot trigger this type of response.

Skin testing identifies antigens causing immediate hypersensitivity reactions, producing an immediate and localized erythema and edema which occurs from increased vascular permeability following skin antigen contact with presensitized, IgE bearing, mast cells/basophils. Patients with severe reactions may be at risk

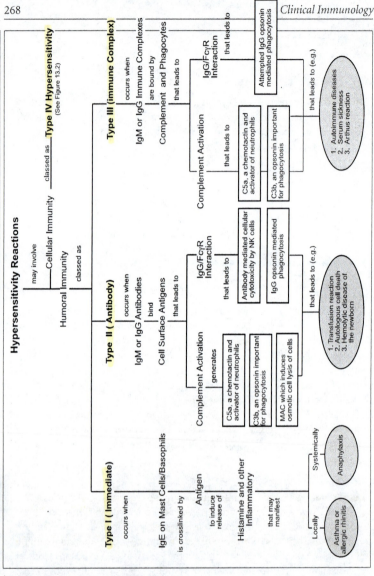

Fig. 13.1. Concept map of hypersensitivity reactions that involve antibody production. Hypersensitivity reactions are exaggerated immune responses detrimental to the host. These reactions are often classified according to the immune mechanisms involved in the response. Types I, II, and III represent exaggerated humoral immunity.

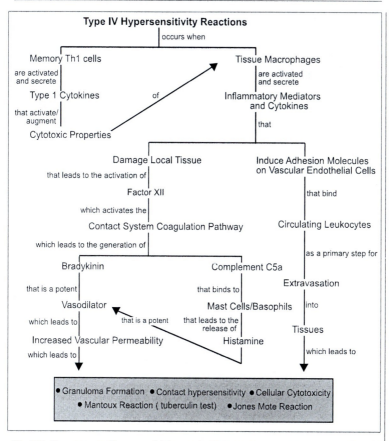

Fig. 13.2. Concept map of hypersensitivity reaction Type IV. Hypersensitivity reaction Type IV is a cellular immune response involving specific, memory CD4+ T cells, and macrophages.

when tested in this manner. For these individuals, an in vitro, antigen specific, radioallergosorbent (RAST) test is used. RAST measures quantitatively the allergen-specific IgE antibodies present in serum. In this test an allergen is bound to an insoluble surface (e.g., cellulose disk) and incubated with the patient's serum, allowing antibodies to bind immobilized antigen. Detection of bound antibodies follows incubation with radiolabeled (or immunofluorescent) anti-Fc(ε) antibodies. One limitation of this test is that IgE bound to mast cells is not estimated, potentially leading to false negative results. Also IgG antibodies specific for the antigen may competitively bind the allergen, preventing detection of IgE.

Clinical manifestations

Clinical manifestations of immediate hypersensitivity reactions include allergic rhinitis, asthma, and anaphylaxis.

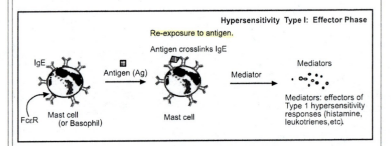

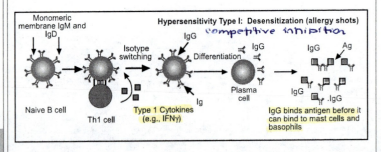

Fig. 13.3. Hypersensitivity Type I: sensitization phase, effector phase, and desensitization. Type 2 cytokines induce isotype switching to IgE. IgE binds to FcεR present on mast cells or basophils. Re-exposure to antigen induces crosslinking of IgE, bound to mast cells and basophils and release of histamine and other inflammatory mediators. Local reactions induce allergic responses, while systemic reactions induce anaphylactic shock. Desensitization involves induction of isotype switching to IgG by B cells following antigen recognition in the presence of T cell derived Type 1 cytokines and appropriate costimulatory molecules. On subsequent exposure to antigen, circulating IgG binds the antigen before it binds to IgE present on mast cells and basophils.

Allergic rhinitis
Allergic rhinitis refers to inflammation of the nasal mucus membranes, sneezing, nasal congestion, and watery discharge from the eyes following antigen exposure.

Asthma
Asthma can be triggered by extrinsic antigens (immediate hypersensitivity), or by nonimmune mechanisms such as infection, exercise and cold air. Wheezing occurs when respiratory passages narrow (bronchoconstriction) following mediator release.

Anaphylaxis
Anaphylaxis is a systemic, potentially fatal, reaction that affects both the cardiovascular and respiratory systems, leading to cardiac arrhythmia, and hypotension.

Therapy
Treatments for patients susceptible to hypersensitivity reactions include (i) minimizing the exposure to the antigens that trigger the reaction, (ii) pharmacological intervention, and (iii) desensitization.

Pharmacological
Prophylactic pharmacological interventions include antihistamines or sodium cromoglycate. Anti-histamines are H1-histamine receptor antagonists that competitively inhibit binding to H1-binding sites. Sodium cromoglycate stabilizes the mast cell and basophil membranes, decreasing the release of inflammatory mediators following crosslinking of cell bound IgE by antigen. Epinephrine administration is NOT prophylactic but is an important antidote following exposure to agents triggering severe, life-threatening, immediate type hypersensitivity reactions (anaphylaxis). Epinephrine provides transient protection (for 30-90 minutes). Steroids are also administered, to control the persistent/recurrent symptoms over the four to eight hours postexposure (during which the inciting agent is generally cleared from the body). Individuals known to be at risk for anaphylaxis often carry injectable epinephrine.

Desensitization
Desensitization, or "allergy shots", refers to controlled immunization with antigen in a manner designed to stimulate the production of IgG antibodies instead of IgE, following promotion of naïve CD4+ T cells to differentiate to a Th1 phenotype. The cytokine profile of Th1 cells generates IgG antibodies, rather than IgE (Fig. 13.3). Circulating IgG antibodies should neutralize the antigen before it reacts with the cell bound IgE. Prolonged immunization is essential to expand this newly polarized Th1 cell subset, and even in desensitized individuals the original Th2 and IgE clones persist.

Type II: Antibody-mediated Hypersensitivity Reactions

Sensitization phase
The sensitization phase of Type II hypersensitivity reactions is marked by the production of IgG and IgM antibodies specific for a cell surface antigen (Fig. 13.4). The eliciting antigens are either constitutive components of the cell, or exogenous antigens (e.g., drugs or drug metabolites) that have bound to cell surface molecules. Consequently, any cell may be a target.

Effector phase
Unlike Type I hypersensitivity reactions, Type 2 hypersensitivity reactions need not "await" re-exposure to antigen because the antigen is not eliminated during primary exposure to the immune system. Destruction of cells expressing antigen/antibody (IgM or IgG) complexes occurs when the classical pathway of complement is activated, leading either to osmotic lysis of cells by the membrane attack complex, or opsonin-mediated phagocytosis when C3b is deposited on the target cell. Cell bound IgG can also serve as an opsonin for phagocytosis.

Cell destruction may also occur by antibody dependent cell mediated cytotoxicity (ADCC). ADCC occurs when natural killer cells expressing the FcγR bind IgG, initiating secretion of the cytotoxic molecule, perforin, that induces osmotic cell lysis (Fig. 13.4). Continued exposure to antigen induces higher titers of high avidity antibody (Chapter 8). Re-exposure to antigen (e.g., to a drug bound to a cell) results in more exaggerated effector responses. When the antigen is a constitutive component of the cell, ongoing cell destruction occurs.

Clinical manifestations
Clinical manifestations of Type II hypersensitivity responses include (i) transfusion reactions; (ii) hemolytic disease of the newborn, primarily due to Rh incompatibility; (iii) autoimmune reactions to cellular antigens or tissues; and (iv) hyperacute rejection of transplanted tissue. Note that in each case the antibody is directed to a cell surface, not soluble antigen.

Transfusion reactions
Individuals receiving blood transfusions are "matched" to ensure that the recipient does not have antibodies recognizing the glycoproteins, predominantly of the ABO system, on the donor's red blood cells. Naturally occurring IgM antibodies, isohemagglutinins, bind to these glycoproteins on red cells, and activate complement leading to either cell lysis or opsonin-mediated (C3b) phagocytosis. Isohemagglutinins develop as a result of immunization by gut commensal organisms that have surface antigens identical to the AB antigens present on human red blood cells. Individuals inherit genes leading to the expression of the glycoproteins designated A and/or B. Some individuals do not express either A or B and are classified as the "O" blood phenotype.

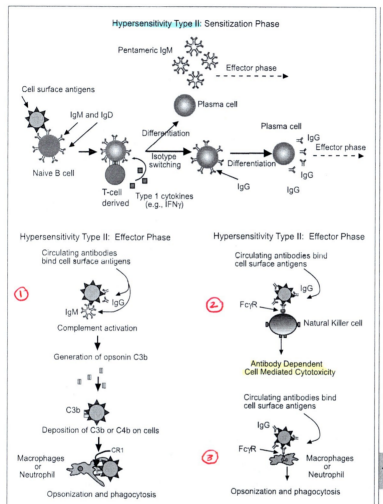

Fig. 13.4. Hypersensitivity Type II: Sensitization phase and effector phase. B cells are activated and differentiate to plasma cells secreting IgG and IgM in standard fashion. Various fates await the cell bearing the surface antigen. (i) Complement activation may occur when antibody binds the antigen. Anaphylatoxins and opsonins are generated and phagocytes are recruited. Opsonin-mediated (C3b) phagocytosis occurs following binding of deposited C3b by CR1 on the phagocyte. (ii) IgG is an opsonin for phagocytosis of target cells following binding via FcγR and (iii) Natural killer cells destroy target cells via ADCC following recognition via FcγR.

ABO Blood Type	Cell Surface Antigens	Isohaemagglutinins
A	A	anti-B
B	B	anti-A
AB	AB	—
O	—	anti-A and anti-B

Blood phenotype "O" individuals, lacking A or B antigen on their cell surface, are universal donors, because their blood cells are not agglutinated when transfused into recipients whose serum contains high titers of anti-A or anti-B ("B" or "A" positive recipients respectively). Although the serum from "O" individuals contains both anti-A and anti-B isohemagglutinins, so little serum is transfused from donor to recipient that the risk associated with transfer of small amounts of antibody present in the "O" individual, which might react with recipient cells, is minimal. The use of washed donor red cells further excludes problems associated with serum transfer. Blood group "O" recipients can only receive blood from other "O" individuals because they have both anti-A and anti-B antibodies. Following the same line of reasoning AB phenotype individuals (no anti-A or anti-B antibodies) are often referred to as universal recipients.

Hemolytic disease of the newborn

Hemolytic disease of the newborn is generally caused by a Rh blood group incompatibility between a Rh negative (Rh-) mother and her Rh positive (Rh+) fetus after the mother has developed anti-Rh IgG antibodies. The presence of anti-Rh antibodies requires prior exposure to Rh antigens. This occurs after the mother has had a previous Rh+ child, becoming sensitized to Rh+ red blood cells entering her circulation at birth, or even during the current pregnancy itself if (clinically insignificant) placental bleeding occurs. Previous blood transfusions could also lead to the production of Rh antibodies.

The mother's anti-Rh IgG antibodies present a problem for the Rh+ fetus because they cross the placenta, bind to the Rh antigen on the fetal red blood cells and cause their hemolysis either by complement-mediated cell lysis or opsonin-mediated (IgG and/or C3b) phagocytosis.

Currently, passive anti-Rh Ig (RhoGam) is given to Rh- mothers immediately postpartum or after any vaginal bleed. The Rhogam is thought to neutralize the Rh antigen before the mother generates an immune response and develops anti-Rh antibodies. Most individuals are Rh positive (85%).

Autologous cell destruction

In Goodpasture's syndrome, glomerular and pulmonary basement membranes are a site of immune mediated damage due to the formation of antibodies to membrane antigens common to both the kidney and the lungs. In insulin dependent diabetes, antibodies develop that recognize pancreatic islet cells, leading to their destruction. Antibodies bound to the cell surface antigens activate complement, leading to osmotic lysis of the autologous cells and opsonin-mediated phagocytosis. Phagocytosis by neutrophils activates the respiratory burst, leading

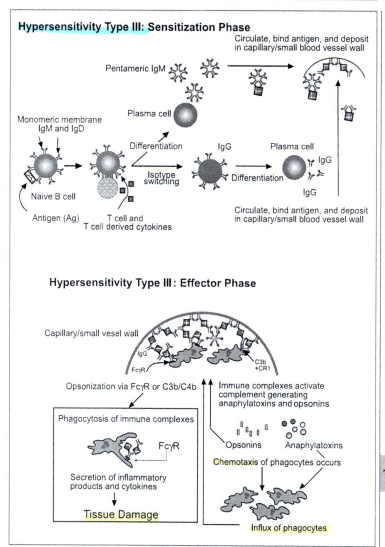

Fig. 13.5. Hypersensitivity Type III: sensitization phase and effector phase. B cells are activated and differentiate to plasma cells secreting IgG and IgM in standard fashion. Circulating IgG and IgM antibodies bind antigen, forming circulating immune complexes that deposit on capillary walls and trigger complement activation. Anaphylatoxins and opsonins are generated. Anaphylatoxins induce chemotaxis of phagocytes. Phagocytosis of immune complexes via FcγR or CR1 triggers the production of inflammatory mediators including reactive oxygen and nitrogen intermediates, causing local tissue damage.

to secretion of reactive oxygen intermediates and the proteolytic enzymes, elastase and collagenase which cause local tissue damage.

Type III: Immune-Complex Mediated Hypersensitivity

Sensitization phase

Unlike Type II hypersensitivity reactions, the sensitization phase of Type III hypersensitivity reactions is characterized by IgM and IgG antibodies binding to soluble antigens with subsequent formation of immune complexes (Fig. 13.5). Persistent immune challenge, in some autoimmune diseases or under conditions of chronic antigen exposure (e.g., chronic parasitemia), induces the formation of immune complexes in excess of the capacity of normal immune clearance mechanisms (in the reticuloendothelial system).

Effector phase

Immune complexes formed in excess are deposited in the capillary walls where they stimulate complement activation (Fig. 13.5), generating anaphylatoxins and the C3b opsonin. One of the anaphylatoxins, C5a, is chemotactic for neutrophils and so neutrophils are recruited to the site where the immune complexes are localized. In addition, C5a binds to mast cells/basophils causing the release of vasoactive amines and associated increases in vascular permeability. As immune complexes filter between the contracted endothelial cells they become trapped in the vessel wall. Recruited neutrophils are activated as they try to phagocytose the immune complexes, following recognition of IgG Fc regions, or the deposited C3b opsonin. Activated neutrophils secrete inflammatory mediators, including reactive oxygen intermediates and the proteolytic enzymes elastase and collagenase. The latter enzymes damage the endothelium, exposing the subendothelium which now serves to activate the intrinsic coagulation pathway, leading to the generation of kallikrein and bradykinin. Bradykinin is a potent vasodilator. The combined effects of histamine and bradykinin on vascular permeability cause increased vascular permeability (Fig. 13.6). In addition, platelets bind to the subendothelium, interact with immune complexes, and aggregate at these sites. If uncontrolled, these events lead to formation of microthrombi, platelet activation and aggregation, vascular occlusion, and tissue necrosis.

Clinical manifestation

Localization of immune complexes

In systemic lupus erythematosus (SLE), complexes are mainly deposited in the kidney glomeruli to cause glomerulonephritis; in rheumatoid arthritis they are deposited in the joints; in farmer's lung they are deposited in the lung. Different hypotheses may help to explain the localization of complexes to these sites. It has been suggested that the kidney basement membrane acts to "trap" polyanionic antigens in a nonspecific manner so that the presence of excess antibodies that recognize these polyanionic antigens (anti-DNA antibodies in SLE) leads to immune complex deposition in the kidney basement membrane.

Hypersensitivity Reactions

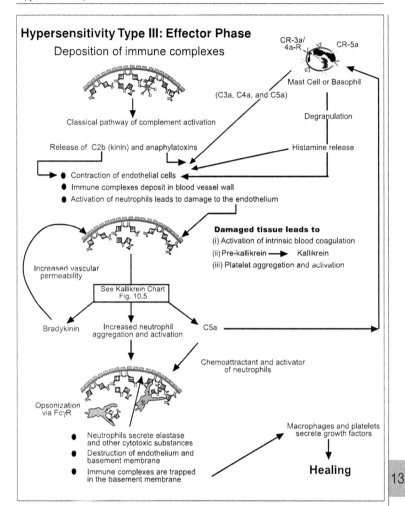

Fig. 13.6. Role of antibodies, complement, mast cells, neutrophils, and intrinsic coagulation pathway in hypersensitivity Type III reactions. Complement activation by the alternative or classical pathways generates anaphylatoxins. Anaphylatoxin binding to mast cells or basophils causes degranulation, histamine release, and increased vascular permeability. The generated proteolytic fragments C5a and bradykinin increase vascular permeability. In addition, C5a is a chemoattractant for, and activator of, neutrophils. Following their recruitment to the site of inflammation, neutrophils secrete enzymes that destroy the endothelium and basement membrane.

Systemic lupus erythematosus

Systemic lupus erythematosus (SLE) is an autoimmune disease in which antibodies are formed to soluble antigens (e.g., double-stranded and single-stranded DNA, histones etc.). Although immune complexes are deposited predominantly in the renal glomeruli, they are also found in other basement membranes, including the membranes lining the lungs, skin, blood vessels and even the central nervous system. Multiple manifestations of localized (in the kidney) and disseminated (throughout all affected organs) disease often occurs.

Serum sickness (systemic)

This was originally identified in some patients who had been passively immunized with horse serum containing anti-diphtheria toxin antibodies (as treatment for diphtheria), with fever, edematous rashes, enlarged lymph nodes and swollen joints occurring one to two weeks after treatment. Patients produced antibodies to soluble horse serum protein antigens, with subsequent formation of large numbers of immune complexes which were deposited in the vasculature (blood vessel wall), causing complement activation, neutrophil recruitment, vasculitis, and the symptoms described above. A second injection of the horse serum could lead to anaphylaxis and death. In North America, one clinically useful passive heterologous antibody preparation (polyclonal antibodies made in nonhuman species) is an anti-snake venom toxin for victims of snakebites. Clinicians must weigh the cost/benefit of its use in selected patients.

Arthus reaction: localized

This localized immune complex reaction manifests as cutaneous vasculitis and necrosis. Following prior exposure to antigen and the formation of circulating IgG antibodies to the antigen (i.e., sensitization phase), the Arthus reaction is observed after subcutaneous, or intradermal, injection of the same antigen.

TYPE IV. CELL-MEDIATED HYPERSENSITIVITY

Sensitization phase

Type IV hypersensitivity reactions are mediated by immune cells, not antibodies. During sensitization naive CD4+ T cells (Thp) are activated and differentiate to Th1/Th2 cells secreting cytokines (Chapter 9). Th cells clonally expand, with some becoming memory cells, providing immunosurveillance as they circulate via blood and lymph. Type IV hypersensitivity reactions are subclassed as:

i. chronic Type IV hypersensitivity (e.g., granulomatous inflammation)
ii. acute Type IV hypersensitivity (e.g., the Mantoux reaction)
iii. contact hypersensitivity (e.g., poison ivy dermatitis)
iv. cutaneous basophil hypersensitivity (e.g., Jones Mote reaction)
v. cellular cytotoxicity (e.g., CD8+ mediated destruction of virally infected cells).

Hypersensitivity Reactions

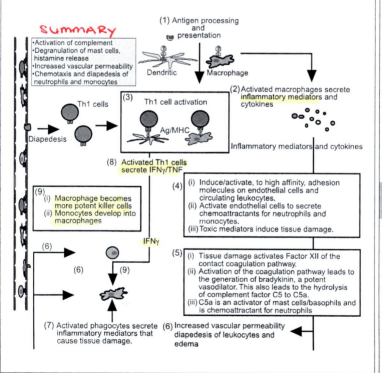

Fig. 13.7. Hypersensitivity Type IV: sensitization phase and effector phase.

The pathophysiology of these disorders often differs significantly from that seen in Types I-III reactions (above). Furthermore, the populations at risk, and the treatment of the disorders are also different.

Effector phase

This occurs following re-exposure to antigen and activation of the memory Th1 cells (Fig. 13.7). The antigen may be re-introduced topically via the skin, or intradermally. In other cases, the antigen may represent the persistent intracellular existence of a microbe, as occurs with *Mycobacterium sp*. Tissue damage is caused by inflammatory mediators and cytokines secreted by activated neutrophils and tissue macrophages following phagocytosis. The following events occur:

i. Memory Th1 cells traffic through tissues and are activated when they contact antigen presented by dendritic cells or macrophages. IFNγ, secreted by activated Th1 cells, is a potent activator of tissue macrophages.

ii. Activated macrophages secrete cytokines (e.g., IL-1 and TNF) and chemokines that induce/activate adhesion molecules on the endothelium and circulating leukocytes. Some cytokines induce secretion of chemokines attracting neutrophils and monocytes to the inflammatory site.

iii. The inflammatory mediators alter the vascular permeability of the endothelium, and cause local tissue damage. Tissue damage activates **Hageman factor (Factor XII)** of the intrinsic coagulation pathway, leading to the generation of kallikrein and bradykinin. Kallikrein hydrolyzes complement component C5, generating C5a, an anaphylatoxin and a chemotaxin for neutrophils. C5a induces the degranulation of basophils/mast cells, leading to the release of histamine and an increase in vascular permeability. Bradykinin, itself a potent vasodilator, combined with histamine causes edema.

iv. Adhesion molecules on the endothelium cause circulating leukocytes to adhere to the activated endothelium. Activated neutrophils (see iii) secrete enzymes that degrade the basement membrane. The increase in vascular permeability, along with a degraded basement membrane, fosters leukocyte transmigration to the site of inflammation, a process called diapedesis.

v. Neutrophils phagocytose antigen and secrete inflammatory mediators that cause local tissue damage.

vi. IFNγ, from activated Th1 cells, promotes differentiation of monocytes to macrophages, and activates mature macrophages to kill intracellular organisms. In addition, activated macrophages secrete products including IL-1 and TNF, that stimulate processes producing inflammatory mediators that cause bystander tissue injury.

Regulation of the response

Simple antigen elimination can dampen immunoreactivity. Additional regulation of Th1 responsiveness is provided by Th2 cell derived IL-4/IL-10 cytokines, probably necessary because uncontrolled Th1 responses produce nonspecific inflammatory mediators that can cause bystander normal tissue destruction. There are pathologic clinical scenarios where uncontrolled Th1 activation (**tuberculoid**

Hypersensitivity Reactions

leprosy), or conversely, uncontrolled Th2 activation occurs. In one example of the latter, **lepromatous leprosy**, the failure of Th1 activation, in turn, results in a failure to eradicate the parasite.

Clinical manifestations

Chronic: granulomatous inflammation

Often the persisting antigens in these cases are microorganisms existing within the macrophage, where they have escaped intracellular enzymatic and biochemical destruction following phagocytosis. Examples include *Mycobacterium leprae* and *Mycobacterium tuberculosis*. The chronically infected and activated macrophages often fuse to form multinucleated giant cells, and the surrounding chronic lymphocyte/monocyte activation leads to tissue changes that manifest in **granuloma formation**. Granulomas form in the lung in tuberculosis, while in **sarcoidosis**, granulomas develop in the lymph nodes, bone, skin and lungs. The inciting agent for sarcoidosis remains unknown, as is the case for another granulomatous disorder, associated with **Crohn's colitis** (in the intestinal tract). In each instance it has long been suspected that the responsible agent is a (unidentified) mycobacterium.

Acute: Mantoux reaction

In the tuberculin test, a protein isolated from cultures of *Mycobacterium tuberculosis*, purified protein derivative (PPD), is injected intradermally to assess prior exposure to this bacterium. Intradermal **PPD** is sequestered by antigen presenting cells and, in previously sensitized individuals, is presented to trafficking Th1 cells. Activated Th1 cells secrete cytokines (IFNγ, TNF) that activate tissue macrophages initiating the effector phase described above, which causes a local area of cytokine-induced erythema and induration reaching a maximum at 24-48 hours. Unlike edema there is no pitting when pressure is applied to this region. This reaction is referred to as a **delayed type hypersensitivity reaction (DTH)**.

Contact hypersensitivity

Poison Ivy dermatitis is the prototypic form of an epidermal disorder triggered by activation of specifically sensitized memory Th1 cells, often in response to a hapten (e.g., urishiol from poison ivy). The urishiol is absorbed, and combines with a protein carrier molecule. Haptens are too small to generate immune responses unless bound to a protein (Chapter 1). The effector phase occurs on second exposure to the contact antigen and manifests as erythema and swelling. The cytokine-mediated inflammatory response is essentially the same as that described above. However, the antigen presenting cells are **Langerhans cells**, and the **keratinocytes** serve as the source of inflammatory cytokines.

Cutaneous basophil hypersensitivity

Also known as the **Jones Mote Reaction**, this reaction is (experimentally) induced by repeated intradermal injections of soluble antigen mixed with adjuvant.

The reaction has been called a ***cutaneous basophil hypersensitivity*** owing to the large number of basophils which accumulate in the lesion. **Adjuvants** promote (quantitatively and sometimes qualitatively) the immune response to a given antigen which will develop, less vigorously, in their absence (Chapter 12).

Cellular cytotoxicity
Activated memory Th1 cells secrete IL-2, the cytokine required for the differentiation of pCTL to mature CTL. Mature CTL can kill virally infected autologous cells that express antigen/MHC class I on their surface. CD8+ T cell cytotoxicity is important for control of viral infections e.g., cytomegalovirus (CMV), herpes simplex viruses I and II (HSV-I, HSV-II).

SUMMARY

Hypersensitivity reactions are exaggerated immune responses that are detrimental to the host. They are generally classified, using a system devised by Gell and Coombs, according to the immune mechanisms involved in the response. Four types of hypersensitivity reactions, Types I to IV, have been designated. Regardless of the immune mechanisms involved, hypersensitivity reactions can be divided into two phases, a sensitization phase and an effector phase.

Sensitization for Type I immediate hypersensitivity reactions occurs when antigen exposure leads to the production of IgE and subsequent binding to FcεR on mast cells and basophils. The effector phase of Type I hypersensitivity reactions is caused by inflammatory mediators, (histamine, prostaglandins, leukotrienes, and platelet activating factor) released from mast cells and basophils following antigen binding to cell bound IgE. Skin testing identifies antigens causing immediate hypersensitivity reactions. Patients with severe reactions may be at risk when tested in this manner, and for these, an antigen specific radioallergosorbent (RAST) test is more appropriate. Clinical manifestations of immediate hypersensitivity reactions include allergic rhinitis, asthma, and anaphylaxis. Treatments include (i) minimizing the exposure to the antigens that trigger the reaction, (ii) pharmacological intervention, and (iii) desensitization.

The sensitization phase for Type II hypersensitivity reactions is marked by the production of IgG and IgM antibodies specific for cell surface antigens, either constitutive components of the cell or exogenous antigens (e.g., drugs or drug metabolites) that have bound to cell surface molecules. Destruction of cells expressing antigen/antibody (IgM or IgG) complexes occurs when the classical pathway of complement is activated leading either to osmotic lysis of cells by the membrane attack complex or opsonin-mediated phagocytosis. In addition to phagocytosis and complement mediated cell lysis, cell destruction may occur by a process termed, antibody dependent cell mediated cytotoxicity (ADCC). Clinical manifestations of Type II hypersensitivity responses include (i) transfusion reactions, (ii) hemolytic disease of the newborn due to red blood cell incompatibility (primarily Rh incompatibility), (iii) autoimmune reactions to cellular antigens or tissues and (iv) hyperacute rejection of transplanted tissue.

Hypersensitivity Reactions

Unlike Type II hypersensitivity reactions, the sensitization phase of Type III hypersensitivity reactions is characterized by the formation of IgM and IgG antibodies to soluble antigens with subsequent formation of immune complexes. Persistent immune challenge induces the formation of an excess of immune complexes which overwhelm the normal clearing mechanisms of the reticuloendothelial system. Immune complexes are deposited in the capillary walls where they serve as the stimulus for complement and phagocyte activation, both of which activate processes causing tissue damage.

Type IV hypersensitivity reactions are mediated by immune cells, rather than by antibodies. The sensitization phase of Type IV hypersensitivity is initiated when naïve CD4+ T cells (Thp) are activated leading to their preferential differentiation to Th1 cells secreting Type 1 cytokines. On re-exposure to the eliciting antigen, activation of the memory Th1 cells occurs. One manifestation of a chronic Type IV hypersensitivity response is granuloma formation caused by chronically infected and activated macrophages that fuse to form multinucleated giant cells surrounded by activated lymphocytes and monocytes. Granulomas form in the lung in tuberculosis, while in sarcoidosis, granulomas develop in the lymph nodes, bone, skin and lungs. Type IV hypersensitivity responses form the basis for the Mantoux test, used to investigate prior exposure to *Mycobacterium tuberculosis*. Poison ivy dermatitis is the prototypic form of contact hypersensitivity, induced by the contact antigen urishiol.

CLINICAL CASES AND DISCUSSION

Clinical Case #25

A 19-year male is rushed to your emergency department from a local Chinese restaurant after becoming acutely "ill" while eating. He is pale, cool, clammy, and has a low blood pressure. There is no medic-alert bracelet to be seen. You find he has wheezes throughout his lung fields, with poor air intake. His sister who is with him says this has never happened before, and no one in the family has ever been like this.

Questions and Discussion: Case #25
1. *List the six likely key features we need to bear in mind in discussing this case.*
   young male
   acute illness while eating in a Chinese restaurant
   pale, cool, and clammy
   respiratory wheezing
   first time occurrence
   low blood pressure
2. *Explain the physiological basis for being "pale, cool, and clammy"?*
The patient is not perfusing his peripheral tissues with blood. In trauma cases with blood loss, peripheral vessels constrict to conserve what blood remains for circulation to the central key organs (brain/heart etc.). When vasodilators (complement components, histamine etc.) are released in large quantities, blood pressure

falls and flow to the periphery also ceases. The "sweating" represents the body's adrenergic response trying to counter this vasodilatation.

3. An acute illness suggests an ingested toxin (poison), or something the body releases which produces these changes. What stimuli could trigger these symptoms?
   i. Some fish (scombroid) produce large amounts of histamine causing a rapid "vascular collapse", associated with blood vessel dilatation, low blood pressure etc. This is one possibility.
   ii. A more common problem than that attributable to ingestion of scombroid would also cause massive endogenous histamine release, namely a food allergy.

4. What is the significance of the family history, and being told "this is the first time?"
   A first time presentation in a 19-year-old, with no family history, implies inherited genetic causes are unlikely.

5. Name an immunodeficiency disorder that might cause a spontaneous syndrome like this.
   C1 esterase deficiency occasionally presents in a similar fashion. Vasodilators are released by uncontrolled complement activation with proteolytically derived C5a inducing degranulation of mast cells and histamine release. Appropriate action would involve replacement of the C1 esterase inhibitor protein and a medic-alert bracelet (below).

6. How would one test for C1 esterase deficiency?
   A variety of ELISA assays exist specific for individual complement components. If you suspect such a defect you order the lab to test for the serum level of that specific component.

7. A Chinese restaurant is an environment rich in shellfish and nuts, TWO OF THE MOST POTENT MEDIATORS OF FOOD ALLERGIES. Would this reaction occur the first time this individual eats such foods?
   This reaction depends upon *re-exposure* of *previously sensitized* individuals, so he must have eaten similar foods before without a response.

8. This patient is in shock. What is this generally called? What is appropriate treatment?
   Anaphylactic shock (immune-mediated). This could proceed to a total respiratory arrest in minutes, so urgent action is needed. Epinephrine provides intense α-adrenergic stimulation in seconds to minutes, lasting for 30-90 minutes.

9. There are many ways to treat immediate hypersensitivity reactions, which act by different mechanisms and have different times of onset. What are they?
   i. Epinephrine is used for immediate and urgent action (see #8).
   ii. Anti-histamines block binding to histamine (type 1) receptors, countering the action of histamine. Their time to action is 5-30 minutes, lasting for up to 2-4 hours.
   iii. Steroids (e.g., prednisone) are potent anti-inflammatory agents whose mode of action is unclear. Their effect begins in 4-8 hours, and lasts up to 24 hours.
   iv. Desensitization therapy involves prolonged exposure to the inciting agent, under controlled conditions, over months to years, in the hope that the

Hypersensitivity Reactions

immune system develops a nonpathological immune response (e.g., produce IgG not IgE antibodies to the inciting antigen).

10. After epinephrine would you provide additional therapy from the list provided in the answer to #9?

Steroids should also be given to control the problem longer term. Recall that epinephrine only provides protection for 30-90 minutes. Anti-histamines would also be a reasonable adjunctive treatment. What is quite UNACCEPTABLE, of course, is to opt for desensitization at this time (and watch the patient die).

11. There are other reasons for choosing steroids, related to the kinetics of hypersensitivity reactions. What are they?

There is a "second peak" of mediator release, occurring some 6-8 hours after the first response, caused by persistent antigen which restimulates new potential effector cells migrating to the area of antigen contact. Steroids provided early will begin to be effective just at the time this problem appears.

12. Food allergies will often present as nausea, stomach cramps and diarrhea. Why?

Histamine release in the gastrointestinal tract stimulates smooth muscle H-1 receptors that cause contractions in the intestinal wall. Other mediators are released which (transiently) alter membrane fluid exchanges, causing the watery diarrhea.

13. What should you advise about longer-term care for this problem?

Many allergic reactions are inconvenient, but not life threatening. Welts after insect bites (local histamine release to insect saliva) and orbital edema on exposure to cat/animal dander are two such reactions.

Other allergies kill people! Included in these are certain food allergies (nuts/shellfish) and some allergies to insect stings (yellow jackets).

14. People with allergies to nuts and shellfish or insect stings should carry three things. What are they?

1. An epi-pen (to deliver immediate epinephrine in the event of exposure).
2. Benadryl (to be taken after #1, en route to the hospital).
3. A medic-alert bracelet (in case they cannot communicate their significant medical history).

Clinical Case #26

A young male comes to your Denver office in February complaining of fatigue since early December. He has been a patient of yours for years and you last saw him in June. Blood work at that time was normal. You find he is quite anemic (Hgb 8.0:normal lab range 14-16). He has not traveled out of the country and has no other ailments except a chronic cough with fever (37.5-38°C for 2 weeks). He is not on any medications.

Questions and Discussion: Case #26

1. List the six likely key features we need to bear in mind in discussing this case.
   young male
   fatigue ~ two months
   blood work 8 months earlier was normal

blood work shows he is now anemic
chronic cough
low grade fever for two weeks

2. Why is the fact that he is not on medication a significant negative?
Drugs can often produce anemia if they bind to red blood cells, acting as haptens to elicit the production of anti-drug antibodies. These antibodies bind to the cell bound drug, causing complement activation, the formation of the membrane attack complex, and lysis of red cells (Type II hypersensitivity reactions).

3. Why is the fact that he has not traveled out of the country significant?
Unusual travel might be associated with infections. Many viruses, e.g., dengue, parvovirus, cause anemia and/or thrombocytopenia, resulting from viral lysis of cells. In the case of parvovirus, this is related to viral attack on myeloid stem cell progenitors from which erythrocytes develop.

4. The chronic cough suggests something in the lungs and so you order a chest x-ray. This reveals patchy "hazy" infiltrates, but no consolidation/masses. What does this suggest?
The absence of consolidating processes confirms that we are unlikely to be dealing with an acute (localized) bacterial pneumonic picture. The "hazy" infiltrates are features of disseminated viral type infections or of microorganisms causing chronic, disseminated infection in the lungs. This picture can also reflect the anatomy of the inflamed lung itself, including the blood flow to it and interstitial leakage of fluid from capillaries into the tissue.

5. In the summer this patient's blood work was normal. Yet a few months later in winter, he is anemic. This is a seasonally related anemia. What blood work or investigations might you order and why?
You order serology for antibodies to the so-called Ii antigens. Mycoplasma infections are capable of causing atypical (chronic) pneumonias. In response to the infection the host mounts an antibody response to Ii antigens which crossreact with antigens (glycophorin) on the surface of normal red cells. Mycoplasma infections are also associated with the production of cold agglutinins (antibodies which preferentially agglutinate, in the cold), so titers of cold agglutinins should also be ordered. All of this data is explained on the basis of a cold-hemolytic disease, secondary to mycoplasma infection, which is associated with anti-Ii antibody, leading to lysis of red cells. As advice, tell the patient to keep warm (especially the periphery e.g., nose/toes/hands) and provide treatment for the mycoplasma infection (erythromycin).

6. What other autoimmune disorders present with this kind of peripheral circulation problem. Why?
Reynaud's phenomenon (cyanosis in the toes/hands) is common in vasculitis. Damage to peripheral nerves controlling the small blood vessels causes the latter to spasm. Waldenström's macroglobulinemia also presents this way. Here high levels of IgM, poorly soluble in the cooler areas of the body, produce increased viscosity in the blood, slower blood flow in the periphery, and, in turn, cyanosis.

TEST YOURSELF

Multiple Choice Questions

1. A 19-year-old female with multiple episodes of sexually transmitted diseases presents to the emergency room bleeding per vagina. Her last period was 13 weeks ago. She is known to be Rh -ve. Ectopic pregnancy is diagnosed and she undergoes emergency surgery. This mother is at risk of developing:
    a. Type II Hypersensitivity, following sensitization from a possible Rh+ve fetus (now aborted)
    b. a transfusion reaction now, from spillover of fetal blood into the maternal circulation
    c. serum sickness from spillover of fetal blood into the maternal circulation
    d. a delayed type (Type IV) hypersensitivity reaction to fetal red blood cells
2. A positive Mantoux skin reaction involves the interaction of:
    a. antigen, complement, and lymphokines
    b. antigen-antibody complexes, complement, and neutrophils
    c. memory T cells, cytokines, and macrophages
    d. IgE antibody, antigen, and mast cells
    e. antigen, macrophages, and complement
3. Your patient has several attacks of sneezing, runny nose and itchy eyes every spring, due to allergy to some plant pollen. On the basis of skin testing, an allergist suggests a course of desensitization. The theory behind "desensitization" is that the dose of antigen and the mode of injection will lead to the generation of activated
    a. Th1 cells and secretion of Type 1 cytokines
    b. Th2 cells and the secretion of Type 2 cytokines
    c. tissue mast cells and histamine release
    d. basophils in the circulation and histamine release
    e. B cells and isotype switching to IgE
4. While jogging in the park on a warm day, a young man was stung by a wasp. Ten minutes later he felt dizzy and began to itch under his arms and on his scalp. He broke out in hives and felt tightness in his chest, so he headed for the hospital, but collapsed on the seat of the taxi. In the emergency room his pulse was barely detectable. Which of the following treatments is most appropriate now?
    a. cromolyn sodium
    b. epinephrine
    c. penicillin
    d. antihistamines
    e. anticoagulant

5. A 28-year-old female complains of fatigue, shortness of breath on exertion and general loss of appetite over the last 8-10 months, following a flu-like illness. Routine blood work shows a significant anemia (hemoglobin less than 50% normal) and a positive Coomb's test. A likely diagnosis is:
   a. Type I hypersensitivity
   b. Type II hypersensitivity
   c. Type III hypersensitivity
   d. Type IV hypersensitivity

Answers: 1a ; 2c ; 3a ; 4b ; 5b

Short Answer Questions
1. Explain the sequence of events causing pathophysiology in Type I hypersensitivity reactions.
2. Which hypersensitivity reactions are T-cell mediated and how do they occur?
3. How does immune complex deposition in glomeruli lead to nephritis?
4. What is plasmapheresis and when is it useful therapy?
5. What is the immune basis for transfusion reactions?

Autoimmunity

Objectives	289
Autoimmunity	290
General Features	290
Tolerance Induction	290
Loss of Self Tolerance	293
Immunopathology of Autoimmune Disorders: Autoreactive Antibodies	296
Immunopathology of Autoimmune Disorders: Cell-mediated Immunity	299
Immunotherapy of Autoimmune Disease: Suppression	301
Immunotherapy of Autoimmune Disorders: Cytokine Modulation	306
Summary	307
Clinical Cases and Discussion	308
Test Yourself	312

OBJECTIVES

The autoimmune disorders are readily understood from discussions on the development and induction of antigen specific immunity (both B- and T-cell immunity). As noted in earlier chapters, the developing immune system produces populations of cells with an infinite array of recognition receptors, which do not recognize self components as foreign. Where such cells do develop, a "back-up" system must be in place to suppress their function. This avoids any functional consequences from AUTOimmune reactivity. A failure at these stages results in disease.

In general, B-cell stimulation is dependent upon T cell help so, in its absence, efficient B-cell immunity does not develop. However, a number of T-cell functions develop in the absence of B cells. Multiple mechanisms exist to regulate the function of self-recognizing T lymphocytes, including peripheral deletion mechanisms, induction of anergy, and active suppression. Because T cells see antigen in the presence of host MHC, and in association with costimulatory molecules, a break-down in the normal regulatory processes (which keep self-recognizing cells *unresponsive*) can often be traced to altered expression of costimulatory molecules, MHC, or even of apoptosis, controlling the lymphocyte's demise.

The reader will find our discussion subdivided into consideration of diseases where immunopathology results from autoantibodies (and/or complement activation), and those where cell-mediated immunity is the primary problem. Note that after destruction of host tissue (following T-cell-mediated immunity), the host may make an antibody response to newly available self molecules, and this presence of autoreactive antibodies in some diseases has sometimes confused the issue over causality in some autoimmune disorders.

Clinical Immunology, by Reginald Gorczynski and Jacqueline Stanley. 2001 Landes Bioscience

Understanding the etiology of the disease is important for planning treatment. While, nonspecific immunosuppression "works" for all autoimmune disorders, the adverse side-effects (acquired immunodeficiency diseases, cancer, drug toxicity) can make the treatment worse than the disease. Effort has been spent attempting to develop specific treatments for the different disorders. Without a better knowledge of the autoantigen itself this is often unsuccessful. However, even such subtle manipulations as altering the balance of T-cell cytokine production (from Type 1 to Type 2 cytokines) can sometimes have profound effects on autoimmune diseases.

AUTOIMMUNITY

GENERAL FEATURES

Immunological **tolerance** is a state of unresponsiveness to a challenge, which would have been expected to elicit measurable immunity. **Self tolerance** refers to immunological unresponsiveness towards one's own self antigens. Deletion or inactivation of T- or B-cell clones whose antigen receptors recognize self-antigen (tolerance induction) often occurs during lymphocyte maturation in primary lymphoid tissues. Some self-reactive clones exist in the periphery, implying that tolerance to self-antigens can be induced by peripheral mechanisms. Operational tolerance can merely reflect sequestration of self-antigens, such that they are not accessible to the immune system (e.g., lens crystallin in the eye). Tolerance is "broken" (more appropriately, *immune responses develop*) when the sequestered antigens are exposed to the immune system. Loss of self-tolerance leads to autoimmunity. The spectrum of autoimmune diseases range from organ specific (e.g., **Hashimoto's thyroiditis**) through diseases representing a mixture of organ specific and systemic symptoms (e.g., **rheumatoid arthritis**) to diseases with non organ specific autoimmune reactivity (e.g., **systemic lupus erythematosus**).

TOLERANCE INDUCTION

Central tolerance induction
Central tolerance induction of T and B cells occurs during maturation in the thymus and bone marrow, respectively (Fig. 14.1). T-cell tolerance induction results from negative selection in the thymus. Clonal elimination or functional inactivation occurs when the avidity of T-cell receptors (TCRs) for antigen/MHC complexes exceeds a predetermined threshold leading to delivery of an activation-induced death signal (Chapter 7). For B cells, tolerance induction occurs at the immature B-cell stage, when they express monomeric IgM, and not IgD. Tolerance induction of B cells leads either to clonal anergy or apoptosis.

Peripheral tolerance induction
Peripheral mechanisms for tolerance induction include (i) deletion (activation induced cell death); (ii) suppression by T-cells (T-cell derived factors); (iii) lack of

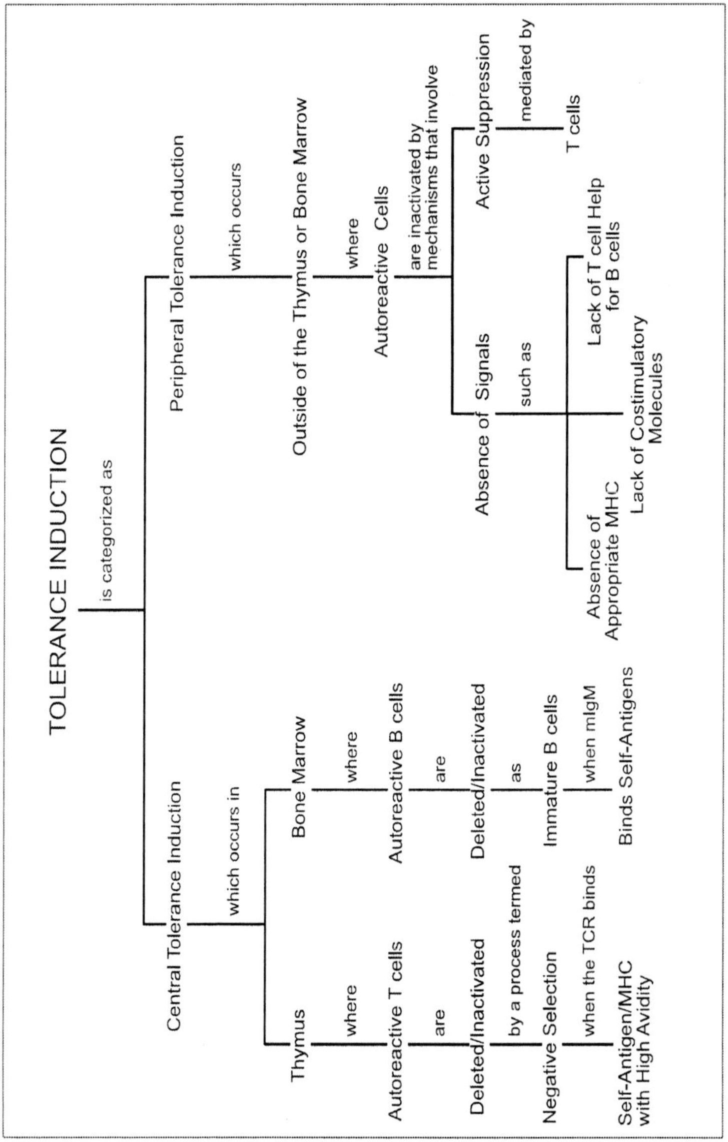

Autoimmunity

TOLERANCE INDUCTION

is categorized as

- **Central Tolerance Induction** — which occurs in
  - **Thymus** — where
    - **Autoreactive T cells** are
      - **Deleted/Inactivated** by a process termed
        - **Negative Selection** — when the TCR binds
          - **Self-Antigen/MHC with High Avidity**
  - **Bone Marrow** — where
    - **Autoreactive B cells** are
      - **Deleted/Inactivated** as
        - **Immature B cells** — when mIgM
          - **Binds Self-Antigens**

- **Peripheral Tolerance Induction** — which occurs
  - **Outside of the Thymus or Bone Marrow** — where
    - **Autoreactive Cells** are inactivated by mechanisms that involve
      - **Absence of Signals** such as
        - **Absence of Appropriate MHC**
        - **Lack of Costimulatory Molecules**
        - **Lack of T cell Help for B cells**
      - **Active Suppression** — mediated by
        - **T cells**

Fig. 14.1. Concept map illustrating mechanisms of tolerance induction. Self-tolerance represents immunological unresponsiveness to one's own antigens. Auto-reactive T- or B-cell clones are deleted, or inactivated by central mechanisms in the thymus and bone marrow, respectively. Peripheral tolerance induction must also occur because some self-reactive cells exist peripherally.

T-cell help for B-cell activation; (iv) absence of appropriate major histocompatibility complex (MHC) molecules for antigen presentation; and (v) absence of costimulatory molecules (Fig. 14.1).

(i) Peripheral deletion
Some clonal deletion clearly occurs in the periphery. As an example, following exposure to superantigen, peripheral T cells clonally expand and subsequently undergo apoptosis. The individual is then refractory (tolerant) to further exposure to the same superantigen, though recovery can occur as new cells generate from the thymus (Chapter 1). Similar phenomena occur in transplant models following donor-specific pretransplant transfusion. Here individuals receiving a tissue/organ transplant are pretreated with whole blood from the tissue/organ donor, along with other immunosuppressive manipulations, to ensure graft rejection does not develop (Chapter 17). Sometimes tolerance to the graft is associated with an expansion followed by deletion of the specific anti-graft T cells. Often no recovery of immunity to the tolerizing antigen occurs, leaving the individual functionally tolerant.

(ii) Suppression by T cells (or T-cell derived factors)
Many immune responses implicated in autoimmune responses are a function of Th1 type (Type 1 cytokine producing) cells (Chapter 9). Given the data suggesting a reciprocal relationship between Th1 and Th2 cells, mediated by the cytokines they produce, it is thus not surprising that Type 2 cytokine producing cells have themselves been implicated in suppression of immunity (Th1 type) or functional tolerance induction. Other activated CD8+ cells can also suppress immune responses, perhaps through a Fas:Fas ligand type interaction. Finally, CD8+ cells with antigen-specific suppressive properties have been described. These suppressor cells have been referred to as "veto cells".

(iii) Lack of T-cell help for B-cell responses
Understanding peripheral B-cell tolerance to T-independent antigens involves clarifying the mechanisms by which T cells become incapable of providing "help". T-cell help requires T-cell/B-cell cognate interaction and T-cell derived cytokines. Without T-cell help, activated B cells become anergic if they have been stimulated by self-antigen. This scenario is observed whenever deletion of self reactive T cells occurs centrally in the thymus, or even when peripheral inactivation occurs. Thus, B-cell tolerance can exist even without deletion of self reactive B-cell clones.

(iv) Lack of appropriate MHC molecules
T-cell stimulation requires (self) antigen presented in the context of appropriate MHC molecules and costimulation (below). Autoreactive T cells with TCR specific for distinct tissue antigens will not be activated if the antigen is not presented in the context of MHC. Even shed antigen (presented on professional APC) induces T cells specific for antigen-MHC, and T cells do not "see" this form of

Autoimmunity

antigen (in association with MHC) on MHC-negative tissue. This helps explain why tolerance can "break" following inflammation and increased expression of MHC on tissue cells.

(v) Lack of costimulatory molecules
T-cell activation is initiated following TCR triggering along with costimulatory molecule interactions. Major costimulator molecules are believed to be members of the B7 family (with coreceptors CD28, CTLA4 on T cells) and CD40 (with CD40 ligand) the coreceptor on T cells. CD28 is constitutively expressed on more than two thirds of CD4+ T cells and on about half of the cytotoxic T cells. B7, which exists in two homologous forms B7-1 and B7-2, is generally expressed only on activated antigen presenting cells. The notable exception to this is the expression of B7-2 on resting dendritic cells. Inducible B7-2 and CD40 is detected six hours after activation of antigen presenting cells, while inducible expression of B7-1 occurs about 24 hours after activation. CD28 (and CTLA4) binds to both B7-1 and B7-2. In the absence of CD28/B7 and CD40/CD40L interactions during TCR engagement, as occurs for antigen presented by nonprofessional antigen presenting host cells, the T cell becomes anergic.

LOSS OF SELF-TOLERANCE

Autoimmunity, following loss of self-tolerance, can occur as follows (Fig. 14.2):
(i) genetic defects leading to defects in lymphocyte regulation,
(ii) loss of apoptotic stimuli,
(iii) antigen related mechanisms,
(iv) hormonal influences and
(v) superantigen related mechanisms.

Antigen-related mechanisms
Antigen-related mechanisms include (i) **molecular mimicry** following infection, (ii) **cross reactivity** with a microbial epitope (iii) release of previously sequestered antigen, and (iv) altered antigen-presentation by nonprofessional antigen presenting cell.

Molecular mimicry
Loss of tolerance caused by molecular mimicry occurs because host tissues share an antigenic epitope, often identical over only a sequence of a few amino acids, with an infecting virus or bacteria. Activation of lymphocytes in response to microbial antigen produces clones of cells recognizing and interacting with self-tissues leading to a loss of tolerance. Presumably lymphocytes specific for that self antigen were not deleted (but were unresponsive for any/all of the reasons outlined above). As example, short amino acid sequences in myelin basic protein are identical to sequences in an adenovirus (type 2) protein, while other sequences are homologous to sequences in hepatitis B protein.

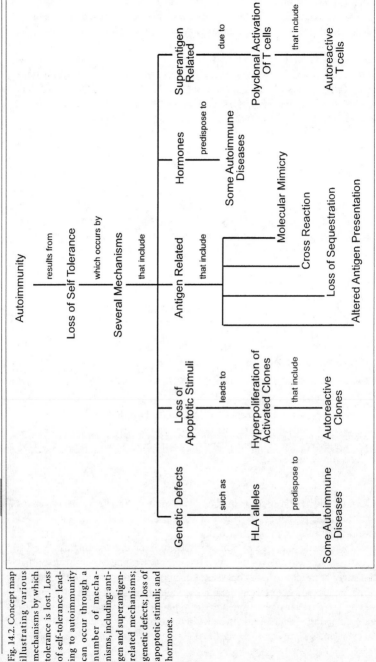

Fig. 14.2. Concept map illustrating various mechanisms by which tolerance is lost. Loss of self-tolerance leading to autoimmunity can occur through a number of mechanisms, including: antigen and superantigen-related mechanisms; genetic defects; loss of apoptotic stimuli; and hormones.

Cross-reactivity
Loss of self-tolerance may occur when host tissues display an epitope cross reactive with one present on the microbial antigen surface. An example is the cross-reactivity between HLA-B27 epitopes and epitopes on Klebsiella antigens, which is believed to underlie the HLA-B27 association with the autoimmune disease ankylosing spondylitis. Ninety percent of the individuals who present with this disease have the HLA-B27 allele, while only 7% of the normal population express it. The possibility has not been excluded that HLA-B27 association with ankylosing spondylitis reflects the fact that this HLA allele is expressed in *linkage disequilibrium* with a gene that encodes *the molecule* important for disease development.

Loss of antigen sequestration
Tolerance is "broken" if the immune system comes in contact with previously sequestered antigens, e.g., lens crystallin in the eye. When ocular damage (inflammation) occurs an immune response can develop to this previously sequestered antigen, resulting in ocular pathology.

Altered antigen presentation
This refers to the presentation of antigen/MHC by cells not normally expressing MHC (see sections (iv) and (v) above), and may be one of the most important mechanisms for autoimmunity. Lymphocytes specific for any tissue antigen pose no "danger" to the immune system unless the conditions for their activation are met, including presentation in association with MHC (class I or II) and costimulatory molecules. Cells in tissues expressing nonstimulating levels of MHC are unable to present those tissue antigens in immunogenic form. If increased expression of MHC occurs (e.g., following inflammation and IFNγ production, a known inducer of class I and II MHC), the tissue antigen may now be seen with sufficient avidity to cause activation of (self-reactive) T cells and autoimmunity.

Superantigen-related mechanisms
Superantigens activate entire sets of T cells whose T-cell receptors share a common variable region segment, typically in the TCR β chain, regardless of the overall antigen specificity of the cells—so-called oligoclonal expansion (Chapter 1). T-cell activation by superantigens is independent of the costimulation needed for activation by antigens recognized by the TCR α/β chains (Fig. 14.2). Oligoclonal activation and clonal expansion of quiescent and potentially autoreactive lymphocytes may induce autoimmunity.

Defects in lymphocyte regulation
A number of genetic defects can lead to autoimmunity, including defects in the normal regulation of lymphocyte development and activation (e.g., defects predisposing to low (regulatory) Th2 cytokine production-see below/Chapter 9). Autoreactive T cells can be activated as "bystander" cells during normal immunological responses to chronic infection, without necessarily being engaged optimally via their TCRs. Over time selection may result in expansion of high avidity (pathogenic) clones.

Loss of apoptotic stimuli
Autoreactive T-cell clones activated as "bystanders" during normal immunological responses to infection, generally die by apoptosis (programmed cell death) shortly after resolution of infection. Apoptosis following antigenic stimulation is mediated via interaction of two activation-induced proteins, Fas and Fas ligand (FasL). In the absence of Fas/FasL interaction, activated clones escape programmed cell death and continue to proliferate. Gene defects in either Fas or FasL are associated in animal models with glomerulonephritis and lymphadenopathy (uncontrolled proliferation of cells within lymphoid tissue).

Hormones
Hormones can influence the development of autoimmune disorders. The ratio of females to males presenting with Hashimoto's thyroiditis is 50:1. For systemic lupus erythematosus the ratio is 10:1. In contrast the incidence of ankylosing spondylitis is higher in males (male:female ratio, 9:1). The specific role of hormones on the development of disease is unknown.

IMMUNOPATHOLOGY OF AUTOIMMUNE DISORDERS: AUTOREACTIVE ANTIBODIES

Immunopathology generally reflects the presence of autoreactive antibodies, or the activation of T cells secreting type 1 cytokines, which activates phagocytes. A list of the more common autoimmune diseases, along with some characteristics of each disease, is illustrated in Table 14.1.

Autoreactive antibodies to cell bound antigens
Autoreactive antibodies bind to cell surface antigens and activate mechanisms leading to cell destruction (Fig. 14.3). Mechanisms of cell destruction are similar, whether the cell is in circulation (e.g., red blood cell in **cold agglutinin disease**), or a component of solid tissues (e.g., pancreatic islet cells, or gastric parietal cells, **in insulin-dependent diabetes mellitus** and **pernicious anemia**, respectively).

Complement-mediated cell lysis
Autoreactive antibodies, bound to cell surface antigens, stimulate activation of the classical complement pathway and generation of the membrane attack complex (MAC) destroying cells by osmotic lysis. The normal complement regulatory mechanisms are overwhelmed due to the unlimited source of antigen, and hence antibody.

Complement-mediated phagocytosis
In addition to MAC formation, complement activation also generates several proteolytic fragments including C3b and C5a. C3b is an opsonin that facilitates phagocytosis when it binds to cell surfaces; C5a is chemotactic for and an activator of neutrophils. Activated macrophages and neutrophils release cytokines, proteases, and inflammatory mediators that destroy the local tissue (Chapter 10). A vicious cycle begins, with more leukocytes recruited and activated to secrete cyto-

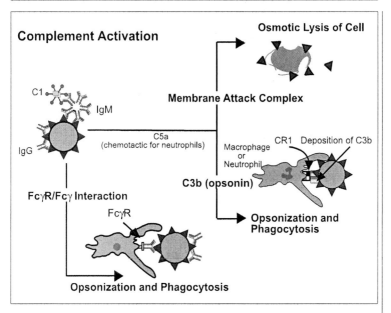

Fig. 14.3. Autoreactive antibodies bind to cell surface proteins and initiate cell damage. Large immune complexes are deposited and trapped in tissues. Complement activation generates the complement fragments C3b and C5a. C5a is chemotactic for, and an activator of, neutrophils. The opsonin, C3b, deposited on complexes, induces activation of and opsonin-mediated phagocytosis by neutrophils. Neutrophils release toxic products locally and induce damage to basement membranes.

toxic molecules and proteases into the local microenvironment causing more tissue damage.

Antibody-mediated phagocytosis

When IgG binds to a cell surface antigen the Fc portion of the antibody undergoes a conformational change allowing it to interact with Fcγ receptors (FcγR) present on neutrophils and macrophages. For tissue bound cells, tissue macrophages are activated as they attempt to phagocytose these cells. Secretion of toxic products and local tissue damage follows as described above.

Blocking or stimulation of receptors

Autoreactive antibodies may be specific for cell surface receptors. Pathology can result, not primarily from phagocytic or complement-mediated damage as described above, but following modification of cell bioactivity as a result of binding to the receptor.

Autoreactive antibodies to soluble antigens

When autoreactive antibodies are specific for soluble antigens, large immune complexes (between soluble antigens and antibodies) are formed in serum. Under normal conditions, the number and size of these immune complexes are sufficiently small that they are eliminated by the clearance mechanisms of the reticuloendothelial system (phagocytic macrophages in the spleen and liver). When the size and number of the immune complexes overwhelm these clearance mechanisms, complexes are deposited and trapped in tissues (Fig. 14.4).

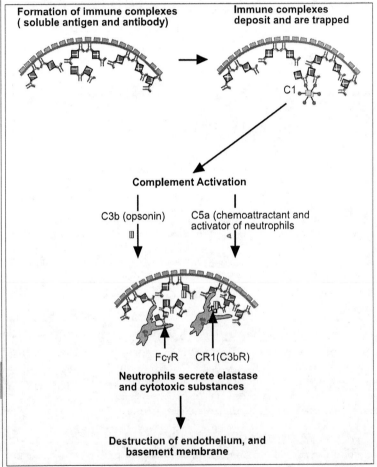

Fig. 14.4. Formation and deposition of large immune complexes initiates tissue damage. Autoantibodies bind to cell surface antigens and activate mechanisms leading to cell destruction. These mechanisms include complement-mediated cell lysis by the membrane attack complex and C3b and IgG opsonin-mediated phagocytosis. Macrophages and neutrophils, activated by C5a, release cytokines, proteases, and toxic reactive oxygen and nitrogen intermediates.

C3b and IgG opsonin-mediated phagocytosis

IgG or IgM, when bound to antigens, stimulates the activation of complement, leading to the deposition of the opsonin, C3b, on the complexes and to the release of C5a, which is chemotactic for and an activator of neutrophils. The presence of IgG and C3b on the immune complexes induces activation of recruited neutrophils leading to local inflammation (see above). In **systemic lupus erythematosus** (SLE), immune complexes are deposited and trapped in the basement membranes of glomeruli, joint synovia, skin/endothelium.

Antibodies block function of soluble proteins

Some autoreactive antibodies bind to soluble proteins, inhibiting their function. Autoreactive antibodies to **intrinsic factor** (IF) block its binding to vitamin B12. Under normal conditions, intrinsic factor (secreted by the stomach) complexes with ingested vitamin B12. This complex binds to a receptor in the intestinal mucosa, releasing vitamin B12, which is then transported to the blood stream. Antibodies that block the vitamin B12 binding site of intrinsic factor leave the individual unable to absorb vitamin B12 causing pernicious anemia. **Pernicious anemia** may also be caused by destruction of gastric parietal cells that secrete intrinsic factor (Table 14.1).

IMMUNOPATHOLOGY OF AUTOIMMUNE DISORDERS: CELL MEDIATED IMMUNITY

For some autoimmune diseases, cell mediated immunity is the primary cause of observed pathology (Fig. 14.5). The additional presence of autoreactive antibodies in some diseases may confuse the issue. Studies with experimental animals, in which disease is transferred by cells, and not by serum, have been used to verify the role of leukocytes in pathology. Autoimmune disorders of T-cell etiology include **Hashimoto's thyroiditis** and **multiple sclerosis**.

Role of CD4+ T cells

A number of factors (Fig. 14.2) can cause loss of tolerance in and activation of CD4+ T cells. When the autoreactive CD4+ T cells are of the Th1 phenotype they will secrete Type 1 cytokines, IL-2, IFNγ, and TNF. While IL-2 is a growth factor for T cells, INFγ and TNF can activate tissue macrophages in the absence of microbes (see below). In addition to the tissue damage mediated by inflammatory mediators, the persistence of antigen and polarization of the CD4+ T-cell response to a Th1 phenotype secreting Type 1 cytokines overrides normal regulatory mechanisms (Th2 cells and Type 2 cytokines) that might dampen the response. Unregulated Type 1 cytokine secretion contributes to the inflammation and tissue damage seen in histological sections from thyroid tissue of patients with Hashimoto's thyroiditis.

Role of tissue macrophages

Activated macrophages can also secrete cytokines, proteases, and inflammatory mediators into the local microenvironment causing tissue damage. The response is amplified because the secreted products lead to the recruitment and

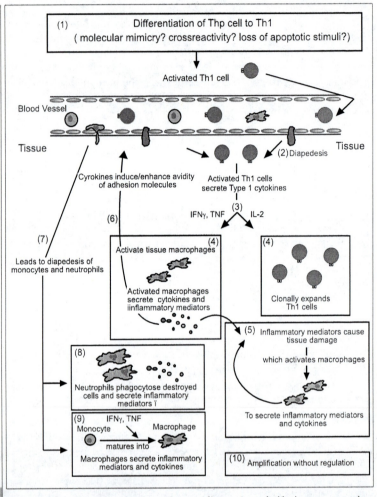

Fig. 14.5. Cell mediated immunity in autoimmune diseases. Loss of self-tolerance can produce activation of CD4+ T cells that secrete Type 1 cytokines, IL-2, IFNγ, and TNF. IL-2 is a growth factor for T cells. IFNγ and TNF can activate tissue macrophages in the absence of microbes. Activated tissue macrophages secrete cytokines, proteases, and toxic reactive oxygen and nitrogen intermediates locally, causing tissue damage. The secreted products recruit and activate monocytes, neutrophils, and lymphocytes, amplifying the response.

activation of monocytes, neutrophils, and lymphocytes into the tissues. Cell damage releases numerous previously sequestered antigens to which the host can now generate antibodies. In the continuing presence of antigen, immune complexes are formed and cause damage as described above.

Immunotherapy of Autoimmune Disease: Suppression

The spectrum of immunotherapy for autoimmune diseases includes the following (i) nonspecific immunosuppression, (ii) specific immunosuppression and (iii) cytokine modulation.

Nonspecific immunosuppression
Nonspecific immunosuppression does NOT reflect suppression of antigen-specific T- or B-cell clones. Nonspecific suppression can be general, or it may include classes or subclasses of cells.

Anti-inflammatory agents
Anti-inflammatory agents, nonsteroidal anti-inflammatory drugs (NSAIDs) and prednisone, methotrexate, and imuran are general nonspecific anti-inflammatory agents. One of the mechanisms by which the nonsteroidal anti-inflammatory drugs mediate their effects is through inhibition of products of the arachidonic acid pathway (prostaglandins, leukotrienes).

T-cell (but nonantigen) specific agents
T-cell specific agents include cyclosporin, antibodies to CD3, antibodies to the interleukin-2 receptor (IL-2R), and antibodies to the TCR beta chain variable segments. These T-cell specific agents inhibit primarily the CD4+ T-cell population such that IL-2, the T-cell growth factor, is not transcribed, secreted, or bound by its receptor. In each case, the goal is to prevent the amplification of the response by inhibiting the proliferation and clonal expansion of those T cells that would secrete more IL-2, IFNγ, and TNF, and perpetuate the response.

Antigen specific immunosuppression

Anti-TCR antibodies
Anti-TCR antibodies recognizing unique sequences in the variable region (anti-idiotypic antibodies) have proven successful in **experimental allergic encephalitis**, an animal model for **multiple sclerosis**. Anti-idiotypic antibodies target only the clone of T cells binding the relevant autoantigens, and immunity to other pathogens is unaffected. While intriguing because of their exquisite specificity, these may not be routinely useful clinically (each patient will likely have a unique idiotype). Evidence for limited expansion of the *same* TCR-bearing T cells would imply a useful role for anti-Vβ TCR antibodies.

Anti-MHC antibodies or peptide antagonists
Anti-class II MHC antibodies prevent CD4+ T-cell activation because the antibody binds to the peptide/class II MHC complex blocking its binding to the TCR. While this inhibits the recognition of all antigenic peptides that bind to a particular class II MHC allele, most individuals express other allelic forms of class II MHC due to the codominant expression of the MHC proteins.

Table 14.1(A). Spectrum of autoimmune disorders

Autoimmune Disease	Ratio F/M	HLA Association	Antigen	Primary Pathology Initiated by	General Features
Systemic Lupus Erythematosus	10:1	HLA-DR2 HLA-DR3	Ds-DNA	Immune Complexes (IC)	• Systemic and multiorgan (NON organ specific) • IC are formed in serum and trapped in basement membrane of glomeruli, skin/endothelium, synovia of joints, kidney • Anti-DS-DNA and anti-leukocyte antibodies • Anti-phospholipid antibody (also termed, "lupus anti-coagulant) • Polyclonal B-cell activation • Etiology unknown
Rheumatoid Arthritis	3:1	HLA-DR1 HLA-DR4		Cell Mediated and Immune Complexes	• Mixture of organ specific and systemic symptoms • Joint involvement; lung, cardiac, skin, and CNS pathology • Excessive Type 1 cytokines • Rheumatoid factors—IgM (or IgG/IgA) to the Fc of IgG. These are not essential for disease, may enhance IC • Some association with Epstein Barr virus (EBV), and human T lymphocyte virus I (HTLV-I)
Hashimoto's Thyroiditis	50:1	—		Cell Mediated	• Organ specific—thyroid • Anti-thyroglobulin and anti-microsomal antibodies are secondary to gland destruction (use for diagnosis) • Manifests as goiter and/or hypothyroidism • Peaks at 3rd or 4th decade

Table 14.1(B). Spectrum of autoimmune disorders

Autoimmune Disease	Ratio F/M	HLA Association	Antigen	Primary Pathology Initiated by	General Features
Multiple Sclerosis	2:1	HLA-DR-2		Cell Mediated	• Organ specific: brain and spinal cord • Antibodies to myelin basic protein (MBP) secondary to cell death • Oliogoclonal, not polyclonal antibodies in cerebral spinal fluid • Some evidence for previous infection with paramyxovirus • Regions further away from equator have greater incidence • Predominantly a Caucasian disease • Evidence that environmental factor triggers disease (virus?) • Treatment with IFNβ (inhibits IFNγ expression of MHC class II)
Scleroderma	3:1	HLA-DR3 (weak)		Cell mediated	• Multi-organ: primarily in the skin/ectodermal tissues, but can cause multi-organ pathology as a result, e.g., GI tract, heart, lung • Skin fibroblasts reproduce faster and secrete more collagen
Goodpasture's Syndrome	1:4 Two peaks, young, and elderly	—	Basement Membrane Antigens	Antibodies to Cell Surface Antigens	• Organ specific (lungs and kidneys) • Anti-glomerular basement membrane antibodies (anti-GBM) • Shared antigens between the lung (alveolar) and the glomerular basement membrane • Linear deposition of IgG and complement

Table 14.1(C). Spectrum of autoimmune disorders

Autoimmune Disease	Ratio F/M	HLA Association	Antigen	Primary Pathology Initiated by	General Features
Addison's Disease	2:1	—	Cytoplasmic cortical antigens and/or ACTH* receptors	Antibodies	<ul><li>Organ specific: adrenals</li><li>Chronic hypoadrenalism</li><li>Some evidence for association with *M. tuberculosis* infection</li><li>Antibodies to adrenal cell microsomes</li><li>Cortex involvement (not medulla)</li><li>Adrenocorticotrophic hormone* (ACTH)</li></ul>
Insulin-dependent Diabetes Mellitus (IDDM)	5:1	HLA-DR3 HLA-DR4	Islet cells Insulin	Antibodies to cell surface antigens	<ul><li>Organ specific—pancreas</li><li>Impending diabetes associated with antibodies to glutamic acid decarboxylase (ongoing trials to treat early with immunosuppression before development of diabetes)</li><li>Environmental trigger (viruses? e.g. Cocksackie virus B4)</li></ul>
Pernicious Anemia				Antibodies cell surface antigens and/or Intrinsic Factor (IF) blocking antibodies	<ul><li>Cell specific; defective red blood cells due to malabsorption of vitamin B12.</li><li>Antibodies bind cell surface antigens and destroy parietal gastric cells that secrete intrinsic factor (IF) or</li><li>Antibodies bind to IF and prevent binding of vitamin B12</li><li>Leads to megaloblastic anemia</li></ul>
Grave's Disease	8:1	HLA-DR-3 HLA- BW35		Antibodies to receptor	<ul><li>Organ specific: thyroid</li><li>Antibodies to the TSH (thyrotropin) receptor stimulate thyroid hormone synthesis</li><li>Get unregulated secretion of thyroxin which leads to hyperthyroidism</li></ul>

Autoimmunity

Table 14.1(D). Spectrum of autoimmune disorders

Autoimmune Disease	Ratio F/M	HLA Association	Antigen	Primary Pathology Initiated by	General Features
Myasthenia Gravis	4:1	Complex/Age Dependent	Acetylcholine Receptor	Antibodies to receptor (blocking antibodies)	• Tissue specific: nerve and muscle—with systemic effects • Neuromuscular transmission disorder • Antibodies are inhibitory and block acetylcholine binding • Some evidence for prior infection with poliovirus
Ankylosing Spondylitis	1:9	HLA-B27 (98%)			• Tissue specific—with systemic effects • Joints • Some evidence for prior infection with *Klebsiella pneumoniae* • There is NO rheumatoid factor
Acanthosis Nigricans				Antireceptor antibodies	• Antibodies to the insulin receptor, with systemic effects • Block binding of insulin to the insulin receptor • Name of disease originates from hyperpigmentation in the flexer and intertriginous areas ???
Cold Agglutinin Disease			Glycophorin or Ii	Antibodies to cell surface antigens	• Only manifests at temperatures below 37°C • Occurs only at the extremities (nose, fingers, toes) when the individual is exposed to cold temperatures • Treatment—keep patient warm and extremities well protected

Peptide antagonists are synthetic molecules, differing from the putative autoantigen only at those amino acids that confer a signaling function after engagement of the TCR. Binding of the antagonist functionally neutralizes autoantigen specific TCRs, without activating the T cells. This approach successfully treats experimental allergic encephalitis (above). Clinically, some information on the putative autoantigen is a prerequisite, in order to synthesize potentially inhibitory ligands.

IMMUNOTHERAPY OF AUTOIMMUNE DISORDERS: CYTOKINE MODULATION

Type 2 cytokines

Pathology associated with multiple sclerosis, (MS), and Hashimoto's thyroiditis, (HT), to name but two diseases, often results from unregulated production of Type 1 cytokines. Under normal circumstances, naive CD4+ T cells differentiate to both Th1 and Th2 cells with one response predominating. Where pathology is attributable to cytokine secretion by Th1 cells, there is a rationale for administration of Type 2 cytokines (e.g., IL-4, TGFβ and IL-13) since these cytokines dampen further Th1 development (Chapter 9). In experimental conditions this has not been as effective as would have been expected with the exception of the use of IL-4 in mice suffering from insulin-dependent diabetes mellitus (**NOD mice**).

Anti-cytokine antibodies

Monoclonal antibodies to cytokines themselves may be effective in some autoimmune diseases. TNF is found at elevated levels in inflamed joints where it causes activation of inflammatory cells within the joint and upregulates expression of a number of so-called adhesion molecules and their counter-receptors (ICAM/LFA-1 etc) which play a role in regulating migration of inflammatory cells to the joint synovium. Ongoing clinical trials are examining the use of antibodies to TNF to "shut-down" the stimulation of inflammatory cells within the rheumatoid joint by released TNF. Human trials with rheumatoid arthritis patients have met with some success.

Induction of Type 2 cytokines

Oral feeding of antigen promotes "tolerance" to diseases associated with Type 1 cytokines. One explanation suggests increased production of TGFβ, IL-10, and IL-4 which "switches" Th cells to a Th2 phenotype (Chapters 9). Immunologically, TGFβ inhibits the proliferation of T cells, B cells, and natural killer cells by inhibition of cycle progression. Clinical trials in which patients with multiple sclerosis are orally fed brain extract are in progress and have met with some success. Note that current (experimental) data suggests that the mechanism of regulation involved after oral feeding of antigen is quite complex, with local (mucosal) increased expression of MCP-1, decreased expression of IL-12, and thus dampening of Type 1 cytokine production (Chapter 9). These data in turn suggest that later trials might also include manipulation of chemokine production. This therapy requires some knowledge of the relevant antigen.

Summary

Tolerance is a state of nonresponsiveness to a molecule (i.e., antigen). Self tolerance, therefore, refers to the state of immunological nonresponsiveness that exists in the presence of self molecules, (i.e., self antigens). Those T-cell or B-cell clones whose antigen receptors recognize self-antigen are said to be autoreactive or self-reactive. Deletion, or inactivation, of these self-reactive clones (tolerance induction) is believed to occur during lymphocyte maturation in primary lymphoid tissues. Some self-reactive clones, however, have been identified in the periphery suggesting that tolerance to self-antigens must also be acquired by peripheral mechanisms. Tolerance induction of T cells and B cells occurs during maturation in the thymus and bone marrow, respectively. For T cells, tolerance induction is the result of negative selection in the thymus. In the process of negative selection, potentially self-reactive thymocytes are clonally eliminated or functionally inactivated. For B cells, tolerance induction occurs at the immature B-cell stage and leads to either clonal anergy or apoptosis. Peripheral mechanisms for tolerance induction include (i) suppression by T-cell derived cytokines, (ii) lack of T-cell help for B-cell activation, (iii) absence of appropriate major histocompatibility complex (MHC) molecules for antigen presentation, and (iv) absence of costimulatory molecules. Loss of self-tolerance leading to autoimmunity has been postulated to occur via a number of mechanisms. These include (i) genetic defects leading to defects in lymphocyte regulation, (ii) loss of apoptotic stimuli, (iii) antigen related mechanisms, (iv) hormonal influences and (v) superantigen related mechanisms.

Immunopathology of autoimmune disorders is triggered by the presence of autoreactive antibodies or by the activation of T cells that secrete Type 1 cytokines leading to the activation of phagocytes. Diseases arising from a breakdown in tolerance are termed autoimmune diseases. Autoreactive antibodies may be generated that recognize antigens present on the cell, while other autoreactive antibodies may recognize soluble antigens. Autoreactive antibodies binding to cell surface antigens activate mechanisms that lead to the destruction of the cell. Mechanisms of cell destruction are similar, whether the cell is in circulation, or whether the cell is a component of solid tissues. When autoreactive antibodies are specific for soluble antigens, large immune complexes (between soluble antigens and antibodies) are formed in serum. Under normal conditions, the number and size of these immune complexes are sufficiently small and so these would be eliminated by the normal. However, when the size and number of the immune complexes overwhelm the clearance mechanisms, complexes are deposited and trapped in tissues causing immunopathology. For some autoimmune diseases, cell mediated immunity is the primary cause of observed pathology. The additional presence of autoreactive antibodies in some diseases may confuse the issue. Studies with experimental animals, however, in which disease is transferred by cells, and not by serum, have been used to verify the role of leukocytes in pathology of some autoimmune disorders.

The spectrum of immunotherapy for autoimmune diseases includes the following (i) nonspecific immunosuppression, (ii) specific immunosuppression and (iii) cytokine modulation. Nonspecific suppression refers to the suppression of immune responses, rather than suppression of a specific T-cell or B-cell clone. Nonspecific suppression can be very general or it may include classes or subclasses of cells. Specific suppression targets clones of cells, or small subsets of a larger population. Much of the pathology associated with autoimmune disorders is the result of unregulated production of Type 1 cytokines. Therapies designed to shift the response to the production of Type 2 cytokines induce tolerance by regulating (inhibiting) the secretion of Type 1 cytokines. Tuning down Th1 cell stimulation, not surprisingly, is of benefit.

CLINICAL CASES AND DISCUSSION

Clinical Case #27
Brenda is a 25-year-old, married, black female. She is adopted. Over the last 5 months she has noticed increasing swelling in her legs, and she has had intermittent severe headaches, unrelated to menses. Also, she has noticed that her urine is dark and "frothy", which when tested indicated the presence of protein (creatinine) and red blood cells. Despite her and her husband's wishes, she has been unable to conceive for 5 years, and has had 3 spontaneous first trimester abortions.

Questions and Discussion: Case #27
1. List the six likely key features we need to bear in mind in discussing this case.

Young female
Adopted
Swelling in her legs
Intermittent severe headaches
Protein and red blood cells in urine
Three spontaneous abortions

2. What is the significance of this leg swelling and urinary problems in an otherwise healthy 25-year old?
Leg swelling in an otherwise healthy individual makes one wonder about renal problems. In the absence of infection this suggests noninfectious inflammation "higher up" the urinary tract (in the kidney).

3. Name one **noninfectious inflammatory disorder of the kidney** and the stimulus/mediator of inflammation.
Glomerulonephritis is caused by immune complex deposition in glomeruli. Immune complexes activate complement, producing C3b, an opsonin, and C5a, which is both chemotactic for and an activator of neutrophils. Neutrophils attempt to phagocytose the immune complexes and secrete toxic inflammatory mediators and proteases into the local microenvironment, producing tissue damage (see Fig. 13.3). C5a induces histamine release from connective tissue mast

cells, leading to increased vascular permeability and trapping of immune complexes in the basement membrane.

4. What might you expect to see if serum C3 levels were measured?

Following complement activation, C3 convertase degrades C3, so one would expect to see decreased C3 levels, relative to normal controls. Levels may be concordant with disease activity.

5. What might you expect to see if a biopsy of renal glomeruli were performed and incubated with immunofluorescent antibodies binding the Fc region of IgG or IgM?

IgG and IgM bind to immune complexes. You would expect to see staining indicating antibodies in the basement membrane/endothelia.

6. Severe intermittent headaches might be a forerunner of a central nervous system (CNS) malignancy. Assuming this is NOT the case, are there immunological reasons for headaches?

In the absence of other causes (both nonlife threatening (e.g., migraine) and otherwise (tumor)), headaches can be caused immunologically by inflammation within blood vessel walls in the CNS. This vasculitis (cerebritis) follows immune complex deposition on basement membranes/endothelia, with complement activation (as described in #3) and subsequent changes in vessel permeability with edema/release of inflammatory mediators.

7. What might you expect to see if you performed a biopsy of blood vessels within the CNS and incubated the tissue with immunofluorescent antibodies to the Fc region of IgG or IgM?

Again, because immune complexes are deposited in the blood vessel walls, one would expect to see immunofluorescent staining.

8. CNS inflammation can often cause very significant CNS pathology. Seizures have been described in this scenario. Neuropsychiatric testing often reveals significant deficits (e.g., in memory, intellectual ability). Are these permanent?

Generally not, if aggressive treatment with potent anti-inflammatory agents and/or immunosuppressive agents is used (e.g., imuran, cyclophosphamide). Presumably the deficits seen reflect transient neurological "stunning" from inflammation.

9. Are there any immunological causes of spontaneous abortions?

In a number of autoimmune diseases autoantibodies are formed. IgG antibodies can cross the placenta and interfere with fetal well-being.

10. In systemic lupus erythematosus (SLE), which is associated with immune complex deposition disease and renal failure (glomerulonephritis), what antibodies might cross into the fetus?

In SLE, anti-platelet, anti-leukocyte and anti-DNA antibodies are common. In addition, the so-called lupus anti-coagulant (a misnomer, because it is a cause of thrombosis!) is an anti-phospholipid autoantibody that causes spontaneous abortions after placental passage.

11. What would you expect to find if you ordered detailed analysis of the mother's serum immunoglobulin and a routine CBC (complete blood count)?

One would expect to find evidence for different autoantibodies, including lupus anti-coagulant. Autoantibodies are often directed towards platelets and white/red blood cells leading to thrombocytopenia, leukopenia and anemia.

12. What is a Coomb's test?

The direct Coomb's test measures anti-red blood cell antibodies bound to the red blood cell. The indirect Coomb's test measures the presence of serum antibodies to an antigen present on a particulate antigen (e.g., Rh antigen on red blood cells).

13. Not uncommonly we see a TRANSIENT neonatal "heart block" (a cardiac arrhythmia caused by autoantibodies) in offspring of SLE mothers. Why is it transient?

The effect is transient because the fetus is not the source of the autoantibody, the mother is. When this antibody is "diluted out" postpartum (3-6 months) by the baby's own antibody, the problem resolves. Recall the half-life of IgG is about three weeks.

14. Why are we given information on this lady's age/sex/ethnicity and family tree?

At the age of 25 years congenital defects are unlikely to make their first appearance. Because she is adopted we cannot trace potential genetic susceptibility for her disease. However, SLE is one disorder in which data indicate that black females have increased susceptibility.

15. Do you know of any other genetic relatedness in this disorder?

There is a known independent genetic association with HLA-DR2 and HLA-DR3. Adding further evidence for genetic susceptibility is the greater concordance (similarity) in monozygotic versus dizygotic twins (30% vs < 10%). There is also a correlation with complement C2 and C4 genes and TNF receptor genes.

Clinical Case Case #28

GK is a 35-year-old farmer from the American Midwest. He complains of weight loss (10 Kg over 4 weeks), intermittent fever, dark colored urine and, recently, coughing up blood in his sputum. There is no history of travel out of the country, and his past medical history is otherwise quite unremarkable. Routine blood work is essentially normal as is a chest x-ray (CXR).

Questions and Discussion: Case #28

1. We need to bear in mind the following in discussing this case.

Mature, male, farmer from American Midwest
Weight loss
Intermittent fever
Dark colored urine
Blood in sputum (hemoptysis)
Normal blood work and chest x-ray

2. *What are the significant negatives?*
This patient has no history of travel out of the country nor prior medical abnormalities.

3. *Unintended weight loss of 10 Kg in 4 weeks is significant.* We are told he is a farmer, has had an intermittent fever, and now has hemoptysis. A number of diseases present in this manner, and so our approach must be one of elimination. The fact that this patient is a farmer may be significant. Name one disorder and one infectious disease to which farmers may be susceptible.

Farmer's Lung is a hypersensitivity reaction triggered by antigens in the grain (Chapter 13). This commonly presents with low-grade fever, dyspnea, and hemoptysis. Farmers are also subject to aspergillosis, a chronic fungal infection, resulting from exposure to mouldy grain in silos-this can present with hemoptysis.

4. *The patient has dark urine.* Urinalysis revealed blood, casts (complex arrays of molecules/tissue detritus, which represent an outline or "cast" of a component of the urinary tree), and proteins. All of these reflect a generalized failure of the filtration apparatus of the glomerulus itself. Explain why the two disorders (in #3 are not a consideration for this farmer.

Neither disorder would cause this kind of renal problem because the damage they cause is primarily to a different organ system (the lung). So, unless he has two diseases, we need to rethink.

5. *Tuberculosis (TB) could present this way,* particularly in severe cases with extrapulmonary TB and with a unintended weight loss of 10 Kg in 4 weeks. In extrapulmonary TB with renal involvement you might expect the patient to be chronically febrile (albeit low-grade). There is nothing here in his lifestyle to suggest a high risk for TB. What lifestyles predispose to tuberculosis? What test could confirm that TB is not a likely possibility and what control would you use?

In Western countries, street individuals or those living in crowded, relatively unsanitary conditions are at high risk. This man is a Midwest farmer and so is not considered at risk. Recall that his chest x-ray is normal. However, a purified protein derivative (PPD) test could eliminate TB as an option. The test for tuberculosis is an injection of a purified protein derived from *Mycobacterium tuberculosis* culture supernatants, termed purified protein derivative (PPD). It is injected (subcutaneously) on one arm while on the other arm, injection of killed yeast organisms, *Candida albicans*, serves as a positive control. The general population has been exposed to the latter organism, and in immunocompetent individuals a response, manifest as swelling and redness at the site of injection, is observed. A negative PPD test in the presence of a positive yeast test is a reliable negative result. However, a negative PPD test and a negative yeast test is not interpretable.

6. *Goodpasture's syndrome is an antibody-mediated autoimmune disorder which manifests as lysis of cells, bleeding, and the symptoms described above. How could you test for this?*

Individuals with Goodpasture's syndrome have antibodies to cell surface antigens on the basement membrane of lungs and kidneys. Therefore, test for anti-basement membrane antibodies. See Figure14.4 for mode of cell destruction.

7. What if, in addition, he complained of painful nodules on his arms, with some necrotic lesions, and you notice a loss of motor nerve function in the foot/ankle. Would this change your thoughts and actions?

Yes...we now would wonder whether we were dealing with a vasculitis, resulting from the trapping of immune complexes in the membrane. This is distinct from Goodpasture's disease, in which the antibodies are directed **TO** basement membrane antigens. Compare Figs. 13.3, 13.4. Vasculitis causes disease in a systemic/multi-organ fashion.

8. Differences in the etiology of Goodpasture's syndrome versus vasculitis lead to different pathology and different treatment. What is effective treatment for each disorder?

Goodpasture's syndrome can be treated effectively in the acute phase with plasmaphoresis since the "culprit" is autoreactive antibody to basement membrane. Plasmaphoresis filters blood to remove plasma/protein components, returning washed cells to the patient. Nonspecific immunosuppression is also given to stop further B-cell and T-cell activation leading to antibody production and inflammation.

Immune complex vasculitic disorders would be treated by drugs designed to shut off antibody production (e.g., cyclophosphamide). Plasmaphoresis is not as effective since the disorder is more chronic in nature and generally does not present as an acute, potentially life-threatening, complaint (unlike the lung injury in Goodpasture's). For vasculitis, plasmaphoresis does not treat the cause, but only a symptom, so it is used only where the symptom poses significant problems. In both cases definitive treatment (immunosuppression) is aimed at the cause of the disorder (aberrant production of autoantibodies).

TEST YOURSELF

Multiple Choice Questions

1. A man of 28 years, HLA-B27, attends clinic complaining of swollen, tender knees. Fluid in the knee contained polymorphonuclear leukocytes but no micro-organisms. The pain settled but he returned 5 months later complaining of back pain/stiffness. He had no detectable circulating autoantibodies but ossified ligaments in the pelvic region. He most likely suffers from?
    a. Ankylosing spondylitis
    b. Rheumatoid arthritis
    c. Systematic lupus erythematosus
    d. Multiple sclerosis
    e. Chronic granulomatous disease

2. You have a muscle biopsy from a patient with myasthenia gravis. Immunohistochemical staining shows linear deposition of antibodies along the muscle cell membrane in the region of the nerve/muscle junction. These antibodies are:
    a. Anti-nuclear
    b. Anti-glomerular basement membrane

c. Anti-myelin basic protein
d. Anti-acetylcholine receptor

3. A 57-year-old female complains of cold intolerance and undue fatigue. Her hemoglobin is 13 gm/dL (normal is 12-14 gm/dL). Tests indicate autoantibodies to thyroglobulin and to microsomal antigens from thyroid epithelial cells. This patient likely has:
   a. Rheumatoid arthritis
   b. Goodpasture's syndrome
   c. Hashimoto's thyroiditis
   d. Systemic lupus erythematosus
   e. Myasthenia gravis

4. Eve is patient of yours you believe has multiple sclerosis (MS). A sample of her CSF (fluid obtained by lumber puncture) reveals oligoclonal banding. Which of the following is true?
   a. Oligoclonal bands detect a single unique antibody directed to myelin antigens in the CSF.
   b. Oligoclonal banding detects antibodies responsible for all manifestations of MS.
   c. Oligoclonal bands provide useful information to support the diagnosis of MS.
   d. Oligoclonal bands are a common manifestation of an X-linked immune deficiency disorder.

5. A 34-year-old female complains of palpitations, sweats, and an increased appetite for the last 3 months. Her mother has diabetes and experienced an early menopause. Both are HLA-DR3+. Blood work reveals high levels of thyroid stimulating immunoglobin (antibody that mimics the action of TSH). The likely diagnosis is:
   a. Factitious disease, caused by self-treatment with thyroxin (thyroid stimulating hormone)
   b. Early ovarian failure
   c. Type I diabetes (diabetes mellitus)
   d. Hashimoto's thyroiditis
   e. Grave's disease

Answers: 1a; 2d; 3c; 4c; 5e

Short Answer Questions:
1. Name several mechanisms involved in self tolerance.
2. How does immune complex deposition lead to inflammation?
3. How might some autoimmune disorders be linked with MHC?
4. How does T-cell cytokine production alter autoimmune processes?
5. What are antagonist peptides?

Immunodeficiency Disorders

Objectives	314
Immunodeficiency Disorders	315
General Features	315
Primary Immunodeficiency Disorders	315
Primary Immunodeficiency Disorders: Progenitor Cells	315
Primary Immunodeficiency Disorders: T Cells	319
Primary Immunodeficiency Disorders: B Cells	320
Primary Immunodefieciency Disorders: Phagocytic	323
Primary Immunodeficiency Disorders: Other Leukocytes	323
Primary Immunodeficiency Disorders: Complement	323
Secondary Immunodeficiency Disorders	327
Secondary Immunodeficiency Disorders: Acquired	329
Secondary Immunodeficiency Disorders: Abnormal Production of Immune Components	330
Summary	330
Clinical Cases and Discussion	331
Test Yourself	335

Objectives

Individuals whose immune system is operationally defective are, by definition, immunodeficient. Conventionally we classify these as primary (i.e., genetically predetermined) or secondary (e.g., to environmental insults) disorders. The purpose of the following chapter is to familiarize the student with various presentations of immunodeficiency disease. These diseases, in general, are readily understandable in terms of current thinking concerning: (a) the regulation of ontogeny of the immune system, and (b) the different mechanisms used by the immune system for host defense. As an example of the latter, if cytotoxic T cells are so important for eradication of virally infected cells, we might expect that T-cell deficiencies will be recognizable by an increased susceptibility to viral infections.

The net outcome (in terms of disease susceptibility) is a little more complicated than this simple example however, because the immune system itself has great redundancy built into it. Without such redundancy, defects in one pathway might leave the developing organism totally unable to survive in a hostile (immunologically speaking) world. Note that some immunodeficiency diseases are associated not necessarily with a clear "lack" of one immune component, but with overproduction of some components (at the expense of normal immune homeostasis). In such cases, the diseases that result can reflect both immune impairment and other concomitant physiological disruptions (e.g., a susceptibility to strokes

Clinical Immunology, by Reginald Gorczynski and Jacqueline Stanley. ©2001 Landes Bioscience

in those patients with overproduction of serum proteins, and thus a hyperviscosity syndrome).

IMMUNODEFICIENCY DISORDERS

GENERAL FEATURES

Dysfunction in components of either innate or adaptive immunity causes **immunodeficiency disorders**. These disorders are classified as either *primary* or *secondary*, depending on whether the dysfunction is inherited or acquired (Fig. 15.1). Inherited, or primary disorders, may arise from defects in either cellular or humoral components of immunity, with some defects being more common than others (Fig. 15.2). In the absence of medical intervention (e.g., gene therapy), primary disorders are permanent. In contrast, acquired, or secondary disorders, may be transient or permanent depending on the factor inducing the immunosuppression. Secondary disorders are extrinsic and may result from the effect of drugs (alcohol), infection (human immunodeficiency virus (HIV)), or other miscellaneous (unknown) etiologies (e.g., insulin dependent diabetes mellitus (IDDM)), or from abnormal production of immune components.

PRIMARY IMMUNODEFICIENCY DISORDERS

Host defense in response to a particular microbe does not necessarily result from engagement of all components of immunity. Consequently, different defects lead to increased, but selective, susceptibility to microbes reflecting the particular aspects of immunity required to eliminate the organism. An understanding of the mechanisms by which the immune system eliminates microbial intruders enables us to predict the organisms to which increased susceptibility will occur given a specific defect (Chapter 11). Additionally, an awareness of the developmental pathways of hematopoietic cells enables us to predict the components of immunity that will be affected by a particular developmental block. An overview of the hematopoietic development pathways of cells that participate in immunity, and the disorders associated with blocks in these developmental pathways, is illustrated in Figure 15.3. **Primary immunodeficiency disorders** may arise from defects in progenitor cells (15-18%), phagocytes (20%), B cells (50%), T cells (10%), or complement (2-4%).

PRIMARY IMMUNODEFICIENCY DISORDERS: PROGENITOR CELLS

Progenitor cell disorders represent some 15-18% of all immunodeficiency disorders. Stem cell and lymphoid progenitor cell defects represent two major classes of progenitor cell disorders (Fig. 15.3, Table 15.1).

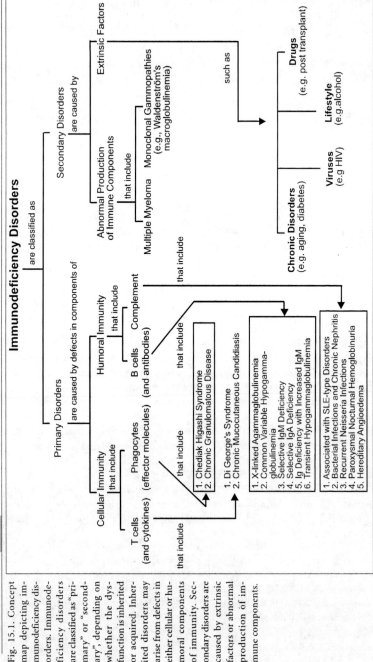

Fig. 15.1. Concept map depicting immunodeficiency disorders. Immunodeficiency disorders are classified as "primary" or "secondary", depending on whether the dysfunction is inherited or acquired. Inherited disorders may arise from defects in either cellular or humoral components of immunity. Secondary disorders are caused by extrinsic factors or abnormal production of immune components.

Immunodeficiency Disorders

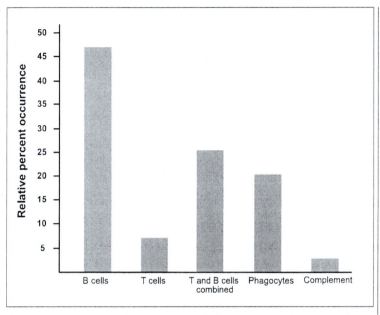

Fig. 15.2. Relative prevalence of primary immunodeficiency disorders. Defects in B cells, T cells, phagocytes, and complement lead to immunodeficiency disorders.

Stem cell

Individuals with no pluripotent stem cells (**reticular dysgenesis**) are deficient in all lymphoid and myeloid cells and are anemic. These individuals have increased susceptibility to all infectious agents. Therapy for this disorder is bone marrow transplantation.

Lymphoid progenitor cell

A defect in lymphoid progenitor cells results in **severe combined immunodeficiency** (SCID), a disorder with a profound deficiency of both T cells and B cells, and increased susceptibility to all infectious agents. Absence of the gene product of JAK-3 (Chapter 6) has been shown recently, in some cases, to be a cause of SCID, offering hope for a future gene therapy approach to treatment. SCID can also arise secondary to a deficiency of the enzyme adenosine deaminase (ADA) in leukocytes. Adenosine deaminase is required for purine metabolism, and is most active in lymphocytes, particularly T lymphocytes. In the absence of this enzyme, toxic metabolites accumulate, DNA synthesis is impaired, and clonal expansion does not occur. Clinically the patients differ from those with only a lymphoid progenitor deficiency, reflecting the other developmental pathways (non-immunologic) also affected in ADA. Therapy for both disorders is bone marrow transplantation. For SCID, secondary to a deficiency in ADA, regular injections of adenosine deaminase linked to polyethylene glycol (PEG-ADA) are often effective.

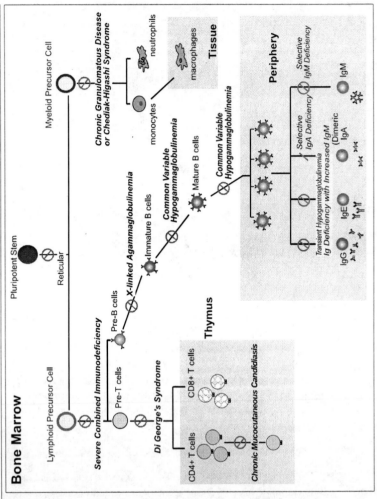

Fig. 15.3. Immunodeficiency disorders associated with developmental blocks at various sites. Developmental blocks occurring during lymphoid cell differentiation/maturation cause specific disorders.

Immunodeficiency Disorders

Table 15.1. Primary immunodeficiency disorders involving progenitor cells

Disorder	Level of Defect	Comments
Reticular Dysgenesis	Hematopoietic stem cells	• Autosomal recessive • Deficiency of T cells, B cells, and phagocytes
Severe Combined Immunodeficiency	Adenosine deaminase (ADA)	• Autosomal recessive • Highest activity in lymphocytes • Metabolites deoxyATP and deoxyadenosine ↑ • These metabolites inhibit ribonucleotide reductase • Treat with polyethylene glycol-ADA (PEG-ADA) • Treat with gene therapy

Gene therapy has been used successfully in patients for whom PEG-ADA is ineffective and no suitable bone marrow donor is available.

Primary Immunodeficiency Disorders: T Cells

T-cell disorders comprise approximately 10% of all primary immunodeficiency disorders and are frequently associated with susceptibility to infection by viruses, intracellular bacteria and fungi. Two distinct categories of T-cell disorders, **Di George's syndrome** and **chronic mucocutaneous candidiasis** have been described (Fig. 15.3, Table 15.2).

Di George's syndrome (congenital thymic aplasia)

Di George's syndrome results from defective embryogenesis leading to a reduced and defective (or absent) thymus. Consequently, the individual has few or no circulating T cells. These individuals have increased susceptibility to viral, fungal, and intracellular bacterial infections. Therapy for this disease is transplantation of functional components of a fetal thymus (tissue fragments placed under a renal capsule). Individuals usually improve with age, perhaps due to the activation of an extrathymic maturation site with increasing age. This disorder affects both males and females.

Chronic mucocutaneous candidiasis

Antigen-specific T-cell defects (especially of CD4+ cells) represent another group of T-cell disorders. One example is chronic mucocutaneous candidiasis, in which individuals lack T cells with receptors specific for the *Candida* antigen. There is a failure, during thymopoiesis, to generate T cells with TCRs specific for *Candida* antigen, so these individuals have increased susceptibility to *Candida* (yeast), but not to other organisms.

Table 15.2. Primary immunodeficiency disorders involving T cells

Disorder	Level of defect	Comments
Di George's Syndrome	Thymus	• Congenital thymic hypoplasia • Congenital abnormality in organs derived from the 3rd and 4th pharyngeal pouches • Hypoparathyroidism • Cardiac abnormalities • Distinctive facial features • Eyes widely separated; ears low; upper lip shorter • Most improve with age
Chronic Mucocutaneous Candidiasis	"Hole in the repertoire" to *Candida albicans*	• Affects both males and females • Suffer from various endocrine dysfunction • Normal T-cell response to other antigens • Normal B-cell immunity to *Candida albicans*

PRIMARY IMMUNODEFICIENCY DISORDERS: B CELLS

B-cell disorders are the most common immunodeficiency disorders, representing approximately 50% of all clinical cases. Some reflect defects in the actual number of mature B cells present, while others represent defects in antibody production with normal numbers of B cells (Fig. 15.3, Table 15.3). These disorders lead to recurrent infections with encapsulated pyogenic bacteria (e.g., *Hemophilus influenzae, Streptococcal pneumoniae*). The major role of B cells in eliminating these organisms is the production of IgG for activation of complement or as an opsonin for facilitated phagocytosis. Since encapsulated organisms are resistant to nonopsonin mediated phagocytosis, Ig deficient individuals are susceptible to recurrent infections by these bacteria.

X-linked agammaglobulinemia

X-linked agammaglobulinemia (XLA) results from a developmental block in B-cell differentiation from a pre-B cell to an immature B cell. Developmental arrest results from a signaling defect in the protein tyrosine kinase (btk) producing a gross deficiency in B-cell numbers and low or undetectable serum immunoglobulin (Ig). This deficiency becomes apparent at approximately 6 months of age when most of the maternally derived antibodies are degraded. The frequency of this disorder in the population is of the order of 1/100,000. Treatment is lifelong monthly infusion of antibodies.

Immunodeficiency Disorders

Table 15.3. Primary immunodeficiency disorders involving antibodies and B cells

Disorders	Antibody Deficiencies	Level of Defect	Comments
X-Linked Agammaglobulinemia	All Igs	Pre-B cells	• Bruton's agammaglobulinemia • Lack of circulating B cells • Lack of germinal centers in follicles • No tonsils; small lymph nodes • Intact cellular immunity • Manifests at 5-6 months • Recurrent bacterial infection
Transient Hypogammaglobulinemia	IgG, IgA, IgE	Lack of Th cells help (cytokines)	• Manifests at 5-6 months • Normal number of B cells in blood • NOT X-Linked
Common Variable Hypogammaglobulinemia	All Igs	Immature B cells or lack of antigen induced differentiation	• Onset occurs at any age • Affects males and females equally • Associated with HLA-B8 and HLA-DR3 • May develop autoimmune disease (e.g., pernicious anemia)
Selective IgA Deficiency	IgA	Unknown	• Autosomal inheritance • Common in Caucasians (1/700) • Increased in incidence of celiac disease • Susceptible to immune complex diseases
Selective IgM Deficiency	IgM	Unresponsive to, or lack of T-cell help	• Autosomal recessive • Have normal membrane IgM/IgD • Do not differentiate into plasma cells
Ig Deficiency with Increased IgM (Hyper IgM Syndrome)	IgG, IgA, IgE	Isotype switching CD40/CD40L interaction is lacking	• X-linked disorder • Many IgM antibodies are autoantibodies

Transient hypogammaglobulinemia of infancy

In this disorder there is a transient deficiency of immunoglobulin (IgG, IgA, and IgE) production thought to result from decreased production of Th cytokines needed for B-cell development and isotype switching. Patients usually recover with only antibiotic therapy, though in severe cases, treatment with immune globulin (for particular infections) is administered. As with x-linked agammaglobulinemia, this disorder presents at approximately 6 months as maternal passive immunity wanes, and an increased susceptibility to bacterial infections becomes evident.

Common variable hypogammaglobulinemia

In **common variable hypogammaglobulinemia** there is defective antibody production following infection. In contrast to XLA, individuals have normal numbers of peripheral blood B cells. There may be a developmental block at the immature B-cell stage, or alternatively defective antigen-induced differentiation in B cells. Aberrant antibody production is sometimes observed in this disorder with the presence of autoantibodies causing autoimmune manifestations of disease (e.g., thrombocytopenia). Treatment depends on the severity of the disorder, but generally involves the injection of immune globulin. This disorder is seen in males and females of all ages.

Selective IgA deficiency

Individuals with **selective IgA deficiency** show an increased incidence of recurrent sinopulmonary infection, in association with an increased incidence of coeliac disease. In most cases, individuals with IgA deficiency are asymptomatic. These individuals need antibiotic treatment for infection, not passive immunoglobulin. The reason for this is that there are only low levels of IgA in serum; it does not get to target sites; and recipients quickly form antibodies to donor IgA. This disorder is relatively common in Caucasians, with a prevalence of approximately 1 in 500-1000.

Selective IgM deficiency

In **selective IgM deficiency** patients present with increased infections by polysaccharide-encapsulated organisms (e.g., *Hemophilus influenzae*, *Streptococcus pneumoniae*). Encapsulated organisms are often T-independent antigens, triggering activation of naive B cells and differentiation to IgM secreting plasma cells with little or no isotype switching to IgG. Selective IgM deficiency produces enhanced susceptibility to encapsulated organisms.

Immunoglobulin deficiency with increased IgM

Immunoglobulin deficiency with increased IgM results from a defective CD40 (B cell) /CD40L (T cell) interaction (Fig. I5.4), such that isotype switching does not occur. Activated B cells differentiate only to IgM secreting plasma cells, with increased production of IgM and a deficiency of isotypes, IgG, IgA, and IgE. A frequent clinical presentation is recurrent bacterial/viral infections, with no evidence for classical immunological "memory" for the infecting organisms.

Immunodeficiency Disorders

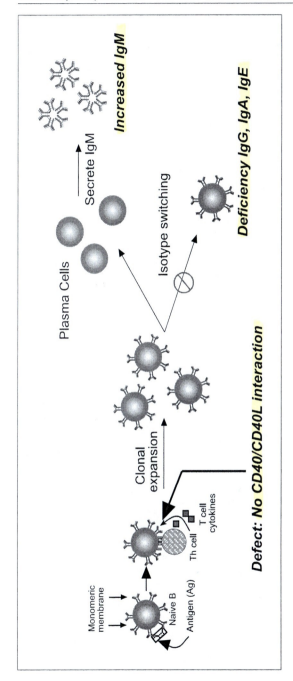

Fig. 15.4. Ig deficiency with increased IgM due to the absence of CD40/CD40L interaction. Immunoglobulin deficiency with increased IgM results from defective CD40 (B cell) /CD40L (T cell) interaction, with failure of isotype switching from IgM to the isotypes, IgG, IgA, and IgE (Also known as Hyper IgM Syndrome).

Primary Immunodefiency Disorders: Phagocytic

Phagocytic defects represent approximately 20% of immunodeficiency disorders resulting from either intrinsic or extrinsic causes. Intrinsic factors are functional defects in phagocytes themselves, affecting the generation of intracellular "killing" pathways, e.g., a deficiency in enzymes producing reactive oxygen intermediates. Extrinsic factors affect phagocyte function indirectly, e.g., absence of activating cytokines such as interferon gamma (IFNγ). Individuals with these disorders have recurrent bacterial and fungal infections and need anti-fungal and anti-bacterial agents as treatment. Long-term treatment such as bone marrow transplantation may be considered.

Chediak- Higashi syndrome

Chediak-Higashi syndrome is associated with defective viral and intracellular bacterial immunity. It is recognized by the accumulation of large cytoplasmic granules in phagocytes whose transport function and fusion to lysosomes is defective. Consequently, phagolysosomes (phagosomes fused with lysosomes) have decreased myeloperoxidase and other lysosomal enzymes required for microbial destruction. Natural killer (NK) cell function is also impaired in these individuals, most likely because exocytosis of granules is required for NK mediated cell killing (Fig. 15.3, Table 15.4).

Chronic granulomatous disease

Chronic granulomatous disease (CGD) is characterized by a dysfunction of the NADPH oxidase enzyme complex in phagocytes. Because NADPH oxidase is required for the production of reactive oxygen intermediates that normally destroy microbes, this defect leads to recurrent and uncontrolled bacterial and fungal infections. Individuals with CGD are not overly susceptible to infections with hydrogen peroxide producing, catalase negative, bacteria because the hydrogen peroxide these bacteria produce in the phagolysosome is cytotoxic. In both normal and CGD phagocytes, IFNγ enhances the production of reactive oxygen intermediates and is used as therapy as CGD (Fig. 15.3; Table 15.4).

Primary Immunodeficiency Disorders: Other Leukocytes

Other leukocyte defects have been identified which are much rarer than the B-cell or T-cell disorders considered above. Amongst these is the so-called **leukocyte adhesion deficiency** (LAD) disorder (Fig. 15.5), in which impaired trafficking of leukocytes to sites of infection leads to increased pustular infections. Bone marrow transplantation is the treatment of choice for this disorder. In the future, gene therapy may be an option.

Primary Immunodeficiency Disorders: Complement System

Complement system defects comprise some 2-3% of immunodeficiency disorders and are frequently associated with bacterial infection and autoimmunity.

Table 15.4. Primary immunodeficiency disorders involving phagocytes

Disorder	Defect	Comments / Treatments
Chediak-Higashi	Accumulation of large cytoplasmic granules whose transport function and fusion to lysosomes is defective—affects phagocytes, and NK cells	• Decrease in myeloperoxidase and/or lysosomal enzymes • Short term treatment: anti-fungal and anti-bacterial agents • Long term treatment: bone marrow transplant
Chromic Granulomatous Disease	NADPH oxidase	• Decrease in H_2O_2 and superoxide radicals • Short term treatment: anti-fungal and anti-bacterial agents • Long term treatment: bone marrow transplant

Table 15.5. Primary immunodeficiency disorders involving complement

Deficiency	Associated Disorder	Comments / Treatment
C1,C2,C4	Immune complex disorder (SLE-like)	Primary effect on classical pathway; failure to clear complexes leads to chronic inflammation (like SLE).
C3	Recurrent bacterial infection Chronic nephritis (results from deposition of C3 nephritic factor)	C3 defect predisposes to failure to activate alternate or classical pathways; antibiotic therapy
C5, C6, C7, C8	Recurrent Neisserial infections	No effective MAC; treat with antibiotics
C1 Esterase Inhibitor	Hereditary angioedema	• Activation of C1, production of vasoactive peptides ↑ • Treatment: infusion of C1 esterase inhibitor
Decay Accelerating Factor	Prototypical disease: paroxysmal nocturnal hemoglobinuria	• Results in increased spontaneous susceptibility of red blood cells to lysis

Several distinct categories have been described, depending upon the complement components that are defective (Table 15.5). They include:

C1 (esterase) inhibitor deficiency

C1 is a complement protein that binds to IgG or IgM molecules bound to antigen. To avoid spontaneous activation of C1, it circulates complexed to the C1 esterase inhibitor protein. A deficiency in C1 esterase inhibitor produces uncontrolled activation of C1, associated proteolysis of C2/C4, and enhanced production of the proteolytic fragments C2b, a vasoactive kinin and C4a, an anaphylatoxin.

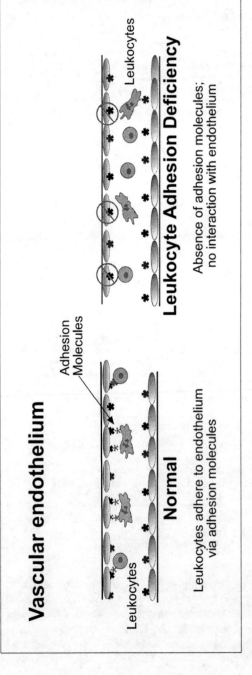

Fig. 15.5. Leukocyte adhesion deficiency disorder prevents leukocyte/endothelium interaction. Leukocyte adhesion deficiency is a disorder in which trafficking of leukocytes to sites of infection is impaired due to a deficiency in adhesion molecules on the leukocytes.

Immunodeficiency Disorders

Both fragments contribute to enhanced vascular permeability and often life-threatening edema, termed **hereditary angioedema** (Fig.15.6). Treatment involves infusion of C1 esterase inhibitor.

C1, C2, or C4 deficiency

The primary role of C1 is to cleave C2 and C4 proteolytically to generate the classical pathway C3 convertase, C4b2a. Deficiencies in C1, C2, or C4 cause diminished C3 convertase production by the classical pathway. This is not usually a serious problem because the alternative pathway can generate an alternative pathway C3 convertase with the same function. Deficiencies of these early complement components often occur in patients with systemic lupus erythematosus (SLE), although the explanation for this association remains unclear.

C3 deficiency

Deficiencies in C3 affect both the classical and alternative complement pathways because C3 is central to both of them. C3 deficiency is associated with an enhanced susceptibility to all bacterial infections because C3 is required for opsonin mediated phagocytosis during innate immunity. C3 deficiency is also associated with chronic nephritis, an immune complex type disorder associated with complement activation resulting from deposition of the so-called, "C3 nephritic factor". C3 "nephritic factor" is an antibody that binds C3, thus explaining both the C3 defect and the glomerulonephritis (associated with high levels of immune complex deposition in the kidney basement membrane).

C5-C9 deficiencies

Individuals deficient in C5-C9 cannot generate the membrane attack complex required for lysis of microbes. These individuals have increased bacterial susceptibility *only* to *Neisseria* bacteria, suggesting that C3 opsonin mediated phagocytosis (not lysis) is the normal role of complement-mediated defense. Susceptibility to *Neisseria* in the absence of a MAC suggests that these organisms are not readily phagocytosed by opsonin mediated mechanisms.

Decay accelerating factor

Decay accelerating factor (DAF) is a regulatory complement protein normally expressed as a transmembrane protein. In red blood cells the complex is attached to the cell surface by a phosphatidylinositol-protein complex. Deficiencies in the enzyme forming this complex lead to a DAF deficiency on red blood cells. Since DAF facilitates decay of the C3 convertase generated by either the classical or the alternative pathway, absence of DAF leads to the activation of the terminal pathway and formation of membrane attack complexes on host cells. Deficiencies in DAF in red blood cells leads to increased spontaneous lysis and the disease entity **paroxysmal nocturnal hemoglobinuria (PNH)**.

Secondary Immunodeficiency Disorders

The etiology of **secondary immunodeficiency disorders** is manifold and spans the gamut from acquired immunodeficiency diseases to abnormal production of

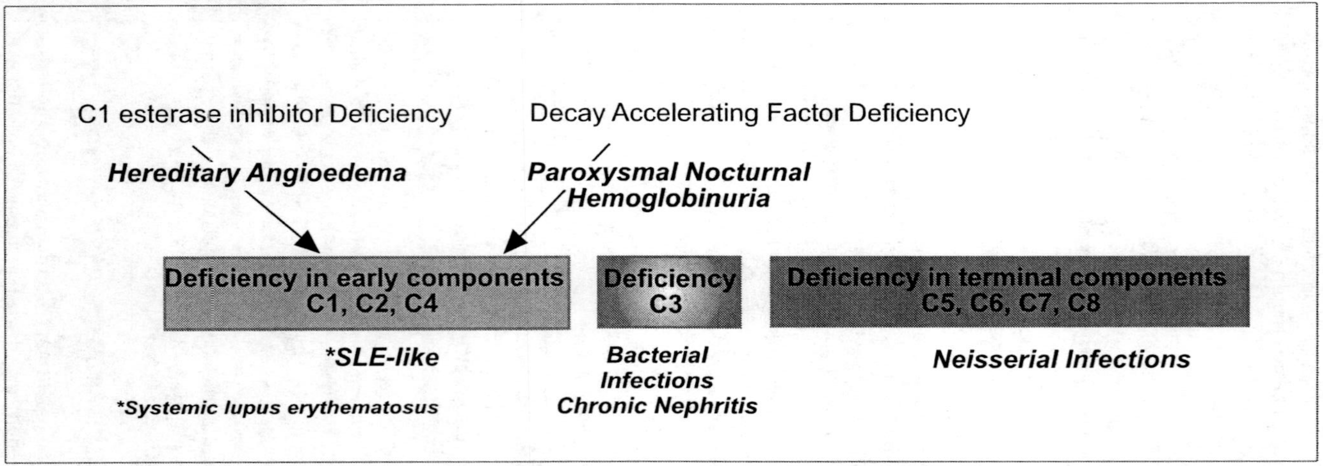

C1 esterase inhibitor Deficiency   Decay Accelerating Factor Deficiency

Hereditary Angioedema   *Paroxysmal Nocturnal Hemoglobinuria*

Deficiency in early components C1, C2, C4   **Deficiency C3**   **Deficiency in terminal components C5, C6, C7, C8**

SLE-like   Bacterial Infections   Neisserial Infections

  Chronic Nephritis

*Systemic lupus erythematosus

Fig. 15.6. Immunodeficiency disorders associated with complement protein deficiencies. Deficiency in C1 esterase inhibitor leads to uncontrolled activation of C1 and generation of vasoactive peptides with enhanced vascular permeability and often life-threatening edema (hereditary angioedema). Deficiency in decay accelerating factor on red blood cells leads to uncontrolled activation of complement because C3 convertases are not rapidly inactivated. The MAC complexes on the surface of red blood cells cause paroxysmal nocturnal hemoglobinuria. Other complement component deficiencies are associated with the specific disorders shown.

immune components (Fig. 15.1). Any B- and/or T-cell malignancy in which random clonal expansion of antigen specific cells occurs (following oncogene translocation/activation) can also cause secondary immunodeficiency disorders.

SECONDARY IMMUNODEFICIENCY DISORDERS: ACQUIRED

Acquired immunodeficiency diseases can result from:
a. virus (e.g., human immunodeficiency virus, HIV)
b. therapeutic drugs (posttransplant immunosuppression; cancer therapy)
c lifestyles (e.g., alcohol)
d other chronic conditions (e.g., diabetes; aging)
e abnormal production of immune components

Viruses

Viral infection of any cell typically leads to the secretion of **interferon alpha** (IFNα) by that cell. IFNα is protective for cells in the local milieu because it induces enzymes that inhibit viral replication. However, IFNα also inhibits the G1 phase of the cell cycle, producing a transient immunosuppression because cells responding to IFNα cannot clonally expand. Exploiting this property, the recombinant form of IFNα is standard treatment for proliferative disorders such as **hairy cell leukemia**. In addition to immunosuppression induced by IFNα, the HIV itself induces immunosuppression in a number of ways, not the least of which is the destruction of CD4+ T cells, cells required for virtually all aspects of immunity. Other viruses encode molecules that have known immunoregulatory properties (e.g., the viral IL-10 like molecule encoded by EBV).

Therapeutic drugs

Cancerous diseases are often treated by administration of cytotoxic drugs intended to kill the tumor cells. These drugs are not cancer cell-specific and other proliferating cells are also destroyed. Cytotoxicity to immune cells causes nonspecific immunosuppression. To combat the risk of graft rejection, transplant patients are intentionally given immunosuppressive drugs, many of which inhibit the secretion of cytokines that enhance immune responses. These patients are thus at risk of the same infectious disorders seen in congenital or acquired T cells defects.

Lifestyle

Alcohol is an immunosuppressant, affecting both cell mediated and humoral immunity, as does severe malnutrition. More specific deficiencies such as zinc, selenium and a variety of vitamin B deficiencies are also immunosuppressive.

Other chronic disorders

Aging is associated with a depression of cellular immunity, multifactorial in origin. One factor is a polarization of Thp to Th2 cells rather than Th1 cells. Type 1 cytokines are required for immune responses to viral, intracellular bacterial and fungal infections. Supporting this hypothesis, experimental administration of Type 1 cytokines to aging laboratory animals increased differentiation to Th1 cells, and reversed susceptibility to viral infections. In addition, dysregulation of apoptosis occurs in aging, which also contributes to the immune defect. Immunosuppression secondary to diabetes has also been well documented, again a result of multiple effects of dysregulated glucose metabolism on cells in the immune system (impaired neutrophil activity; production of nonspecific, poorly characterized, serum inhibitors, etc.)

SECONDARY IMMUNODEFICIENCY DISORDERS: ABNORMAL PRODUCTION OF IMMUNE COMPONENTS

Secondary immunodeficiency disorders are often associated with abnormal production of immune components. Included amongst these are:

Monoclonal gammopathies

In these diseases clonal overproduction of immunoglobulin occurs with relative deficiencies in other (specific antigen-induced) immunoglobulins. One disorder, **Waldenström's macroglobulinemia** (an IgM gammopathy) is associated with a hyperviscosity syndrome and hypogammaglobulinemia. Patients frequently present with vague symptoms which reflect this hyperviscosity e.g., headaches, visual blurring (often mini-strokes) etc.

Multiple myeloma

Multiple myeloma is a disease primarily affecting the elderly, associated with increased urinary excretion of free light chains, **Bence Jones proteins**. In the absence of obvious renal impairment (e.g., with blood in the urine, or progressive weight gain from edema), this disease is quite insidious, and the first manifestation may be a so-called "pathological fracture" of bone, attributed to "leaching" of calcium from bone following chronic inflammation (and IL-6 production).

SUMMARY

Dysfunction in components of innate or adaptive immunity causes immunodeficiency disorders, classified as either *primary* or *secondary*, depending on whether the dysfunction is inherited or acquired. Inherited (primary) disorders may arise from defects in either cellular or humoral components of immunity. Primary disorders are permanent, in the absence of medical intervention such as gene therapy. In contrast, acquired (secondary) disorders, may be transient or permanent depending on the factor inducing the immunosuppression. Host responses to particular microbes do not mobilize all components of immunity. Consequently, different defects lead to selectively increased susceptibility to microbes reflecting the particular immune components required to eliminate the organism.

Primary immunodeficiency disorders may arise from defects in progenitor cells, phagocytes, B cells, T cells, or complement. Individuals with stem cell disorders have increased susceptibility to all infectious agents; therapy involves bone marrow transplantation. T-cell disorders are frequently associated with susceptibility to infection by viruses, intracellular bacteria and fungi. Two distinct categories of

Immunodeficiency Disorders

T-cell disorders, Di George's syndrome and chronic mucocutaneous candidiasis have been described. B-cell disorders are the most common immunodeficiency disorders. Some B-cell disorders reflect defects in the number of B cells (e.g., XLA), while others reflect defective antibody production with normal numbers of B cells (e.g., selective IgA deficiency). These disorders lead to recurrent infections with encapsulated pyogenic bacteria (e.g., *Hemophilus influenzae, Streptococcal pneumoniae*). Individuals with phagocytic defects (e.g., CGD) have recurrent bacterial and fungal infections and need anti-fungal and anti-bacterial agents as treatment. Other leukocyte defects have been identified which are quite rare. Included in these is the so-called leukocyte adhesion deficiency (LAD) in which impaired trafficking of leukocytes to sites of infection leads to increased pustular infections. Bone marrow transplantation is the treatment of choice for this disorder. In the future, gene therapy may be an option. Complement system defects are frequently associated with bacterial infection and autoimmunity.

The etiology of secondary immunodeficiency disorders is manifold and spans the gamut from acquired immunodeficiency diseases to abnormal production of immune components. In principle, any B- and/or T-cell malignancy in which abnormal random (in terms of the antigen specificity of the affected cells) oncogene translocation/activation has been described can be classified as a secondary immunodeficiency disease.

CLINICAL CASES AND DISCUSSION

Clinical Case #29
John, a 14-month boy with severe Gram-positive bacterial pneumonia, is referred to the Children's Hospital by the family physician. This is his third such infection in four months. He has two healthy sisters aged three and five years. The family lost a boy at ten months of age to bacterial pneumonia six years ago. The family doctor has sent along some blood test results which show low serum immunoglobulin (Ig) levels (all classes), few B cells, but normal numbers and functioning of T cells.

Questions and Discussion: Case # 29
1. *Six key features we need to bear in mind in discussing this case are:*
   Gender of the patient/siblings
   Age of the patient and age of deceased sibling
   Susceptibility to what types of infection?
   Low levels serum immunoglobulin
   Few B cells
   Normal numbers and function of T cells
2. *What does the data regarding gender suggest?*
Note there are two affected boys, both at an early age (less than 15 months), but no affected girls in this family. These data suggest an X-linked congenital defect in immune functioning.

3. Although we are not informed of John's resistance to viral infections, what laboratory information suggests he is likely able to mount a normal immunological response to viral infections?

Viral infections are increased in T-cell deficiencies. Because John has a normal number number/function of T cells, he is not likely predisposed to viral infections.

4. *John has a severe respiratory infection, which may be the result of impaired mucosal immunity. Which immunodeficiency disorder would predispose to mucosal infections? What data is provided that suggest this is unlikely the case for John?*

Selective IgA deficiency would predispose individuals to impaired mucosal immunity leading to sinopulmonary infections. However, we are told that John has low levels of all classes of serum Ig and few B cells. This is the picture of a conventional immunoglobulin defect (IgM and IgG), rather than of selective IgA deficiency.

5. Given that the levels of serum Ig are low, that there are few B cells, and that the number/function of T cells is normal, we should be able to rule out several defects. Explain why this information helps to rule out each of the following immunodeficiency disorders: (i) severe combined immunodeficiency (SCID), or Di George's syndrome, (ii) transient hypogammaglobulinemia of childhood, Chediak-Higashi syndrome, chronic granulomatous disease, or (iii) a complement defect.

Severe combined immunodeficiency (SCID) or Di George's syndrome

This is not a progenitor cell defect, such as SCID or Di George's syndrome. Both would present with increased infections, but we would expect some hint at diminished resistance to viral infections as well as susceptibility to bacterial infections. In addition, we would expect evidence for decreased numbers/function of T cells.

Transient hypogammaglobulinemia of childhood

This is unlikely transient hypogammaglobulinemia of childhood. Our logic here is less dogmatic, but we are told of two affected boys and two unaffected girls. We should be thinking of X-linked disorders, which is not the case for transient hypogammaglobulinemia of childhood.

Chediak-Higashi syndrome, chronic granulomatous disease, or a complement defect

This is also unlikely to be chronic granulomatous disease (phagocytes), Chediak-Higashi syndrome (phagocytes or natural killer cell), or a complement defect. The argument against this is still the evidence for X-linkage and the significant negatives (i.e., we are not given any information that would point us in this direction!).

6. With reference to # 5, what tests might you ask for, however, if you were concerned that Chediak-Higashi syndrome, chronic granulomatous disease or a complement defect were possible explanations for this problem?

Natural killer cells can be measured directly using fluorescent antibodies that recognize the CD16 molecule on the cell surface, or by measuring their function in culture assays. Complement defects can be measured by specifically requesting complement levels, or tests for those isolated complement components which are most frequent causes of immunodeficiency disorders (C3, etc.). Chronic granulomatous disease can be investigated by assaying activity of oxidative enzymes that are defective/absent in this disorder (e.g., NADPH oxidase).

7. Note the significant positives that we are given. John has few B cells and low serum Ig levels. What does this suggest?

This is suggestive of an early block in B-cell differentiation (so-called "differentiation arrest"), and is a relatively classic presentation of X-linked agammaglobulinemia.

8. How might a block at a later stage in B-cell differentiation present?

A block at a later stage in B-cell differentiation e.g., isotype switching defects, would lead to increased IgM and decreased IgG, IgA, or IgE.

9. To what are later blocks in B-cell differentiation attributed?

Later blocks in differentiation are associated with defects in antigen dependent differentiation, rather than antigen-independent differentiation, which occurs in the bone marrow during B-cell maturation. Later blocks in differentiation are generally related to altered CD4+ T-cell functions, cytokine production, etc.

10. An example of an immunodeficiency disorder with decreased antigen induced B-cell differentiation is "increased (Hyper) IgM with decreased Ig". What is the underlying mechanism of this defect?

Hyper-IgM syndrome is an interesting example for which the biology is well understood. This syndrome is caused by defective expression of a T-cell molecule, CD40L, that normally interacts with CD40 on B cells during their activation. This signal is required for isotype switching to IgG, IgE, and IgA. In the absence of the CD40/CD40L interaction there is preferential production of serum IgM.

11. What is known to date about the genetic defect in X-linked (Bruton's) agammaglobulinemia?

This seems to be a defect in a tyrosine kinase enzyme (btk) essential for an intracellular pathway involved in signaling for normal B cell development/differentiation.

12. How might this disorder be treated?

Conventional treatment involves the LIFELONG replacement of the defective components (i.e., serum Ig replacement). This is costly, and not without risks. Bone marrow transplantation might be a suitable alternative if rejection could be controlled. Consider some of the pros/cons that enter into your decision concerning the treatment of this disorder.

Clinical Case #30

Ms. Sidhu is an elderly diabetic lady of Asian descent, who complains of a significant weight loss over the last few months, associated with night sweats and a cough with some whitish-yellow sputum. She monitors her own blood sugar, which routinely runs in the range 5-8 mMol, but over the same period this has been fluctuating more widely (4-15 mMol-normal range 4-6). There has been no significant change in her diet and no recent travel. She is currently afebrile, but does not look as well as when you last saw her. Blood work is unremarkable.

Questions for Discussion Case #30

1. List the six likely key features we need to bear in mind in explaining in this problem?

    Blood sugar more difficult to control
    No dietary indiscretion and no travel
    Weight loss/night sweats/productive cough
    Elderly, diabetic
    Afebrile (without fever)
    Asian descent

2. Under what "acute" conditions is blood sugar more difficult to control?

Blood sugar becomes more difficult to control in diabetics under conditions of physical/emotional stress. There is no suggestion of psychiatric disorders (emotional stress), so we should be alert at this stage to a chronic (few months) physical stressor.

3. What possible chronic physical stressors has the physician considered in his interview with the patient?

There was no change in diet and no lengthy travel. Thus, assuming lack of sleep is not an issue, think of malignancy, autoimmunity (besides the diabetes) or chronic infection.

4. With what malignancy would the weight loss, night sweats, and cough be consistent?

The weight loss, night sweats and cough would be consistent with a number of cancers. The cough is suggestive of something going on in the lungs (perhaps lymphoma, lung cancer).

5. With what autoimmune disorder is weight loss, night sweats, and cough consistent?

A **vasculitic type process** might be a consideration here, including that often seen in rheumatoid arthritis, or even the primary vasculitides themselves (leukocytoclastic vasculitis), or disorders directly affecting the lung (**Churg-Strauss; Wegener's granulomatosis**).

6. Weight loss, night sweats, and cough are consistent with infectious diseases. In this regard, what is the significance of the lack of travel?

Diabetics and the elderly represent an important immunodeficiency population. The travel is important here because we can assume we are not meant to focus on bizarre infections of immunodeficient persons, localized to certain "hot spots" (e.g., **blastomycosis** in the Mississippi Valley area of the (USA)).

7. Note that this lady is afebrile right now. What does this suggest regarding the type of infection this patient might have?

We should not be thinking of fulminant (acute) infections, but a "smouldering" (chronic) process. This is consistent with normal blood work. In the presence of acute viral infections expect to see lymphoproliferation; in the presence of bacterial infections expect to see a marked neutrophilia. However, a chronic lung infection might well be a consideration.

Immunodeficiency Disorders

8. **For what chronic infections is this patient susceptible?**
This patient is of Asian descent. This marks a population at risk for certain chronic infectious diseases, including hepatitis and tuberculosis (TB). The immunodeficiency of age is certainly associated with TB.

9. **Given the above consideration, what tests might you now order?**
   a. A chest X-ray
   b. Order serum titers for hepatitis B, hepatitis C etc.
   c. Find out about her previous TB status (if possible).
   d. Order a Mantoux test.

10. **Is a negative Mantoux test by itself sufficient to eliminate the possibility tuberculosis? Explain.**
In the absence of a positive control, it is not possible to interpret a negative Mantoux test because the negative test might represent nonresponsiveness associated with immunodeficiency. A control test (e.g., *Candida*) should be administered on the opposite arm at the same time as the Mantoux test.

TEST YOURSELF

Multiple Choice Questions

1. A 10-year-old girl is hospitalized for persistent fever of eight weeks duration. She had developed measles some nine to ten weeks ago, while vacationing in Asia. Repeating blood cultures were negative. A PPD test was negative in the GP's office, but an infectious disease specialist suggests miliary tuberculosis. Repeat PPD testing using intermediate dose PPD gave a 20 mm induration; chest x-ray showed multiple nodules. The fever resolved after appropriate therapy. Explanations for this course of disease include all except:
   a. Immunosuppression secondary to measles
   b. False "negative" early PPD test—no concomitant test run to ensure patient not anergic
   c. Anergy caused by miliary tuberculosis itself
   d. Area of high TB prevalence accompanied by the measles infection (see (a))
   e. Acute streptococcal infection

2. Fred, a 65-year-old male, previously well, complains of headaches. His "thinking" is slower, and fundoscopic examination of the eyes suggests sluggish blood flow. A serum test shows a "monoclonal spike", IgM type. These data suggest:
   a. SLE
   b. Complement (C3) deficiency
   c. Waldenström's macroglobulinemia
   d. Common variable immunodeficiency
   e. AIDS

3. A four-year-old boy presents with recurrent sinusitis. On physical examination you find he has no lymph nodes or tonsils. There are few circulating B cells.

Cell mediated immunity, as tested in vivo by skin reactivity, is normal. He has three healthy brothers and two sisters. A possible diagnosis is:
   a. Bruton's agammaglobulinemia
   b. Transient hypogammaglobulinemia
   c. Severe combined immunodeficiency
   d. Wiskott-Aldrich syndrome
   e. Selective IgA deficiency

4. A 20-year-old female diabetic, with hypothyroidism and irregular menses complains of a chronic, nonerthymatous, macular-papular rash for six months. There is no family history of immunodeficiency disorders, no history of connective tissue diseases, no travel, and no history of drug abuse. PPD testing is positive (she was exposed to TB when working on an Indian Reservation 4 years ago). Serum Ig and complement levels and white cell counts were normal. She is possibly suffering from:
   a. Selective IgA deficiency
   b. Chronic mucocutaneous candidiasis
   c. Di George's syndrome
   d. SCID
   e. Common variable immunodeficiency

5. An eight-month-old male has had recurrent bacterial infections over the past three months. His sister, age eight years, is well, but an older brother, who was below the 5th percentile for weight, died two weeks ago at two-and-one-half years, after repeated episodes of pneumonia. Other males on the mothers' side have also died early in childhood after lengthy illnesses, but no females (the history of 12 is known) are affected. Laboratory results indicate all of the following except:
   a. Pre-B cells are absent
   b. Absent B cells
   c. Normal T cells
   d. Decreased Ig levels
   e. Normal numbers of plasma cells.

Answers: 1e ; 2c ; 3d ; 4b ; 5e

Short Answer Questions
1. What are the most common primary immunodeficiency diseases of B or T cells?
2. How does the leukocyte adhesion deficiency disorder manifest itself and why does this cause susceptibility to infection?
3. What is the common defect in neutrophils/NK cells in Chediak-Higashi disease?
4. Why do transplant patients often develop cytomegalovirus infections?
5. What are monoclonal gammopathies?

Tumor Immunology

Objectives	337
Tumor Immunology	338
General Features	338
The Concept of Immunosurveillance	338
Tumor Antigens	340
Tumor Immunosurveillance	344
Effector Mechanisms for Elimination of Tumors	345
Evasion of Immune Surveillance	349
Immunology in Diagnosis or in Monitoring Prognosis	354
Novel Therapies: Enhancing Antigen Presentation by Dendritic Cells	355
Novel Therapies: Cytokines and other Molecules Transfected into Tumor Cells Themselves	357
Novel Therapies: Modification of CTL as a Strategy for Enhancing Tumor Immunity	359
Novel Therapies: Monoclonal Antibodies and Immunotherapy	359
Summary	360
Clinical Cases and Discussion	361
Test Yourself	364

Objectives

In this chapter we encounter a dynamic clinical field, that of tumor immunology. Few aspects of clinical immunology are as interesting, though to date the field has yet to realize its expectations. A major stumbling block seems to have been negotiated however, and we are now in a position to characterize molecules on tumors that are used by the immune system to distinguish tumor cells from normal cells. The student will become familiar with terms such as oncofetal antigens, tumor specific antigens and tumor associated antigens.

All of the mechanisms studied to date are implicated in immunity to tumors. However, the growth of a tumor in a host indicates that immunity has failed. Thus active immunotherapy regimes must somehow circumvent this "failure". A number of approaches aimed at improving tumor immunogenicity are under investigation. These mechanisms include alterations in (i) antigen presentation, (ii) the manner of antigen expression on the tumor cells and (iii) the cytokine milieu in which tumor antigen exposure occurs. Artificial ways of producing or modifying tumor specific antibodies and/or cells for use in vivo are also being investigated.

The limitations imposed by using the immune system for immunotherapy of tumors are different from those when using tumor immunology for immunodiagnosis or for monitoring tumor treatment. Examples of these approaches will be given in some detail.

Clinical Immunology, by Reginald Gorczynski and Jacqueline Stanley. 2001 Landes Bioscience

TUMOR IMMUNOLOGY

GENERAL FEATURES

Tumors are growths that may be benign or malignant. Encapsulated tumors whose cells are well differentiated and resemble normal tissues are considered benign. At least some of the cells in malignant tumors are undifferentiated, with high proliferative potential causing persistent tumor growth. The tumor mass is not encapsulated, but has the capacity to invade adjacent tissue locally, and ultimately spread (metastasize) to distant sites. Malignancies are categorized according to the tissue from which they derive. Thus, sarcomas, lymphomas, and leukemias are tumors of mesenchymal origin. Carcinomas are tumors of epithelial origin.

Regardless of the biology of tumor development, eradication of tumors by the immune system requires recognition of something (an antigen) unique to the tumor which is not expressed (or not expressed to the same degree) by normal tissue. In animals it has been found that chemically-induced tumors have unique tumor antigens, such that in a genetically identical group of animals, tumors induced by the *same chemical*, in *different animals*, possess *unique antigens*. In contrast, virally induced tumors in these same genetically identical animals express common tumor antigens (presumably virus-encoded).

THE CONCEPT OF IMMUNOSURVEILLANCE

General features
Many years ago Thomas hypothesized that one role of the immune system lay in immunosurveillance against spontaneously arising tumor cells. Tumors that appear in the normal population represent those that have escaped surveillance for a number of reasons. Amongst these latter are immunosuppression of any form, whether natural or acquired; loss of antigenicity in the tumor (failure to present foreign antigens for recognition and stimulation of protective immunity); and development in immunologically privileged sites. The concepts of immunosurveillance were tested against such predictions with equivocal results.

Spontaneous remission of metaplasia
Data that seemed to support the model arose from incidental autopsies performed on young individuals dying of trauma during the Vietnam War. This revealed a higher incidence of metaplasia (abnormal cell growth, perhaps precancerous lesions), above the incidence of subsequent cancer observed in the general population (when adult). Advocates of a role for the immune system in controlling tumor development suggested that the immune system had "intervened" and destroyed the precancerous cells. Alternatively, the frequency of metaplastic cells may not reflect their tumorigenic potential.

Malignancies in immunosuppressed populations

The incidence of malignancy in an immunosuppressed population (e.g., patients treated with high doses of immunosuppressant drugs following organ transplantation, for autoimmune disorders, or other acquired immunodeficiency disorders (AIDS)) was studied. As hypothesized by Thomas (see above), these individuals had a higher incidence of malignant growth. However, while cancers in the general population are frequently solid tumors, in these individuals only the frequency of lymphomas, skin cancers, and Kaposi's sarcomas was increased. It was argued that these unique tumors arose not from a failure of immunosurveillance but as a direct (toxic) effect of the drugs and/or virus causing immunosuppression. Epstein-Barr virus infection of B cells (causing mononucleosis, a self-limiting disease, in the general population) can lead to B-cell lymphoma (Burkitt's lymphoma) in immunosuppressed individuals. Patients with acquired immunodeficiency syndrome (AIDS) often develop Kaposi's sarcoma, following exposure to herpes simplex virus–6 (HSV-6), which is nontumorigenic in normal individuals.

Refuting a role for the immune system in tumor development

Both natural killer (NK) cells and T cells have been implicated as playing key roles in immunosurveillance of tumor development (see below). One would predict that defects in the function of these cells would lead to increased incidence of tumors. However mice with defects in NK cells (Bg/Bg) or mice that are athymic (Nu/Nu) do not show an increased incidence of malignancy, other than of virally induced tumors. The latter might be expected because these mice have an impaired anti-viral immunity (Chapter 11). These data may not be as damaging to Thomas's hypothesis as was first thought because even in the absence of NK (or T) cells, other arms of the immune system may function normally in immunosurveillance in these mice.

A final argument raised against the concept of immunosurveillance concerns the postulated increased incidence of tumors in privileged sites. One natural site for immunoregulation is in the uterus during pregnancy. The fetus is a foreign growth that is not destroyed by the immune system, perhaps the most successful graft known. There has been no reported increase in the frequency of metastatic growth in the placenta during pregnancy.

Nonimmunogenic tumors

One prediction of Thomas' hypothesis was that the spontaneously arising tumors seen in humans would not be typical of those for which immunosurveillance was effective, but instead represented those for whom it failed. One cause of failure would be a lack of immunogenicity. Indeed spontaneously arising tumors in man are quite nonimmunogenic. This feature has made it extraordinarily difficult both to study immunity to natural tumors, and to consider ways in which this might be manipulated for therapeutic purposes. In recent years, with the advent of more sophisticated molecular biology tools, there is some renewed hope that these negative findings will be "a thing of the past".

TUMOR ANTIGENS

Tumor specific antigens
Proteins specific to a tumor (or tumors) are called **tumor specific antigens** (**TSAs**). If these proteins produce immune responses leading to tumor rejection, they are referred to as **tumor specific transplantation antigens** (**TSTA**) (Fig. 16.1). The mIg present on a B-cell monoclonal tumor, (chronic lymphocytic leukemia (CLL) is an example of a TSTA. In CLL, all the tumor cells are identical, expressing a tumor-unique immunoglobulin molecule on their cell surface. Anti-tumor antibodies should recognize the CLL tumor but not normal host B cells because they express different mIg from that expressed on the clone of B cells comprising the CLL tumor. De novo expression of TSAs in other types of tumors could be manifest if:

i "silent" genes are activated, following altered transcription factor activity or inactivation of tumor suppressor genes (e.g., retinoblastoma and p53). Tumor suppressor genes encode proteins that control cell cycling. In the absence of tumor suppressor proteins, cells proliferate uncontrollably, increasing the mutation frequency and likelihood of malignancy.
ii a mutation in a normal gene sequence leads to the expression of mutant peptides. Point mutations in the ras protein have been observed in tumor cells, and it is conceivable that this mutated ras protein might serve as a tumor antigen. In its active state, p21 ras activates a kinase cascade that leads to increased transcription of several proteins.

The identification of unique TSTAs in human tumors has been fraught with inconsistency. More recently newer molecular biological tools have been brought to bear on this problem, searching tumor cDNA expression libraries with human tumor patient sera or patient's peripheral blood cells for evidence for antibodies or CTL which recognize unique molecules in these libraries (Clinical case #32).

Amongst the serologically detected antigens are **NY-ESO-1**, a novel antigen expressed by a number of human tumors (including melanoma), but not known to be expressed by normal cells (except testis); **galectin 9**, recognized by sera from 50% of Hodgkin's disease patients; a human colon carcinoma antigen 17-1A; and a number of relatively melanoma specific antigens, some of which had been previously identified using more conventional procedures. MAGE-1 to –3 represent melanoma specific antigens identified this way (Fig. 16.1). Tyrosinase and **MelanaA/MART-1** are less melanoma specific (present on normal melanocytes also), but melanoma associated. Several novel antigens identified serologically were subsequently shown to serve as target antigens for CTL, including MAGE-3, recognized by human CTL seeing a MAGE-3 peptide displayed on the cell surface associated with the class I MHC molecule, HLA-A1. CTL are thought to be most important for immunity to melanoma. The potential value of these antigens in immunotherapy is discussed in more detail below.

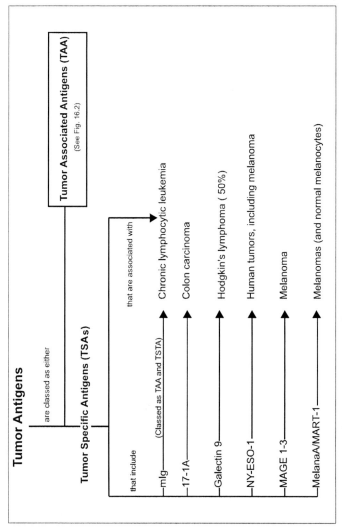

Fig. 16.1. Tumor specific antigens. Proteins specific to a tumor (or tumors) are called tumor specific antigens (TSAs). If these proteins produce immune responses causing tumor rejection, they are called tumor specific transplantation antigens (TSTA).

Tumor associated antigens

Tumor associated antigens (TAAs) can be used to characterize tumors, but are not necessarily unique to the tumor as opposed to other (normal) host tissue (Fig. 16.2). Often these TAAs reflect antigens expressed at stages of normal cell differentiation, although the tumor cell expression is either qualitatively or quantitatively different from normal cells at that particular stage of maturation/differentiation. TAAs have potential use in the diagnosis and monitoring of tumor growth. Because the antigens are not tumor-unique, they have limited immunotherapeutic value for immunization to eradicate the tumor. An important class of tumor associated antigens is the so-called **oncofetal antigens** (see below). As the name implies these are antigens characteristic of tumor cells in mature tissue which were expressed at some earlier (fetal) stage of normal development. Examples are **carcinoembryonic antigen (CEA), alpha-fetoprotein (AFP)**, and **beta human chorionic gonadotropin, (β-HCG)**.

Carcinoembryonic antigens
CEA is an oncofetal antigen initially thought to be relatively unique to tumors of the gastrointestinal tract, particularly colonic carcinomas. It has now been clearly documented that CEA levels are elevated in colon, lung, breast and stomach tumors. Because of these latter associations, CEA levels cannot be used as a specific marker for the detection of colon cancer. Furthermore, while CEA is not significantly expressed in normal healthy adult tissue, high levels are found in cigarette smokers, patients suffering from chronic obstructive pulmonary disease (COPD) and in alcoholic cirrhosis.

CEA is one of a family of cell:matrix adhesion molecules. This is intriguing because the regulation of metastic cancer spread occurs by mechanism(s) which alter the way cells adhere with one another and their environment. Enzyme linked immunosorbent assays (ELISA) are used to measure CEA levels. Like other oncofetal antigens, while CEA has little value for diagnosis it is useful for monitoring the early recurrence of treated tumors before they become clinically detectable or visible using more sophisticated imaging procedures.

Alpha-fetoprotein antigens
AFP is another oncofetal antigen expressed by liver and testicular tumors. It is normally synthesized by the fetal liver, yolk sac and gastrointestinal tract cells, peaking at 15 weeks of gestation, and declining to low normal adult levels by 12 months postbirth. Increased serum levels (often 100-fold or more) are secreted by hepatoma cells and yolk-sac elements in germ cell tumors (teratocarcinomas of the testes/ovary). Increased levels are also seen in cases of pancreatic cancer, gastric and lung cancer patients. In addition, viral and alcoholic cirrhosis of the liver is associated with elevated levels, as are other rare disorders (ataxia telangectasia, hereditary tyrosinemia). Again, the value of ELISA assays for AFP lies in monitoring patients being treated for a known AFP-expressing tumor.

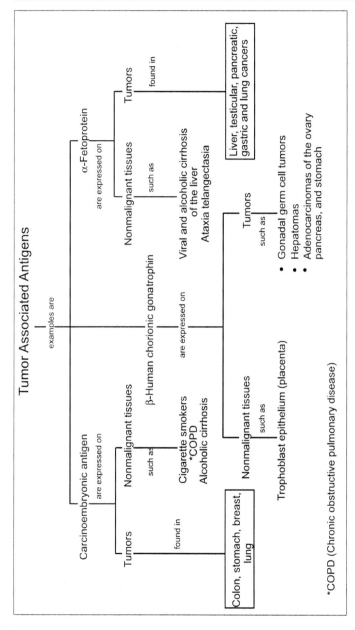

Fig. 16.2. Tumor associated antigens. Tumor associated antigens (TAAs) can be used to characterize tumors but do not necessarily distinguish tumor versus normal host cells. Examples are carcinoembryonic antigen (CEA), alpha-fetoprotein (AFP), beta human chorionic gonadotropin, (β-HCG).

Beta-human chorionic gonadotrophin

Beta-HCG is produced by the trophoblast epithelium of the placenta during pregnancy. Detectable β-HCG in males or nonpregnant females indicates an underlying tumor. Gonadal germ cell tumors, and adenocarcinomas of the ovary, pancreas, stomach, as well as hepatomas, produce this molecule. In those patients with germ cell tumors producing both AFP and β-HCG, discordant reduction in the levels of the two generally reflects the existence and differential eradication, of separate (nonidentical) tumor clones. In patients treated for choriocarcinoma the decline in β-HCG levels represents such an effective way to monitor therapy that a failure to detect a fall in levels or a sudden stop in the decline is often a sufficient reason to alter therapy, without other evidence for tumor recurrence.

TUMOR IMMUNOSURVEILLANCE

The destruction of tumors by innate and acquired immunological effector mechanisms has been demonstrated in vitro. Documentation of the in vivo occurrence of these mechanisms for eliminating spontaneously arising tumors remains poor. Amongst the findings that might constitute such evidence would be the following:

i   the presence of tumor infiltrating lymphocytes, suggesting that lymphocytes have trafficked to the tumor and have been activated at that site. Stronger evidence for their role in controlling tumor development would be the demonstration that these tumor infiltrating lymphocytes are tumor specific.

ii existence of tumor specific cytotoxic cells (cytotoxic T lymphocytes). These have been identified for some tumors (see above) using tumor expression libraries.

iii evidence for local changes in cytokine production (e.g., increased IFNγ) suggestive of local antigen activation. IFNγ is secreted primarily by activated CD4+ Th1 cells and activated NK cells. The presence of IFNγ in the tumor bed would suggest the local activation of these cells.

iv increased lymphocyte proliferation to tumor antigens in vitro. Although this might represent evidence for in vivo antigen exposure (with memory cell development), failure of restimulation in vitro might merely reflect the fact that in vivo activation of cells has already occurred, as in some autoimmune states (e.g., activated cells taken from rheumatoid arthritis patients often cannot be easily restimulated in vitro).

v   evidence for restricted V beta usage in T-cell populations in the host. In some individuals with a high tumor load, analysis of peripheral blood T cells indicates that several T-cell clones have been activated. Further analysis of these clones revealed a similarity in the TCR variable regions between patients. Many T-cell clones use the same beta chain V region but not the same D region or J region (alpha chain variability is not as important in generation of diversity in TCRs-see Chapter 7). Restricted (oligoclonal) expansion of T cells generally reflects in vivo exposure to a similar (defined) set of antigens.

EFFECTOR MECHANISMS FOR ELIMINATION OF TUMORS

The immune system might be engaged to eliminate tumor cells in a number of ways. Evidence exists, in some systems at least, for all of the following in human cancers.

Macrophages (innate immunity)
Resting macrophages are ineffective in tumor destruction. However, stimulation with lipopolysaccharide or IFNγ can induce macrophage activation, and the secretion of cytokines, some of which, at least, are tumoricidal (e.g., tumor necrosis factor (TNF)). Although the mechanism of TNF cytotoxicity is debated, cell death is associated with (or mediated by) apoptosis. Apoptosis is characterized by fragmentation of DNA into units of 200 base pairs (nucleosomes) or multiples thereof. Supporting an in vivo role for macrophages in impeding tumor growth are reports that tumors (especially breast carcinomas) with massive macrophage infiltration have a better prognosis. There is also evidence that tumors with IgG antibodies bound to their cell surface are recognized and destroyed by opsonin-mediated phagocytosis (Fig. 16.3).

Natural killer cells (innate immunity)
Natural killer (NK) cells may recognize tumor cells using the NK receptor, (Fig. 16.4). Tumor cells are destroyed when the NK cell secretes granules containing the protein, perforin. Perforin inserts in the cell membrane to form pores. NK cells also participate in antibody dependent cell mediated cytotoxicity (ADCC), where the NK cell uses its FcγR to recognize IgG bound to tumor cells. Destruction of the tumor cell occurs by osmotic lysis, as described for NK cells recognizing tumor cells by NK receptors. NK cells lyse

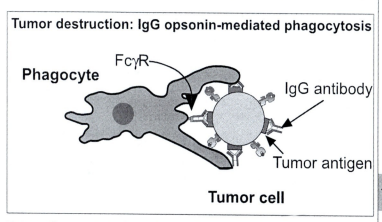

Fig. 16.3. Effector mechanism for elimination of tumors: macrophages. Tumors that have IgG antibodies bound to their cell surface are recognized and destroyed by opsonin-mediated phagocytosis. Macrophages have FcγR and bind IgG Fc regions. The in vivo role of macrophages in regulating tumor growth remains to be elucidated.

NK cells recognize some tumor antigens via the NK receptor to induce their osmotic lysis

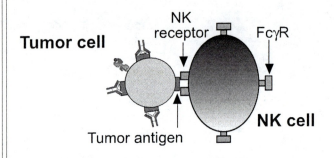

NK cells recognize some tumor antigens via the FcγR to induce their osmotic lysis (ADCC)

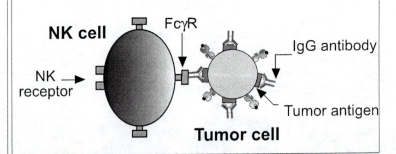

Fig. 16.4. Effector mechanism for elimination of tumors: natural killer cells. Natural killer (NK) cells may recognize tumor cells using the NK receptor, which has broad specificity. Tumor cells are destroyed by osmotic cell lysis when the NK cell secretes granules containing the protein, perforin. Perforin inserts in the cell membrane to form pores. NK cells participate in antibody dependent cell mediated cytotoxicity (ADCC), where the NK cell recognizes the IgG bound to the tumor cell via the FcγR present on the NK cell. Destruction of the tumor cell occurs by osmotic lysis, as described when recognition occurs via the NK receptor.

tumors in an MHC unrestricted manner. Importantly, recognition of tumor antigens by NK cell receptors is inhibited by MHC molecules, and those tumor cells expressing high levels of class I MHC are not killed by NK cells. The receptors mediating this inhibition are the so-called killer inhibitory receptors (KIRs). NK cells may thus mediate surveillance against tumors which down-regulate MHC (and are not detected by CD8+ T cells). Some human anti-melanoma CTL also express KIRs, which thus hampers both CTL and NK mediated tumor killing. The efficacy of NK cell mediated tumoricidal activity is enhanced in the presence of cytokines derived from activated T cells, including IL-2, IL-12, and IFNγ. Incubation of peripheral blood cells with high concentration of IL-2 leads to the generation of lymphokine activated killer cells (LAK). LAK cells are derived from NK cells and show markedly increased ability to lyse tumor cells, relative to NK cells not exposed to high concentrations of IL-2.

B cells and antibodies (adaptive immunity)
Antibodies may play a role in tumor cell destruction, as demonstrated by in vitro studies. The efficacy of antibodies depends on the presence of complement, phagocytes, or natural killer cells. Complement mediated osmotic lysis of tumor cells, following activation by the classic complement pathway, occurs for leukemic cells in culture. Phagocyte-mediated destruction of leukemic cells has been seen where antibodies function as opsonins to enhance phagocytosis. However, there is little evidence for the operation of these mechanisms in vivo in leukemia.

Evidence suggesting a role for antibodies in human tumor immunity comes from the growing body of data using expression library screening (see TSA and Clinical case #32), which documents serum antibodies to unique tumor antigens in many cancer patients. Further evidence for a role for antibodies in regulation of tumor growth comes from immunotherapy studies in patient populations. In colon carcinoma patients, with minimal residual disease after standard (surgical) therapy, infusion of antibody to the colon carcinoma antigen 17-1A reduced mortality and tumor recurrence by some 30% over the following 7 years.

Note that in some cases, antibodies can de detrimental to the ability of the host to control tumor growth locally, if the antibodies mediate a down-regulation and/or loss of adhesion molecules serving to attach the tumor cell to the local matrix. In the absence of this attachment, dissemination (metastasis) of the tumor is favored.

Bispecific antibodies in therapy
An interesting (artificial) antibody mediated immune mechanism of potential value against tumors uses so-called bispecific antibodies, in which one arm of the bivalent antibody molecule is constructed with a site recognizing a tumor antigen, while the other recognizes a determinant on a known effector cell (e.g., CD16 on NK cells). Infusion of such antibodies brings the NK cell into juxtaposition with the tumor, leading to increased killing. This technique was tested in Hodgkin's lymphoma using an anti-CD30 (a molecule expressed at high levels on these lymphoma cells) and anti-CD16. A small response rate (30% improvement) was seen in a phase II trial.

Cytokine-antibody hybrids
In a similar fashion, cytokines (e.g.,IL-2) have been artificially fused (using molecular biology tools) to tumor specific IgG antibodies. The antibody now targets and binds to the tumor bringing IL-2 into close proximity. IL-2 is a *growth factor* for both NK and T cells, and this technique ensures high, biologically active levels

of IL-2 cells with local activation of T cells and NK cells adjacent to tumor cells. Such high concentrations of IL-2 delivered systemically are toxic. Administration of IL-2 in hybrid form reduces the toxic side effects of the cytokine alone (see below) while retaining its anti-tumor efficacy. These studies are in their infancy.

T cells (adaptive immunity)
Some evidence for a potential role for CTL in normal human tumor immunity has come from expression library screening, this time looking for evidence for antigens recognized by CTL in the tumor bearing population (see above). As for expression library screening using sera (see Clinical case #32), an expression library is prepared in which cDNAs, made by reverse transcription of mRNAs in the tumor, are incorporated into a virus vector. The viral vector is used to transfect a host cell population (ex vivo), and then these cells are stimulated to express protein from the cDNAs transfected into them. The tumor proteins are then processed by the proteasome (Chapter 3) and subsequently displayed on the transfected cell surface in association with class I MHC. CTLs from the tumor bearing host are then incubated with these transfected cells to identify CTLs specific for the expressed tumor peptide/class I MHC. Successful stimulation (implying recognition of expressed tumor antigen in transfected cells) is measured by T-cell proliferation or cytokine production.

A number of human tumor antigens have been identified in this fashion. Some of these antigens have been delivered in vivo in adenovirus vectors in an attempt to induce CTL activity and tumor regression. Immunization using adenovirus vectors and a MAGE-3 peptide, known to be presented by human HLA-1A cells, was attempted in patients with metastatic melanoma who had failed conventional therapy. Seven of 25 patients responded to this treatment.

Role of Type 1 cytokines for CD8+ mediated cytotoxicity
Most studies of tumor destruction by T cells have focused on the role of CD8+ cytotoxic T cells. A tumoricidal role for CD8+ T cells in vivo is postulated because tumor specific CD8+ T cells have been isolated from peripheral blood of cancer patients, as well as from excised tumor masses. Because differentiation of pCTLs to mature CTLs requires the presence of IL-2, tumor specific CD4+ T cells are probably required for effective CTL mediated antitumor immunity. One might expect CD8+ T-cell mediated tumor killing to be most relevant for virally induced tumors, and perhaps to be a function of MHC expression on the tumor (needed for effective antigen presentation). Thus locally derived (or exogenously administered) IFNγ should increase MHC expression and augment killing by CTL, with more effective anti-tumor immunity (see below, under immunotherapy).

Role of Type 2 cytokines on efficacy of CD8+ T cells in tumor destruction
Whether the preferential activation of Th2 cells, rather than Th1 cells, affects the course of tumorigenesis or tumor rejection is unclear. At least one study found that CD8+ T cells showed suppressor cell activity, not cytotoxic activity, when stimulated with Th2 cytokines.

Tumor Immunology

Mechanism of CTL destruction of tumors

When the CTL interacts with the tumor cell, the mechanism of subsequent tumor destruction follows the pathway outlined in Chapter 9. Secretion of granules containing the protein, perforin, occurs. Perforin inserts in the cell membrane to form pores, and osmotic lysis results (Fig. 16.5).

EVASION OF IMMUNE SURVEILLANCE

Studies with many cancer patients have shown that tumor specific antibody, CTLs and even active NK cells are present in the face of progressive tumor growth. These data imply both an activation of the immune system in response to tumor antigens and the inadequacy of the immune response for effective tumor growth control. Many studies have tried to identify the mechanisms by which tumors evade immune mediated destruction. These include T-cell related defects or dysfunction (Fig. 16.6) as well as antigen related ones (Fig. 16.7). In addition, a role for secretion of immunosuppressive molecules by the tumors themselves, and a decrease in class I MHC expression provide immune system evasion strategies for some tumors (Fig. 16.8).

T-cell related defects or dysfunction

i The tumor immune response would be dampened if Th cells were not stimulated to release cytokines required for the differentiation of pCTLs to mature CTLs, or if inappropriate subsets of Th cells (e.g., Th2 cells) were activated (Fig. 16.6).

ii Tumors may escape immune detection if the T-cell repertoire does not include a TCR specific for the tumor antigen/MHC complex, i.e., there is a hole in the repertoire (Fig. 16.6).

iii Efficient antigen presentation for immune responses requires appropriate costimulatory molecules on antigen presenting cells. Absence of these (and/or their ligands on lymphocytes) produces ineffective immunization (Fig. 16.6).

iv T cells recognize antigen in association with MHC molecules. An inability of host MHC alleles to bind tumor peptide for presentation by antigen presenting cells, a phenomenon called determinant selection (Fig. 16.6), leads to failed tumor immunity.

Tumor antigen related phenomenon

i Immune responses to foreign peptides are directed to discrete antigenic epitopes. Because there are few antigenic epitopes on most proteins, "mutations of mutations" might allow tumor cells to escape detection due to a loss of antigenicity (Fig. 16.7).

ii Tumors could also escape detection by "antigenic modulation", the decrease/loss of antigen epitopes by endocytosis which follows the formation of antigen/antibody complexes on the tumor cell surface (Fig. 16.7).

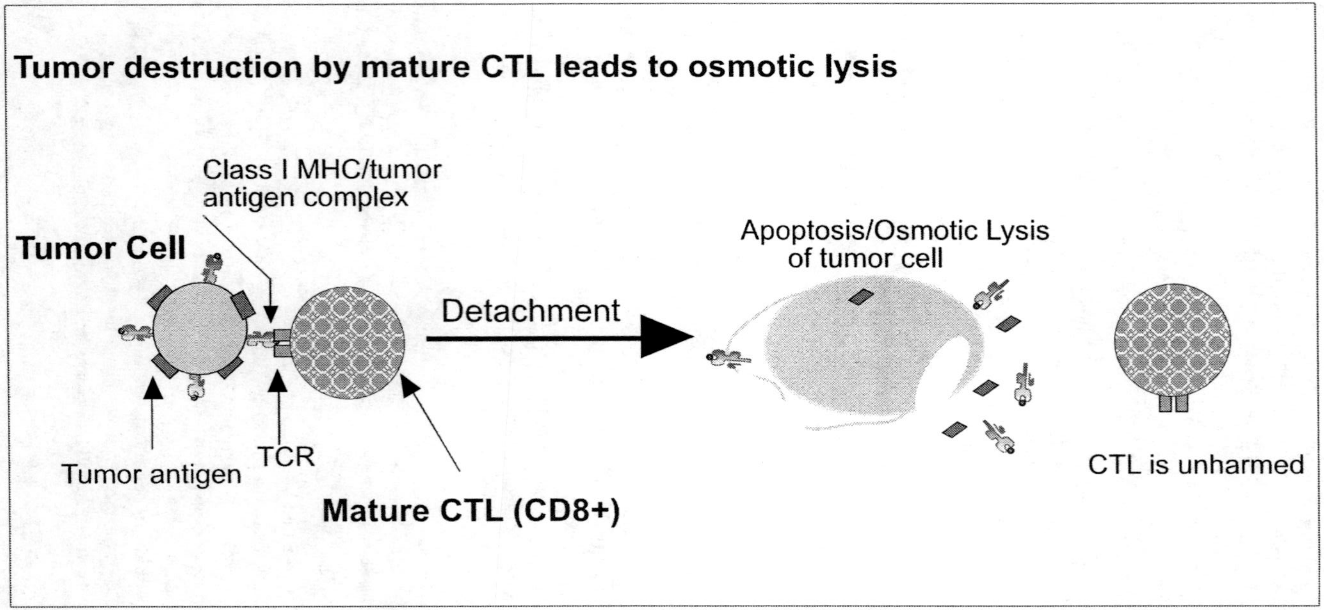

Tumor destruction by mature CTL leads to osmotic lysis

Tumor Cell — Class I MHC/tumor antigen complex — Tumor antigen — TCR

Mature CTL (CD8+) → Detachment → Apoptosis/Osmotic Lysis of tumor cell

CTL is unharmed

Fig. 16.5. Effector mechanism for elimination of tumors: cytotoxic T cells. A tumoricidal role for CD8+ T cells in vivo is postulated because tumor specific CD8+ T cells have been isolated from peripheral blood of cancer patients and from excised tumor masses. Mature cytotoxic CD8+ T cells (CTL) recognize tumor cells expressing antigenic peptides/class I MHC complexes on their cell surface. CTL secrete granules containing the protein perforin which cause osmotic lysis.

Tumor Immunology

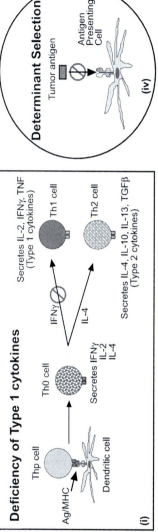

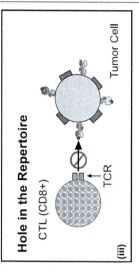

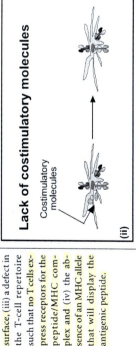

Fig. 16.6. T-cell related defects leading to evasion of immune surveillance by tumors. T-cell related defects leading to tumor cell evasion of immunosurveillance include: (i) a deficiency of Type 1 cytokines required for pCTL differentiation to CTL, (ii) a lack of costimulatory molecules on the cell presenting the peptide/MHC complex on its surface, (iii) a defect in the T-cell repertoire such that no T cells express receptors for the peptide/MHC complex and (iv) the absence of an MHC allele that will display the antigenic peptide.

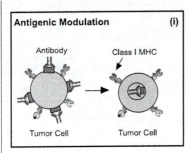
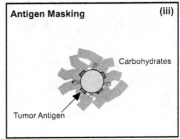
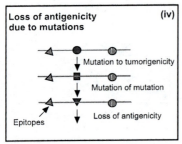
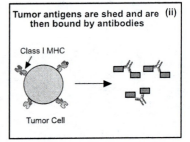

Fig. 16.7. Antigen related phenomenon leading to evasion of immune surveillance by tumors. All of the following prevent tumor antigen recognition: (i) endocytosis following the formation of immune complexes on the tumor cell surface; (ii) antigen shedding and binding by antibodies; (iii) the presence of carbohydrates masking the antigen; (iv) mutation of antigenic determinants on the tumor antigen to a nonimmunogenic form.

iii Tumors may evade destruction by "antigen masking", a phenomenon by which tumor antigens are "hidden" from the immune system by complex carbohydrates on the cell surface (Fig. 16.7).

iv The role of antibodies in tumor destruction in vivo remains elusive. Antibody complexed to soluble tumor antigen (shed from the tumor) might itself play a role in blocking tumor destruction. The exact mechanism(s) for this are not understood, but are thought to involve a role for TCR blockade by the complex (Fig. 16.7).

Down-regulation of class I MHC: Antigen complexes on the tumor cell

Tumor lysis by CTL requires recognition/presentation of a tumor peptide by class I MHC. Cell transformation can decrease expression of MHC, leading to tumor cell survival because of inefficient antigen recognition (Fig. 16.8). Loss of class I MHC expression would be expected to result in increased NK-mediated lysis of tumor cells (above). Because the antigen processing machinery leading to effective antigen presentation is quite complex, it is no surprise to learn that a number of steps interfere with CTL tumor antigen recognition. Defects may occur in the generation of immunogenic peptides in the cytosol (proteasomal defects), or in the "loading" of peptides in the endoplasmic reticulum as a result of

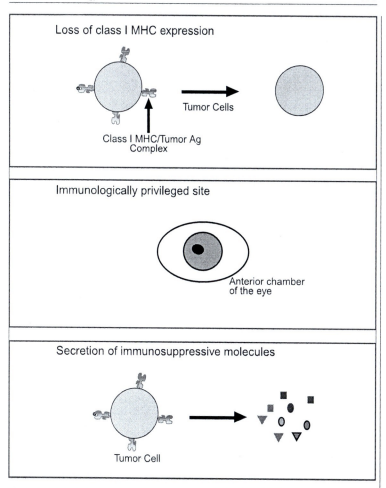

Fig. 16.8. Evasion of tumor surveillance by tumors. Tumor lysis by CTL requires recognition/presentation of a tumor peptide by class I MHC. Cell transformation decreasing expression of MHC can prevent tumor recognition. Antigen sequestration reflects the presence of the tumor in an immunologically privileged site (e.g., the anterior chamber of the eye). Some tumors secrete immunosuppressive molecules to evade the immune system.

defects in the transporter associated with antigen processing (TAP) proteins (Chapter 3).

Apoptosis of CTL and/or dendritic cells
Recent reports in a study of patients with metastatic melanoma have reported all of the above aberrations. More subtle mechanisms by which melanoma cells have been reported to down-regulate CTL recognition include expression of FasL

by metastatic melanoma cells, with subsequent lysis of Fas+ CTL. Apoptosis induced by FasL+ melanoma cells may even extend to host (Fas+) dendritic antigen presenting cells themselves.

Antigen sequestration

The tumor may be in an immunologically privileged site (e.g., the anterior chamber of the eye) (Fig. 16.8) or in host placental tissue (tumors of the female reproductive tract). Multiple mechanisms produce tumor protection in the urogenital tract, including the local hormonal milieu (immunosuppressive), local cytokine production (TGFβ), known immunoregulatory cells (e.g., γδ TCR+ cells) etc.

Secretion of immunosuppressive molecules by the tumor

Tumors often produce molecules which have potent, nonspecific, immunosuppressive properties, e.g., prostaglandin E2 (PGE2) (Fig. 16.8). Other molecules released by tumors (proteinases etc.) serve to degrade the surrounding matrix and enhance metastatic potential.

IMMUNOLOGY IN DIAGNOSIS OR IN MONITORING PROGNOSIS

There are several possible roles for immunology in tumor biology. Immunology can be used in diagnosis, to monitor the prognosis of tumors or efficacy of therapy, or in novel tumor therapies.

Diagnosis of tumors using immunological tools

The use of immunological tools for specific diagnosis of malignancy depends upon the (still unproven) existence of unique antigens on tumors of different histological types. Evidence that these exist is growing, though there is insufficient data to support routine screening for antibodies/CTL to distinct antigens as conclusive evidence for the existence of certain tumors. Individual cases can be cited where existing data implies this sort of technology may be on the horizon. Relatively unique antigens have been described in melanoma (MAGE-1 to 3), in colon carcinomas (17-1A) and in ovarian tumors. CTL specific for MAGE-3 have been identified in HLA-A1 positive patients with melanoma. In rare cases where malignancies exist within the immune system itself, the normal products of the (malignant) immune cell can often assist in diagnosis. Myeloma cells overproduce light chains, which are released at high concentrations into the serum, overwhelming the renal filtration apparatus and spilling into the urine. The existence of these *Bence Jones* proteins in urine (identified by immunoelectrophoresis and/or ELISA) is diagnostic.

Monitoring tumor growth/treatment: Using immunological tools

The use of immunological technologies to guide treatment and/or monitor tumor progress is less demanding than for diagnosis. To screen a large population for the presence of disease, exquisite specificity is needed to avoid inclusion of a large number of false positives (which might go on to much more expensive and unnecessary definitive investigations). However, when the diagnosis is clear and a test that detects the presence of small deposits of malignant cells is needed, sensitivity often becomes more crucial than specificity. Ideally one needs a test with high sensitivity and specificity, but often we sacrifice one for the (greater) benefit of the other. The application of monoclonal antibodies in both diagnosis/monitoring are already routine in clinical laboratories.

Radiolabeled (e.g., with radioactive iodine for detection by gamma-cameras) monoclonal antibodies are valuable to improve sensitivity in imaging studies to detect micro-metastases. This is especially so in scenarios where the primary tumor has been located but there is concern that small deposits of tumor exist elsewhere, below the limits of conventional imaging procedures (CAT scan, MRI etc.). For antibodies to be used to detect micro-metastases, the antibody must either be very specific with high avidity, or its cross reaction with normal tissue must be known. Positive scans can identify regions of tissue where further investigation is needed to ensure absence of metastatic tumor growth.

When antibodies are used to monitor the efficacy of drug therapy on a tumor, high sensitivity is more crucial than specificity. Even antibodies to the oncofetal antigens have proven invaluable in cancer care. As examples, early recurrences in gastrointestinal malignancy are detected by following CEA levels postoperatively. As noted above for choriocarcinoma, the levels of β-HCG represent such a reliable test for recurrence that monitoring by ELISA is used to guide treatment decisions regarding chemotherapy.

Innovative approaches designed to stimulate anti-tumor immunity are being tested in clinical trials. The premise is that tumors have evaded immune mediated destruction because some critical element, required for stimulating an immune response, is lacking. The following are examples of some new strategies for treating cancer.

NOVEL THERAPIES: ENHANCING ANTIGEN PRESENTATION BY DENDRITIC CELLS

The greatest contemporary interest in potentiating immunity to tumors resides in understanding mechanisms to improve the immunogenicity of antigen presented by dendritic cells (DCs). DCs are the most efficient professional antigen presenting cells for induction of primary immune responses.

Role of CD40/CD40L interaction

The interaction between CD40 (on DCs) and CD40L (on helper T cells) is instrumental in effective T-cell activation. In artificial mouse "knockout" studies, mice lacking CD4+ T cells only produced effective anti-tumor responses when anti-CD40 was used as an alternative means to cross-link CD40 on DCs.

Anti-CD40 antibodies are not present in a normal immune response, but the CD40 ligand (CD40L) expressed on (activated) CD4+ T-cells functions in this capacity. DCs activated in response to CD40 crosslinking will display antigen in the context of class II MHC as well as class I MHC, although different peptides are presented. The assumption in this model is that tumor antigens are endocytosed and encounter class II MHC within the endocytic vacuole (Chapter 3), while some tumor antigens are pinocytosed so that they are not contained within an endocytic vacuole. These cytosolic tumor antigens are fragmented by the proteasome complex and then transported into the endoplasmic reticulum where they are loaded onto class I MHC molecules. Activation of DCs by CD40L then enables effective presentation of peptide:class I MHC to CD8+ CTL. Interestingly, preactivated T cells incubated with CD40+ tumor cells often down-regulate CD40L, rendering them incapable of providing the necessary stimulus to DCs and thus resulting in failure to stimulate CTL anti-tumor immunity! This clearly has implications for understanding how we might use this form of therapy in clinical trials.

Role of chemokines and chemokine receptors

Because DCs migrate from peripheral tissues to lymphoid organs to induce immunity, factors controlling migration are important to those interested in manipulation of anti-tumor immunity. This is an expanding new area of clinical research, involving the study of chemokines and chemokine receptors on DCs. To date no clinical trials have used such manipulations in this tumor immunology field.

Role of DCs as adjuvants

Adjuvants enhance the immune response. The use of DCs as adjuvants has, to date, relied on artificial pulsing of (autologous) DCs with tumor lysates, tumor proteins or tumor peptides. However, transfection of cDNA encoding the tumor antigens should be equally, if not more, effective, ensuring that tumor antigens are processed and displayed on the DC cell surface. Reinfusion of the dendritic cells back into the patient leads to the presentation of tumor peptides to the CD4+ T cells, with the expectation that naive cells would differentiate to Th1 cells secreting cytokines required for activation of NK cell and CTL cytotoxicity.

Animal studies have validated the use of such tumor antigen pulsed DC as immunotherapy to protect from tumor growth, a fact confirmed by preliminary clinical trials, especially in cases of minimal residual disease following therapy of a primary tumor. Renal cell carcinoma patients received autologous DCs loaded with a renal carcinoma lysate in a phase I trial with moderate success. Similarly DCs pulsed with melanoma antigens were injected intradermally into patients with metastatic disease with good results. In this case deliberate coadministration of an artificial antigen (keyhole limpet hemocyanin, KLH) known to stimulate Type 1 cytokine (especially IL-2) production was given. The presumption is that the cytokine milieu so produced further facilitated induction of melanoma specific CD8+ CTL with anti-tumor reactivity.

Fusion of DCs with tumor cells

An alternative approach, currently undergoing a phase I/II clinical trial, involves *fusing* DCs with tumor cells to produce a more immunogenic form of tumor (antigen). The hybrid cell would express both high concentrations of class I and class II MHC so that relevant tumor peptides would be simultaneously displayed on the cell surface. These hybrid cells would activate both CD4+ T cells and CD8+ T cells, increasing the likelihood that IL-2 would be available for the differentiation of the pCTL to CTL.

Potential pitfalls
There are some potential pitfalls in the use of immunotherapy to generate tumor protective CTL. Vaccination of experimental animals with DCs pulsed with peptides to adenovirus encoded antigens, in an attempt to induce immunity to (and rejection of) tumors caused by adenovirus transformation of normal cells, enhanced the growth of the adenovirus antigen-expressing tumors. Presumably the immunization protocol led to some form of "tolerance induction" to the adenoviral encoded antigens. In addition, infusion of large amounts of free peptide might result in uptake by class I MHC+ cells that do not simultaneously express costimulatory molecules, again inducing tolerance—not immunity—to the tumor antigen.

NOVEL THERAPIES: CYTOKINES AND OTHER MOLECULES TRANSFECTED INTO TUMOR CELLS THEMSELVES

Clinical trials using granulocyte-monocyte colony stimulating factor
Alternative strategies to those above include modifying weakly immunogenic tumor cells to enhance their ability to present antigens to T cells. In a renal cell carcinoma phase I trial, irradiated tumor cells transfected with granulocyte-monocyte colony stimulating factor (GM-CSF) were injected into patients with late stage disease. GM-CSF is a hematopoietic cytokine, which leads to the differentiation and enhanced production of distinct myeloid cell populations, as well as the activation of macrophages and increased differentiation of Langerhans cells to dendritic cells. Increased infiltration of the injection site with a variety of antigen presenting cells was seen. It was hypothesized that these would stimulate presentation of tumor antigen to the host.

This model is similar to one studied by clinicians working with melanoma patients, where peptide administration of MART-1 melanoma antigen was coupled with local injection with GM-CSF to stimulate the differentiation of dermal Langerhans cells to dendritic cells. In this trial with the MART-1 and GM-CSF, a small response (decreased tumor burden) was seen in 4 of 25 patients.

Clinical trials using interleukin-2
A strategy aimed at enhancing tumor immunity involves the introduction of the IL-2 gene directly into inactivated tumor cells ex vivo and the reintroduction of these modified cells into patients. The assumption is that there are tumor specific naïve CD8+ T cytotoxic cells (pCTL) that have not differentiated to mature CTL capable of destroying the tumor because the IL-2 cytokine has been lacking (see above, use of KLH in a clinical trial with melanoma patients). IL-2 is crucial for this differentiation and is generally derived from CD4+ Th1 cells (Chapter 9). Exogenous IL-2 obviates the need for Th1 cells. In a phase I trial, cells transfected with the IL-2 gene, using an adenovirus vector containing a cDNA insert encoding

for the IL-2 gene, were injected into patients. This led to delayed type hypersensitivity responses (Chapter 13) to melanoma antigen and the development of vitiligo in 3 of 15 patients, providing clear evidence of destruction of melanocytes following this immunization.

Metastatic cells from melanoma patients have been successfully transduced in culture with canary pox virus carrying a number of different human cytokine genes. Local injection into patients of these inactivated and transduced melanoma cells led to infiltration with lymphocytes when the melanoma cells had been transduced with pox virus carrying IL-2. In contrast, local injection of the melanoma cells transduced with a pox virus carrying the GM-CSF gene led to infiltration by macrophages/neutrophils. Thus, this manipulation can "orchestrate" a cellular immune response which occurs independent of the (viral) vector system used.

Clinical trials using IL-12, IL-7, and IFNγ in retroviral vectors

The introduction of cytokine genes, other than IL-2, into isolated and inactivated tumor cells for reintroduction into patients is also being examined. Clinical trials with melanoma patients are underway investigating the effect of transfecting melanomal cells with the interleukin-12 (IL-12) gene. IL-12 enhances Type 1 cytokine production and stimulates growth of NK cells. NK cells, with a relatively broad specificity, will then be activated to destroy the melanoma cells. Production of Type 1 cytokines should provide "help" for differentiation of those pCTL that recognize the tumor antigen, but need IL-2 (a Type 1 cytokine) to become mature CTL.

IL-7 plays a role in the proliferation of pre-T cells, pre-B cells, NK cells, and some mature T cells. IL-7 is also a growth factor for subsets of preactivated T cells (CTL) and natural killer (NK) cells. Introduction of an IL-7 gene into inactivated tumor cells would provide a local source of this cytokine when the CTL, or the NK cell interact with the tumor.

Other groups are studying the effect of introducing the gene for IFNγ into inactivated tumor cells because NK cells are activated by this cytokine, as are macrophages. Recognition of tumor antigen by the NK cell receptor would place the NK cell in the vicinity of the IFNγ-secreting tumor where this cytokine would make the NK cells more potent tumor cell killers. Note that IFNγ also up-regulates the expression of MHC molecules on the tumor cells. This would make the NK cell *less effective* in the destruction of tumors, following the interaction of MHC with the killer inhibitory receptors (KIRs) on NK cells. However, in the presence of increased MHC, T-cell antigen recognition is increased, and presumably CD8+ CTL, specific for the tumor antigen, will develop to kill the tumor cells.

Clinical trials using enhanced expression of class I MHC

Another strategy aimed at enhancing the activation and differentiation of pCTL to CTL is the introduction of class I MHC genes into inactivated tumor cells ex vivo, again returning these cells to the patient. Tumors (particularly melanoma, for which there is evidence that CD8+ CTL provide important anti-tumor immunity) may escape destruction because the concentration of class I MHC on the tumor cell is so low that the activation threshold for pCTL is not reached and differentiation to mature CTLs does not occur. It is assumed that adequate amounts of IL-2 are available for differentiation of pCTLs to CTLs, that tumor specific antigens are present on the tumor, and that there are indeed tumor specific pCTL present in the individual's T-cell repertoire. A related strategy, not yet explored in human tumor biology, involves the introduction of accessory molecules into the inactivated tumor, ex vivo, and reintroduction into the patient to promote better stimulation of T-cell immune responses.

Novel Therapies: Modification of CTL as a Strategy for Enhancing Tumor Immunity

One approach to enhance existing tumor immunity is to remove immune effector cells and expand/modify them in vitro before reinfusion into patients. This technique has been explored, in melanoma and renal cell carcinoma patients using tumor-infiltrating T lymphocytes (TILs) obtained following excision of tumor from patients. TILs are clonally expanded in vitro and reinfused into the patient, often along with IL-2. In a modified version of this strategy the gene for tumor necrosis factor was inserted into the TIL prior to infusion of the genetically modified TILs into the patient. The TILs home to tumors, where they will now secrete tumor necrosis factor, a tumoricidal cytokine. Preliminary phase I/II trials are encouraging. Interestingly both IFNγ and TNF are both known to modify expression of adhesion molecules on cells/vascular endothelium, and this may play an important role in the effects seen.

Novel Therapies: Monoclonal Antibodies and Immunotherapy

Based on the premise that tumors bear tumor specific antigens, it was believed that monoclonal antibodies (Mabs) would serve as "magic bullets" for the destruction of tumors. It was postulated that the specificity of the antibody would ensure that only tumor cells would be destroyed, via the mechanism outlined earlier. Reasons for the failure of these ideas were discussed above.

Monoclonal antibodies are used for ex vivo purging of low levels of tumor cells in bone marrow preparations from lymphoma patients. The patient's bone marrow cells are removed and incubated with tagged tumor specific antibody (e.g., CD30 in the case of Hodgkin's lymphoma). Using the tag (either a fluorescent label or a magnetic label) the (few) tumor cells are depleted from the bone marrow cells. Meanwhile the patient receives exhaustive chemotherapy to destroy the tumor in the host. Finally the purged bone marrow cells are reinfused in the patient for autologous transplantation. Because autologous cells are used, the patient is not at risk of graft versus host disease associated with allogenic transplants (Chapter 17).

Modified antibodies

Other approaches have been used to increase the efficacy of antibody therapy for the in vivo destruction of tumors, as outlined earlier. These include the infusion into lymphoma patients of bispecific antibodies. In other studies cytokines (e.g., IL-2) were fused (using molecular biology tools) to specific antibodies, in the hope of reducing the side effects of infusion of the cytokine alone (see below) while retaining its anti-tumor efficacy. Other approaches have involved designing antibodies, which were radiolabeled (thus serving to carry a toxic level of radioactivity specifically to a tumor site), or labeled with a toxin (e.g., pseudomonas toxin). These studies are still in their infancy.

Idiotypic antibodies

Finally we should consider the special case where, in a tumor of the immune system itself (e.g., of chronic B-cell lymphocytic leukemia (CLL)), the tumor cells carry a unique antigen (the immunoglobulin molecule) which can be used to generate an immune response leading to the destruction of the B cell. There are sites within the variable region that are unique to the mIg on the B-cell tumor. Immunization produces a particular type of antibody (or T cell) immunity referred to as anti-idiotypic. The surface Ig idiotype in this case represents a unique TSTA. However, the very (individual) specificity of the treatment, along with the length of time often needed to produce the anti-idiotypic reagents, results in this form of therapy not being a viable proposition (logistically and financially) for routine medical practice.

Summary

Eradication of tumors by the immune system requires recognition of foreignness on the tumor. In animal model systems, it has been found that chemically-induced tumors have unique tumor antigens, but that virally induced tumors express common tumor antigens.

The concept of immune surveillance was developed to explain a developmental significance for anti-tumor immunity. Definitive proof that this provides a useful way to understand tumor immunity is lacking. There is good evidence that the immune system reacts to the presence of tumor cells in the host. Using a variety of approaches both tumor specific antigens (TSTAs) and tumor associated antigens (TAAs) have been described. TAAs include the so-called oncofetal antigens, molecules that are expressed on normal tissues during certain stages of development and are also later, in adult life, found re-expressed on some tumor cells. Oncofetal antigens are often used to monitor the progress of the tumor.

Activated macrophages, NK cells and CD8+ cytotoxic T cells are all capable of destroying tumors under varying conditions. A role for CD4+ T cells is implied because these processes all require CD4+ T-cell derived cytokines for their effector function. In addition, antibodies have been shown to play a role in facilitating the effector function of both macrophages and natural killer cells.

Studies with cancer patients have shown that tumor specific CTLs are present in many patients, suggesting the activation of the immune system in response to tumor antigens. This is particularly the case for melanoma patients and patients with renal cell carcinomas. However, detectable malignancy in these patients indicates that the immune response is inadequate. A number of T-cell related defects or dysfunctions could contribute to the failure to activate anti-tumor immune T cells, including the absence of CD4+ T-cell cytokines to the lack of costimulatory molecules required for T-cell activation. Tumors may also escape detection because the antigenic sites present on the tumors have been altered, masked, or shed. Finally, tumors may be sequestered, secrete immunosuppressive molecules, or down-regulate their expression of MHC so that they are not detected by cells of adaptive immunity.

Independent of the role of the immune system in the eradication of tumors, components of the immune system can be used in diagnosis of tumors, to monitor the prognosis of tumors, to enhance the efficacy of therapy, or to serve as effectors in novel therapies for tumors.

CLINICAL CASES AND DISCUSSION

Clinical Case #31

A 35-year-old lady has been treated for choriocarcinoma (a germ cell tumor of syncytiotrophblastic cells). She received a prolonged course of methotrexate and was feeling well. She was lost to follow up for 6 months. When you see her she has taken up cigarette smoking again and has redeveloped her chronic cough. Physical exam is normal, except for scattered wheezes in her chest. Her complete blood count (CBC) and electrolytes are normal. She reports amenorrhea for 3 months but denies sexual activity. Her mother experienced early menopause. ↳ absence of menses

Questions and Discussion: Case #31
1. List the six likely key features we need to bear in mind in discussing this case.
   - 35-year-old lady treated for choriocarcinoma
   - prolonged course of metotrexate, but no follow up for 6 months
   - cigarette smoking again, chronic cough, scattered wheezes in her chest
   - physical exam, and blood work are normal
   - amenorrhea for 3 months; denies any sexual activity
   - family history of early menopause.
2. **Which oncofetal marker is monitored in cases of choriocarcinoma"?**
   β-HCG is an oncofetal antigen, expressed by tumor cells in choriocarcinoma. It is such an effective way of monitoring treatment that we pay particular attention to the response of β-HCG levels to therapy of the tumor. We assume her levels were never monitored to baseline.
3. This **patient was found to have elevated** β-HCG levels (55,000 Units in serum). What **complicating factor** must you consider when analyzing the results?
   This lady has amenorrhea and could be pregnant. β-HCG levels are consistent with a 14-week fetus.
4. With reference to #3, how would you proceed?
   Pelvic ultrasound will rule out a uterine pregnancy as the cause of the elevated β-HCG. A 14-week fetus should be easily visible. Nothing was seen.

5. **Why is the chronic cough worrisome in the context of this case? How would you proceed?**
   Dissemination of this tumor to the lungs is common. You order a chest x-ray (CXR). If you have not yet ruled out pregnancy this lady needs a lead shield over the pelvis.
6. **The CXR shows multiple "cannonball" lesions throughout the field. How do you proceed?**
   You now need to check on the details of her first treatment for choriocarcinoma. This is most likely a metastatic recurrence. A biopsy (open lung) may be warranted for confirmation, but probably is not necessary. Note the specificity of β-HCG in this scenario. Adenocarcinomas of the ovary, pancreas, stomach and even hepatomas (rarely) produce this molecule. Germ cell tumors often produce both β-HCG and AFP (alpha feto protein). In patients with germ cell tumors producing both AFP and β-HCG, discordant reduction in the levels of the two generally reflects the existence and differential eradication of two separate tumor clones.
7. **Another commonly used oncofetal antigen in tumorogenesis is CEA (carcinoembryonic antigen). However, CEA has more limitations than b-HCG. Explain.**
   CEA can be used to monitor patients posttreatment to detect early recurrence. However, increased levels of CEA are also common in smokers, in alcoholics (especially with cirrhosis), and with other malignancies including breast, pancreas etc. Thus the differential diagnosis of an elevated CEA would not have been as restricted.

Clinical Case #32
DE is a young (22 years of age) sun-worshiping boy whom you have been following for 3 years for malignant melanoma. He has a particularly aggressive form of the disease, which has not been controlled with frequent rounds of conventional chemotherapy. He reports a total loss of the ability to fix the right eye for lateral gaze. He asks you what is known about more experimental treatments, including antigen immunizations, cytokine therapy etc.

Questions and Discussion: Case #32
1. **List the six likely key features we need to bear in mind in discussing this case.**
   young male
   malignant melanoma
   three years of conventional chemotherapy
   loss of right lateral gaze
   therapy does not control disease
   requests experimental therapy
   DE's melanoma has been refractory to treatment. The additional loss of the right lateral gaze is suspicious for a new (small) lesion in the central nervous system, involving one cranial nerve only (right C-VI). MRI scan suggests a small tumor nidus here. Not surprisingly then, this unfortunate

patient has metastatic disease. This group of patients has formed the cohort for a number of novel medical immunotherapeutic interventions in tumor biology. In the discussion that follows a number of these are highlighted.

2. **What tumor antigen is detected on melanoma cells?**
One of the first tumor specific antigens identified, MAGE-1, was discovered on human melanoma cells. A number of melanoma specific antigens are now known (MAGE 1-3).

3. More recently expression libraries have now been used extensively in attempts to characterize unique tumor antigens. *What is an expression library?*
Expression libraries are made from cDNA molecules derived by reverse transcription of mRNA. These cDNA molecules reflect the sum of all mRNAs expressed in a malignant cell. To generate an expression library, the cDNA is inserted into a viral vector that allows transcription and translation of the gene product. The vectors are expressed in a cell, often a bacterial cell. The sum of the expression products of all transduced cells constitutes the "expression library". Proteins synthesized by transduced cells can be identified using serum antibodies or T cells which are stimulated to produce a measurable function.

4. *What is the advantage of having an expression library to identify and characterize tumor antigens?*
The expression libraries have general applicability and increased sensitivity. They can be used to characterize both Igs and T-cell reactivity. Serum antibodies or T cells from the tumor host are screened for recognition of any antigenic determinants expressed in the library. If these are detected, the antigens are purified. MAGE 1-3 were characterized in this way.

5. *What is the clinical relevance of characterizing a tumor antigen?*
Once a tumor antigen has been identified, it must be characterized to determine which, if any, nonmalignant tissues also express this antigen. This information determines whether the antigen can serve as a diagnostic tool, as a target for antibody therapy, or as a tool for monitoring reccurrence of disease. To do this, antibodies specific for the tumor antigen must be generated and purified, and host tissues tested to see if they bind the antibody.

6. *Assuming that a tumor specific antigen is identified, and an antibody generated that recognizes that tumor antigen, how might these antibodies work therapeutically?*
When the antibody binds to the tumor antigen, the cells may be destroyed by IgG opsonin-mediated phagocytosis. Alternatively, cells may be destroyed by osmotic lysis when FcγRs on NK cells bind the Fc region of the antibody bound to the tumor antigen (ADCC).

7. *Are there ways in which activated CD8+ T cells could be used to destroy tumors?*
Activated CTLs specific for a tumor antigen could destroy tumor cells if the tumor antigen is presented by class I MHC on the tumor cell. The key

step is efficient activation of CD8+ T cells. In one protocol dendritic cells grown in culture are "pulsed" with the tumor specific antigen and reinfused in the patient. There, T cells specific for the tumor antigen are activated and clonally expand. This has been successful in experimental models and in phase I and II clinical trials.

8. Other experimental techniques under investigation suggest inserting several genes into the vector. The genes recommended for therapy are those required for efficient CD4+ T-cell activation in order to provide the necessary cytokines for activation of macrophages and/or CTL. What genes should be included in this hypothetical vector?

   IFNγ is believed to polarize the Thp differentiation to a Th1 phenotype, secreting Type 1 cytokines. Type 1 cytokines, IL-2 and IFNγ, activate pCTL and macrophages, respectively. Additional genes that could facilitate activation of the Thp cell would include B7-1, B7-2, and CD40. These are important costimulatory molecules that might further enhance Thp cell activation and induction of Th1 cells.

9. What are the commonest problems associated with cytokine infusions into patients?

   The most common problem is "capillary leak syndrome", reflecting a nonspecific increase in vessel permeability and chronic edema. This is probably not a factor under physiological conditions of cytokine production because cytokines are usually produced in very high concentrations locally. One approach to circumvent this problem uses the delivery of the cytokine covalently attached to an antibody, which itself recognizes the tumor antigen, thus serving as a specific delivery system for the cytokine.

10. It has also been suggested that we can "clone out" CTL from the patients themselves and manipulate them to carry beneficial cytokine genes. What gene is required?

    The differentiation of pCTL to CTL requires IL-2. If IL-2 is cloned into the host CTL and reinfused into the patient, maturation and differentiation should occur without Th1 cells.

11. Some studies have removed tumor cells, altered them genetically, and then reinfused them into the patient. What genetic manipulation would increase activation of Thp cells?

    Tumor cells can escape immunosurveillance following down-regulation of costimulatory molecules (e.g., B7-1, B7-2, CD40, IL-2 expression etc.) required for T-cell activation. Reinfusion of tumor cells transduced to express these molecules might activate T-cell immunity.

12. All of the above therapies must be studied in randomized, double-blinded trials, particularly in the case of melanoma. Why?

    The incidence of SPONTANEOUS recovery is reportedly high for melanoma patients.

Tumor Immunology

TEST YOURSELF

Multiple Choice Questions
1. A 25-year-old woman was recently diagnosed with choriocarcinoma. She began treatment with Methotrexate, and levels of β-HCG initially fell. You now find the β-HCG levels are rising. Appropriate action would be:
   a. Assume that the new lab tech is having "quality control problems"
   b. Repeat the test at another laboratory (waiting time approximately 1 week)
   c. Wait and see if the next test (due in 1 week) "corrects" this increase
   d. Likely pregnancy so refer to obstetrician
   e. Oncofetal antigen level rising; change treatment
2. A 26-year-old male, nonsmoker, previously well, has a dry nonproductive cough, low-grade fever for 2 weeks and night sweats. He uses no drugs and has not traveled recently. A chest x-ray shows marked hilar lymphadenopathy. Biopsy reveals non-Hodgkin's lymphoma. Which of the following might be associated with this problem?
   a. Low serum IgA
   b. Low serum IgG
   c. CD4+ T cells < 400
   d. Low complement levels
   e. Low serum IgM
3. A 44-year-old male friend is newly diagnosed with CLL. He hears that there may be a new treatment available, using anti-idiotype vaccination. The basis for this treatment is:
   a. Cytokine mediated and nonspecific
   b. Cytokine mediated that therefore specific
   c. Antigen-specific and directed to unique T-cell antigens
   d. Antigen nonspecific and directed to B-cell antigens
   e. Antigen-specific and directed to B-cell antigens
4. The most common type(s) of tumor occurring in immunosuppressed individuals is (are):
   a. Mammary carcinoma
   b. Prostate cancer
   c. Lung cancer
   d. Lymphomas
   e. Hepatoma
5. Elevated CEA will most likely be found in serum in all of the following EXCEPT:
   a. Lung cancer
   b. Hepatoma
   c. Breast cancer
   d. Stomach cancer
   e. Cancer of the colon

Answers: 1e; 2c; 3e ; 4d ; 5b

Short Answer Questions
1. What is immunosurveillance?
2. What mechanisms have been implicated in tumor immunity?
3. How would you search for tumor specific antigens?
4. What are oncofetal antigens?
5. How do tumors evade the immune system?

Transplantation

Objectives *367*
Transplantation *368*
General Features *368*
Classification of Grafts According to Their Source *368*
Classification of Graft Rejection *371*
Genetics of Transplantation *373*
Immunology of Graft Rejection *379*
Tissue Differences in Clinical Transplantation *387*
Graft Versus Host Disease *389*
Immunosuppression in Transplantation *389*
Summary *391*
Clinical Cases and Discussion *392*
Test Yourself *396*

Objectives

Transplantation is a process whereby cells/tissue from one individual (a donor) are transferred to a second individual (a recipient). Given the genetic disparity involved, under most situations the grafted tissue is recognized as foreign and rejected by the recipient's immune system. The immunological processes involved are the subject of this chapter. Rejection is generally a function of the T-cell arm of the immune response, though bystander cells are often recruited following release of mediators from T cells. In unique circumstances (preimmunized recipients or recipients of grafts across a species barrier, xenotransplantation) antibody responses are important.

In clinical practice recipients are prescreened to ensure the best genetic "fit" between donor and recipient. Following transplantation, recipients are treated long term with nonspecific immunosuppressive drugs to prevent rejection. Undesirable side effects of these drugs promote the search to induce specific tolerance (for the graft) in the recipient, eliminating the need for nonspecific immunosuppression.

Bone marrow transplantation is a situation in which both host-anti-graft and graft anti-host (**HvG** or **GvH** respectively) responses are potential problems. It is important to understand the immunology of these reactions, and their immunoregulation. When a bone marrow transplant is performed in cancer patients, often the anti-host immune response plays a positive role in the elimination of host tumor cells.

Clinical Immunology, by Reginald Gorczynski and Jacqueline Stanley. 2001 Landes Bioscience

TRANSPLANTATION

General Features

Transplantation refers to the engraftment of cells or tissues from one individual (donor) to another (recipient/host). Transfusion is a specific case of transplantation, using blood. Because a graft is foreign, the host's immune system will attempt to eliminate this "*intruder*", a phenomenon termed **graft rejection** (Fig. 17.1). For vascularized and nonvascularized (e.g., skin) grafts genetic differences at the **major histocompatibility complex (MHC)**, are mostly responsible for graft rejection processes. **Minor histocompatibility proteins** with allelic forms can also induce graft rejection, with varying degrees of immunological "vigor". Current technology does not permit rapid determination of minor histocompatibility differences between donor and recipient, and the clinician is most concerned with the degree of MHC disparity involved.

The MHC encodes several cell surface proteins. In humans, class I MHC and class II MHC proteins are referred to as **human leukocyte antigens (HLA)**. The existence of multiple MHC alleles in the population is referred to as **polymorphism**. Human class I MHC molecules are encoded by three loci (A, B, and C), whereas the class II MHC molecules are encoded by a "D" locus, subdivided into three loci, DP, DQ, and DR (Chapter 3). Each MHC allele is codominantly expressed, so individuals generally express six *different* class I MHC proteins, and six different class II MHC proteins, unless the parents were genetically related. Given MHC locus polymorphism and codominant expression of inherited MHC proteins of each class, most individuals have a pattern of MHC expression that differs from that present in other individuals, except in the case of identical twins.

Successful organ transplantation depends on suitable MHC matching and life long nonspecific immunosuppressive therapy. Because of the complications of nonspecific immunosuppression, specific tolerance induction to grafts remains an area of high priority in transplantation.

Classification of Grafts According to Their Source

Grafts are classified according to the source of the tissue donor (Fig. 17.2). **Isografts** are grafts between identical twins (**autografts**, e.g., skin, are grafts within the same individual); **allografts** are grafts between members of the same species; **xenografts** are grafts across species.

Iso- (or auto-) grafts

Since there is no genetic disparity in iso/auto grafts, engrafted tissue survives without the need for immunosuppression. Besides the use of organ and bone marrow grafts from identical twins, autografts (bone marrow) are used in rescue therapy for lymphoma and/or some other malignancies (e.g., breast cancer). Patients donate their own bone marrow (which is treated to "purge" it of residual malignant cells), then receive doses of chemotherapy which are "super toxic",

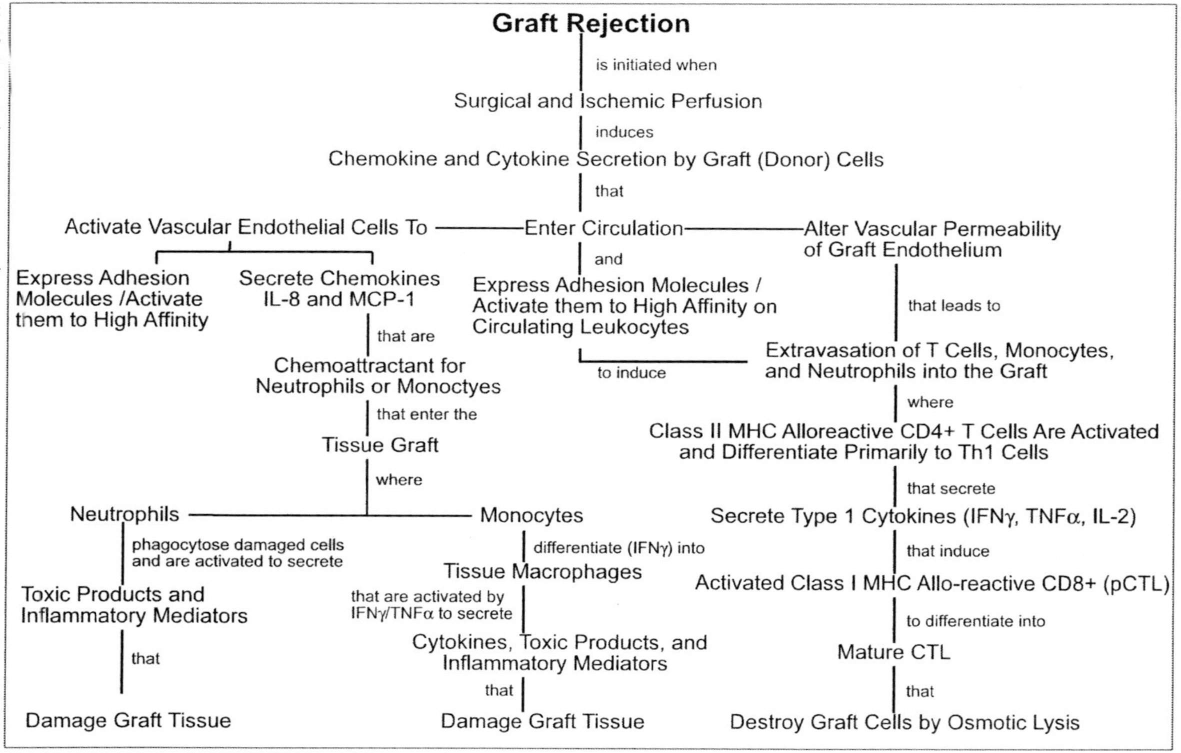

Transplantation

Graft Rejection

is initiated when

Surgical and Ischemic Perfusion

induces

Chemokine and Cytokine Secretion by Graft (Donor) Cells

that

Activate Vascular Endothelial Cells To — **Enter Circulation** — **Alter Vascular Permeability of Graft Endothelium**

and

that leads to

Express Adhesion Molecules / Activate them to High Affinity on Circulating Leukocytes

to induce

Extravasation of T Cells, Monocytes, and Neutrophils into the Graft

where

Class II MHC Alloreactive CD4+ T Cells Are Activated and Differentiate Primarily to Th1 Cells

that secrete

Secrete Type 1 Cytokines (IFNγ, TNFα, IL-2)

that induce

Activated Class I MHC Allo-reactive CD8+ (pCTL)

to differentiate into

Mature CTL

that

Destroy Graft Cells by Osmotic Lysis

Express Adhesion Molecules / Activate them to High Affinity

that are

Secrete Chemokines IL-8 and MCP-1

Chemoattractant for Neutrophils or Monocytes

that enter the

Tissue Graft

where

Monocytes differentiate (IFNγ) into **Tissue Macrophages**

that are activated by IFNγ/TNFα to secrete

Cytokines, Toxic Products, and Inflammatory Mediators

that

Damage Graft Tissue

Neutrophils phagocytose damaged cells and are activated to secrete

Toxic Products and Inflammatory Mediators

that

Damage Graft Tissue

Fig. 17.1. Concept map illustrating graft rejection. Immune recognition and ischemia-reperfusion injury trigger the secretion of chemokines and cytokines, producing the inflammatory/immunological changes of graft rejection.

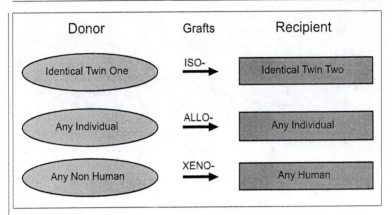

Fig. 17.2. Classification of grafts according to the donor source. Isografts are grafts between identical twins; allografts are grafts within a species; xenografts are grafts across species.

destroying malignant cells but also cells of the hematopoietic system. They then receive their own, autologous, bone marrow. No immune rejection (Host vs Graft, **HvG** or Graft vs Host, **GvH**) should occur. Sometimes a so-called syngeneic GvHD is seen (see later), the immunological basis of which remains unclear.

Allografts

An allograft is a graft between members of the same species. Graft survival is a function of the degree of genetic similarity between individuals and the immunosuppressive treatment used. Most human organ grafts are of this type, and these have met with some success following the advent of modern immunosuppressive drug therapy. Chronic ongoing treatment remains essential for long-term graft survival, bringing with it a multitude of side effects, many life threatening. Considerable effort is directed at understanding how allografts might be manipulated to achieve the same success as the one allograft that occurs *naturally* in mammalian species, namely the fetus. Tolerance established at the maternal-fetal interface has been attributed to multiple factors, including altered MHC expression, altered local cytokine production, nonspecific immunosuppression, etc. All have also been implicated in organ transplantation.

Xenografts

Grafts across a species (e.g., pig to human or nonhuman primate) are highly experimental. A number of advantages accrue to successful implementation of a xenograft program, including, amongst others, a (relatively) unlimited supply of organs; a genetic and pathogen-controlled source of material; and the ability to plan for transplantation so that the recipient's general health is optimal prior to surgery. For man, a nonhuman primate donor might be the best tissue source. Ethical and other limitations make it likely that the pig will be the animal of choice for future work in this field.

Transplantation

A number of ethical and scientific concerns remain, including risks of zoonotic transmission of disease (e.g., retroviral transfer across species). Such transmission can have disastrous consequence, given current data that implicates a monkey to human viral transmission as the etiology of the AIDS epidemic. The risk involved in pig to human transfer may be more apparent than real. While pig retroviruses exist, there has been no reported evidence for transfer to humans following introduction of porcine heart grafts (a procedure in existence for two decades or more). Even if these concerns and risks turn out to be acceptable and/or negligible, there remains the immunological barrier to xenotransplantation. This is a formidable obstacle, with T cells, B cells, complement and the innate immune system all implicated.

CLASSIFICATION OF GRAFT REJECTION

Graft rejection is classified as hyperacute (and delayed hyperacute or delayed accelerated), acute, or chronic (Table 17.1), based on the time over which the rejection process develops and the treatment options available. Both of these are a function of the immunopathological processes involved. Hyperacute rejection, occurring in minutes to hours, is antibody mediated (below); delayed accelerated rejection, occurring over the first 1-3 days post transplant, is a function of antibody/complement-mediated activation of graft endothelium; acute and chronic rejection represent the early and/or chronic effects of triggering of T cell immunity.

Hyperacute Rejection

Preformed antibodies to donor antigens mediate **hyperacute rejection**, occurring in minutes to hours post transplant. The existence of preformed antibodies indicates that the recipient has previously been immunized, intentionally, or unintentionally, against antigens on the donor tissue. For organ allografts the commonest individuals at risk are multiparous women and individuals who have had a previous (unsuccessful) graft. Often the antibody reaction is of such low affinity (or to antigens at low frequency on cells used for tissue typing) that it is "missed" accidentally. Potential donors against whom the recipient has a positive serum reactivity ("panel reactive") are not used as donors. This makes graft procurement for these recipients much more difficult.

Another scenario in which hyperacute rejection is seen, is when a xenograft is used. This reaction reflects the existence of natural antibodies in man to carbohydrates present on the transplanted pig organs. Production of these antibodies is believed to occur following stimulation by endogenous flora in the gastrointestinal tract.

Hyperacute rejection is associated with complement activation, stimulation of the coagulation cascade, thrombosis and rapid graft failure. The only treatment option is graft removal. For xenografts, researchers are exploring the possibility of producing transgenic animals expressing human complement regulatory molecules to inhibit this early activation of the complement cascade (Chapter 5). However the relative failure of these strategies to date suggest that early thrombosis is a

Table 17.1. Classification of graft rejection

Type of Rejection	Time Frame	Mediators	Treatment
Hyperacute	Minutes to hours	Preformed antibodies	• Remove organ !!!!
Delayed Hyperacute	First few days following transplantation	Activators of endothelial cells; also pro-coagulants (including fibroleukin/fgl-2)	• Currently under investigation
Acute	Days to weeks	Cell mediated immunity	• Increase immunosuppression (with caution)
Chronic	Months, to years	Multiple, likely nonspecific growth factor-like mediators (e.g. fibroblast growth factor; endothelial growth factor etc.) leading to an insidious fibrosing/proliferative reaction	• Does NOT respond to increased immunosuppression • Replace organ

function of the activation of other novel prothrombotic molecules as well (e.g., fibroleukin/fgl-2-see Chapter 5). Having overcome hyperacute rejection, the immunological hurdles of acute/chronic rejection will remain.

Acute rejection

The most common type of allograft rejection is "**acute rejection**" occurring in the early period post transplantation (weeks). **Acute rejection** reflects recognition by, and activation of, T cells. Depending on the organ system involved there are a number of ways to monitor for acute rejection. Following a liver graft one could follow serum levels of liver enzymes (reflecting damage to liver cells); for a kidney graft one could follow the ability of the kidneys to filter protein and toxic materials from the blood (i.e., following serum creatinine, which is normally removed by renal filtration). Suspicion of graft rejection often leads to tissue biopsy, examining evidence for immune cell infiltration and/or inflammation. Treatment involves increasing the dose of immunosuppressive agents used. This invariably brings with it an increased risk of infection, malignancy, and drug toxicity, so that the clinician "walks a tightrope" between increasing immunosuppression (to preserve the graft, increasing the risk of side effects) and decreasing immunosuppression (decreasing side effects, but increasing the risk of rejection).

Chronic rejection

Rejection occurring weeks/months/years following transplantation is termed chronic rejection. It is correlated with release of nonspecific growth factor-like mediators (e.g., fibroblast growth factor; endothelial growth factor etc.), which fits the histological picture of chronic fibrosis and hyperproliferation of connective tissue and mesenchymal cells characterizing this process. Because chronic rejection takes this form of an insidious fibrosing/proliferative reaction, with no clear start or end, it is not surprising to find that it is a process that is less amenable to treatment. There are some correlational studies, which suggest that chronic rejection represents the inevitable outcome of multiple episodes of acute rejection. However, other studies suggest that chronic rejection can be seen even in cases where no clear evidence existed for acute rejection. Since both processes are certainly less evident in immunologically compromised animals, current thought is that acute and chronic rejection reflect recognition/operation of different components of cell-mediated immunity. As an example, one school of thought is that acute rejection is more closely associated with Type 1 cytokine production (DTH type immunity), while chronic rejection is more associated with Type 2 cytokine production. This is unquestionably an oversimplification, however, and it is clear that other features are of importance in chronic rejection (e.g., the dramatic increase in levels of non-T-cell derived nonspecific growth factors, such as fibroblast growth factor).

GENETICS OF TRANSPLANTATION

Early studies in mice by Snell, mostly designed to investigate tumor immunity, revealed evidence for a gene complex, on chromosome 17 in mice (6 in man) which regulated the survival of tissue transplanted from one group of genetically identical animals to another. Mice identical at this gene complex accepted grafts from one another, while animals differing at this region rejected them vigorously. This gene complex became known as the major histocompatibility complex (MHC). Later studies revealed that disparity at multiple other loci could also provoke rejection of grafts between individuals matched at the MHC locus. These are known as minor histocompatibility loci (MiH).

Major histocompatibility complex

In humans MHC antigens are also termed human leukocyte antigens (HLA). The gene products of the class I MHC gene loci are HLA-A, HLA-B, and HLA-C, while those of the class II MHC gene loci are HLA-DP, HLA-DQ, and HLA-DR (Fig. 17.3). HLA proteins are highly polymorphic in the population. Genetic differences at any HLA locus contribute to the immunological rejection of a graft. Thus the fewer the number of mismatched loci, in general, the greater the likelihood that the graft will be accepted. HLA matching is an important step for clinical transplantation of tissues (below).

Minor histocompatibility loci

MiH loci encode proteins that serve some (unknown) function in a tissue. MiH antigens have allelic forms i.e., they differ between individuals, and immune recognition of those differences can induce graft rejection, with variable degrees of severity. In human bone marrow transplantation, immune recognition of H-Y (an antigen encoded by a gene in the Y-chromosome) occurs frequently and can cause GvHD. The H-Y epitopes recognized by T cells causing GvHD are under investigation.

Often differences in MiH antigens can lead to graft rejection that is as vigorous as that occurring with MHC differences. This has been confirmed in human bone

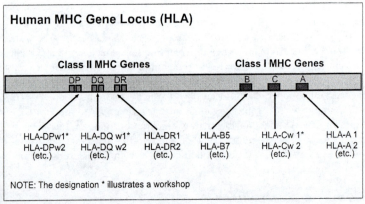

Fig. 17.3. MHC genes are polymorphic. Class I MHC gene loci are HLA-A, HLA-B, and HLA-C. The products of class II MHC gene loci are HLA-DP, HLA-DQ, and HLA-DR. These proteins are highly polymorphic, with multiple alleles encoded by each gene locus.

Transplantation

marrow transplantation when, despite using recipient and donor pairs that were MHC-matched, vigorous rejection, still occurred, reflecting a disparity at unknown MiH loci. The number of MiH loci capable of causing acute rejection is unknown, but there is no *a priori* reason to believe that MHC matching ensures MiH loci matching. Without methods to measure MiH differences, clinical transplantation often occurs in the face of significant immunological *minor histoincompatibility*, which becomes evident "after the fact".

Major histocompatibility typing in organ transplantation

In the absence of techniques to induce graft tolerance it is generally felt that optimal survival depends on minimizing immune recognition of the graft by minimizing the genetic disparity (MHC) between donor and recipient. This implies that total histocompatibility matching (0/6 haplotype mismatches) is the ideal scenario for clinical transplantation. Methods for tissue typing to measure histocompatibility between donor and recipient include serological, mixed lymphocyte reactions, and molecular techniques.

Serological techniques

Until recently, matching by serological techniques (for both class I MHC and class II antigens) was considered the method of choice (Fig. 17.4). Panels of sera reacting with individual HLA haplotypes have been characterized from multiparous females (immunized during pregnancy both by male sperm and by leakage of paternal antigen, positive fetal cells into the mother's circulation). Reactions of tissues of the potential donor and the recipient with these antibodies are compared,

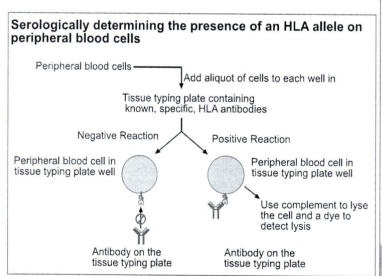

Fig. 17.4. Serological tissue typing. Serological techniques detect HLA antigens (primarily class I MHC) on cells. Antibodies are obtained from multiparous females.

with identical reactivity implying compatibility (serologically). While rapid and simple to use, a major limitation is that we can only identify differences for which sera exist in the "panel" of test antibodies. Nondiscrimination between donor and recipient does not necessarily indicate compatibility! The mixed lymphocyte reaction (MLR), which attempts to mimic in vivo graft rejection using in vitro assays, and molecular techniques, offer alternative approaches to circumvent this limitation.

Mixed lymphocyte reaction

CD8+ T cells (developing into CTL) recognize antigen in association with class I MHC while CD4+ T cells recognize antigen in association with class II MHC molecules (Chapter 9). Predicting CD4+ T cell activation is likely more important for gauging the likelihood of graft rejection because CD4+ T cell derived Type 1 cytokines are required for virtually all aspects of immunity involved in tissue rejection, ranging from "help" for B-cell activation, enhancement of macrophage and natural killer (NK) cell function, and differentiation of pCTL to CTL. The mixed lymphocyte culture reaction (MLR) quantitates CD4+ T cell activation.

Cells from the donor and recipient are cultured together with proliferation of recipient CD4+ T cells occurring only when they "see" a class II MHC difference on stimulating (donor) cells (Fig. 17.5). Proliferation is detected by measuring the amount of radioactive isotope incorporated into responding cell DNA. This assay measures immunological host/graft disparity376 and can have significant value in transplantation. Unfortunately the technique takes approximately 72-96 hrs, which can be a limitation for organ allografts that generally must be used quickly following their availability (preservation times vary for different organs, with lung being short (6-12 hrs), while kidney grafts are well preserved in the cold for 24-48 hrs). The MLR retains clinical use for bone marrow grafts and in cases of living related donors. In the case of the latter it is possible to match donor and recipient with less time constraints, using multiple techniques, and ensure that the donor most MHC compatible with the recipient is used.

Molecular techniques

Tissue matching has been improved using molecular biology tools, including restriction fragment length polymorphism (RFLP), in which DNA fragments are compared after specific enzyme digestion (Fig. 17.6). Genomic DNA extracted from recipient and donor blood cells is digested with a panel of enzymes, each of which recognizes unique sequences of nucleotides in the DNA. If, over a stretch of DNA, a sequence GAATTC occurs only once, the enzyme EcoR1 (which cleaves between G and A in this sequence) will introduce one cut into the DNA strand. Separation on a sizing gel reveals two "bands" of DNA, while uncut DNA migrates as only one larger band. If DNA from different individuals is compared, the likelihood that there will be identity across all DNA for the position of this sequence is very low. Cutting these different DNAs thus gives rise to different size bands in the samples from the two individuals. By comparing the polymorphism in restriction fragment (DNA) lengths in different individuals, using different enzymes,

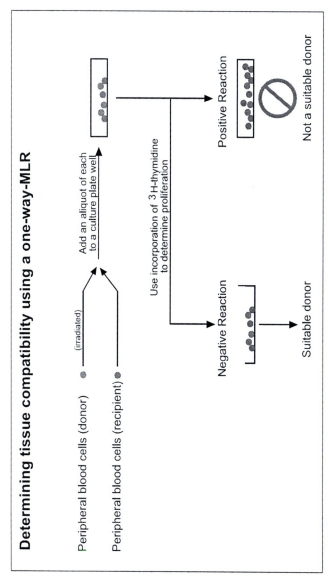

Fig. 17.5. Tissue typing using mixed lymphocyte reactions (MLR). Mismatches at class II MHC loci are measured in MLR by culturing cells from the donor and recipient together. Antigen recognition stimulates proliferation and clonal expansion of T cells, which is measured by quantitating radioactive isotope incorporation into DNA. The donor cells are usually irradiated to prevent their proliferation, ensuring they serve only as antigen to stimulate proliferation in recipient cells.

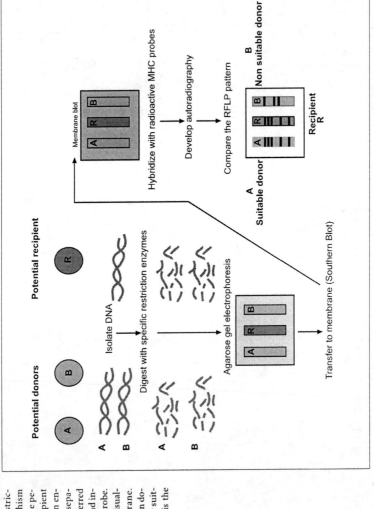

Fig. 17.6. Tissue typing using restriction fragment length polymorphism (RFLP). DNA is extracted from the peripheral blood cell of donor:recipient pairs and digested with restriction endonucleases. DNA fragments are separated by gel electrophoresis, transferred to a membrane (southern blot) and incubated with a radioactive MHC probe. After washing, autoradiography visualizes DNA bands on the membrane. Comparison of the RFLP pattern in donor and recipient estimates donor suitability. Method of choice today is the polymerase chain reaction.

we can estimate how disparate the DNAs are. *The number of such disparities does not predict the severity of rejection between donor/recipient.*

Using polymerase chain reaction (PCR), specific sequences of DNA are amplified using allele-specific primer pairs for known class I (or II) MHC genes. These primer pairs encode DNA sequences present in unique mRNAs. If the pool of mRNAs extracted from a blood sample contains the mRNA for the gene of interest, cDNA for that mRNA is amplified over a million-fold (in the presence of the primer pairs and a polymerase enzyme). The amplified cDNA is readily detected by gel electrophoresis. With different primer pairs for various class I or II MHC alleles we can compare alleles expressed by any donor/recipient pair. The problem of mismatches in unknown genes (for which no primer pairs exist) still remains.

IMMUNOLOGY OF GRAFT REJECTION

Graft rejection is mediated following activation of CD4+ or CD8+ T cells, macrophages, neutrophils, and the vascular endothelium. Cytokines, inflammatory mediators, and toxic products secreted by activated phagocytes contribute to graft rejection (Fig. 17.1). The sequence of cell activation and the interplay between various cells of the immune system that participate in graft rejection follows a general pattern. Early after transplantation, ischemia-reperfusion damage induces chemokine secretion by donor graft cells, e.g., macrophages, vascular endothelial cells (Fig. 17.7), along with secretion of several inflammatory cytokines. This increases vascular permeability and alters expression of adhesion molecules on the vascular endothelium and circulating leukocytes. Several days later, host cells, e.g., monocytes, neutrophils, CD4+ and CD8+ T cells, infiltrate the graft (Fig 17.8). Subsequently monocytes differentiate into macrophages in the presence of IFNγ, which also enhances the phagocytic capability of macrophages. Both host macrophages and neutrophils secrete toxic products and inflammatory mediators that initiate a cycle of ongoing tissue damage (Fig. 17.9). Alloreactive host Thp cells differentiate to Th1 cells secreting IL-2, IFNγ, and TNF, while alloreactive host CD8+ T cells differentiate into mature CTL in the presence of IL-2. These allo-specific CTL destroy allograft cells by osmotic lysis (Fig. 17.10). Ultimate rejection of an allograft reflects a composite of multiple processes, described in greater detail below (see also Fig. 17.11).

Graft invasion by CD4+ T-cells

CD4+ T-cell derived cytokines are required for virtually all aspects of immunity. The significance of T cells in graft rejection is supported by increased survival of allografts in neonatally thymectomized mice and children with Di George's syndrome (thymic aplasia). Both defects lead to a deficiency in CD4+ and CD8+ T cells.

Circulating T cells contact graft antigens as they traffic throughout the body in an immunosurveillance role. T cells enter peripheral tissues via postcapillary venules, migrate through the interstitial fluid to lymph capillaries, re-enter the lymphatic system and pass to the blood via the thoracic duct. When T cells leave the circulation and enter a graft, alloantigen can be seen directly on antigen

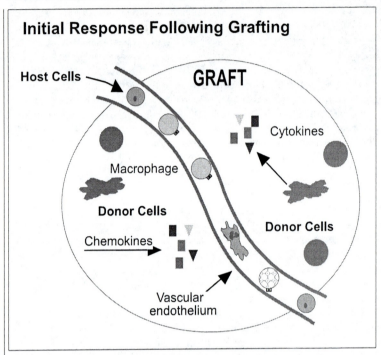

Fig. 17.7. Acute inflammation: 1-48 hours post transplant. Ischemia-reperfusion injury induces chemokine/cytokine secretion by numerous cells, e.g., macrophages, vascular endothelial cells, matrix cells. Increased vascular permeability occurs, as well as altered expression of adhesion molecules on the vascular endothelium and circulating leukocytes.

presenting cells in the tissue (so-called DIRECT alloantigen recognition). High affinity interaction of naïve host CD8 T cells with allogeneic class I MHC on donor tissue occurs, with fewer requirements for costimulation (Chapter 9) than is the case for nominal antigen. Unlike the case for nominal antigen, some degree of DIRECT recognition of allogeneic class II MHC by naïve CD4+ T cells also takes place in the graft itself (and not only in secondary lymphoid tissues), again without requiring engagement of costimulator molecules. In addition to DIRECT recognition, a process of INDIRECT recognition of allogeneic MHC antigens also occurs, particularly for CD4+ T cells. Graft antigen is processed by dendritic cells which migrate to secondary lymphoid tissue and activate, with costimulator interactions, CD4+ T cells. Since CD4 activation "drives" immune rejection, understanding INDIRECT CD4+ T cell recognition is key to understanding graft rejection (Figure 17.12).

Antigenic stimuli that activate CD4+ T cells
Genetic differences at the class II MHC loci between the donor and recipient lead to the most vigorous rejection of grafts, reflecting the higher frequency of

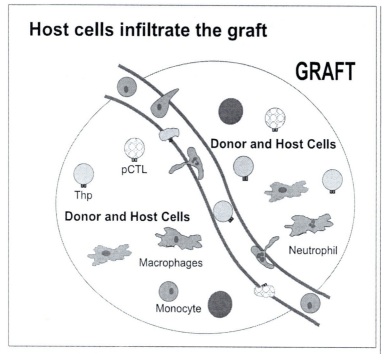

Fig. 17.8. Host cell infiltration into the graft: 1-7 days post transplant. Host cells, e.g., monocytes, neutrophils, CD4+ T cells, and CD8+ T cells, infiltrate the graft following alterations in vascular permeability and expression of adhesion molecules.

T cells (approximately 1%-2% of the total T-cell population) which recognize a given alloantigen. In a typical immune response to a nominal antigen only approximately one in ten thousand to one in a million T-cells of the total T-cell population is reactive with any given (nominal) antigen. The higher frequency of T cells activated after allostimulation is confirmed by in vitro studies, in which the frequency of cells recognizing a given alloantigen was determined directly by limiting dilution studies, and compared with the frequency of T cells existing for a nominal antigen. These results were taken to reflect a different mechanism for recognition of allo-MHC compared with conventional antigen. One explanation suggested that the antigenic determinant(s) of allo-MHC (with/without peptide in the groove) mimicked those produced by an array of self-MHC plus different foreign antigens, i.e., allo-MHC = self-MHC + antigen x and/or self MHC + antigen y, etc (Figure 17.12).

Donor cells that express class II MHC include dendritic cells, B cells, mononuclear phagocytes, and vascular endothelial cells. These cells could process shed donor antigens, and display the allo-antigen peptide fragment on the surface, in the context of the allo-class II MHC (DIRECT allo-recognition). In addition, host

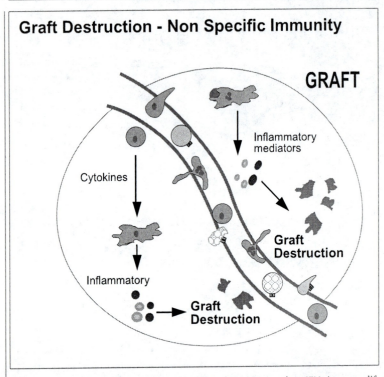

Fig. 17.9. Graft destruction: nonspecific immunity 4+ days post transplant. IFNγ increases differentiation and phagocytic activity of macrophages. Host macrophages and neutrophils secrete toxic products and inflammatory mediators, initiating a cycle of ongoing tissue damage.

antigen presenting cells (still class II MHC positive) could process and present donor antigen, this time in the context of host class II MHC, leading to the activation (INDIRECT recognition) of a different population of CD4+ T cells (Fig. 17.12).

Role of CD4+ T cells in graft rejection

Activated CD4+ T cells secrete many cytokines. Different subsets of cells are implicated in the production of different cytokines. Thus, CD4+ Th1 cells produce IFNγ and IL-2, while CD4+ Th2 cells produce IL-4, IL-5, IL-10 and IL-13. IFNγ stimulates monocytes, macrophages, and natural killer cells, while other cytokines (IL-2, IL-4) play important roles in development/differentiation of lymphocyte responses. IL-2 is a growth and differentiation factor for CD8+ pCTL cells, while IL-4 (IL-5) are growth/differentiation factors for B cells.

Role of macrophages in graft rejection

Tissue macrophages, activated nonspecifically by IFNγ secrete toxic mediators and cytokines (IL-1, IL-12, and TNF) and chemokines (e.g., IL-8) that

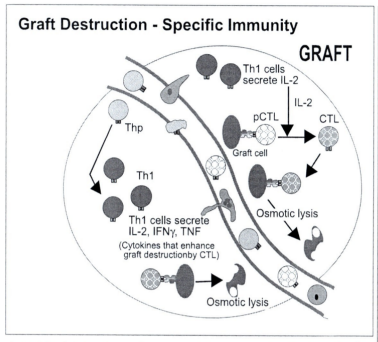

Fig. 17.10. Graft destruction: specific immunity 4+ days post transplant. Host Thp cells differentiate to Th1 cells that secrete IL-2, IFNγ, and TNF in response to allo-class II MHC. Allo-class I MHC reactive host CD8+ T cells (pCTL) differentiate into mature CTL in the presence of IL-2, destroying graft cells by osmotic lysis.

nonspecifically enhance the inflammatory response and contribute to "bystander" tissue injury in the engrafted tissue. Activated macrophages secrete IL-12, a molecule involved in stimulating the activation of natural killer cells, as well as in the differentiation of CD4+ T cells to Type 1 secreting cells that also secrete IFNγ. Macrophage-derived cytokines (IL-1, TNF) enter the circulation, change the adhesive properties of circulating leukocytes, and induce fever by acting on the hypothalamus.

Role of vascular endothelial cells

Vascular endothelium expresses molecules (selectins) that slow down circulating leukocytes, causing them to roll on the endothelium present at the site of inflammation. Macrophage-derived cytokines (TNF, IL-1) and chemokines (IL-8) induce either de novo expression and/or activation to a higher affinity of integrins on the endothelial cells and/or circulating leukocytes. Integrins induce strong adhesion between the leukocyte and the vascular endothelium. Trapped leukocytes are activated to secrete metalloproteinase enzymes that disrupt the integrity of the basement membrane resulting in the extravasation of leukocytes from the circulation into the graft bed.

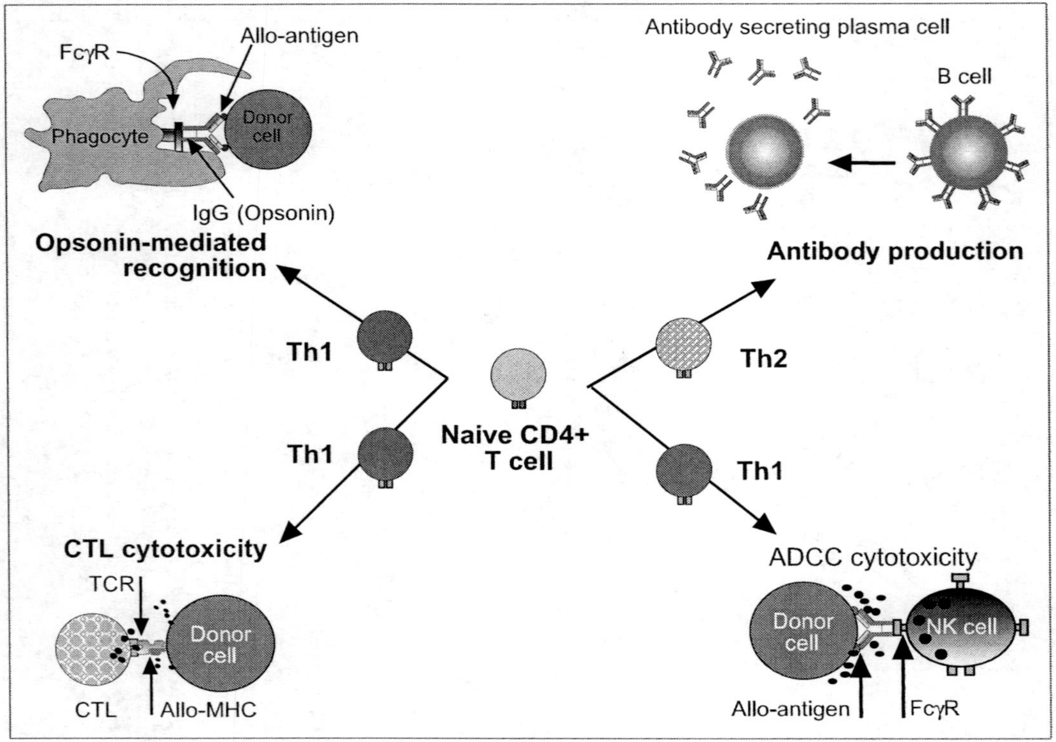

Fig. 17.11. Key cells in graft rejection. CD4+ T cells secrete cytokines required for virtually all aspects of immunity. Macrophages recognize graft cells with bound IgG antibodies, initiating opsonin mediated phagocytosis that is enhanced in the presence of IFNγ. Natural killer cells are cytotoxic for graft tissues when IgG is bound, causing osmotic lysis by perforin. IFNγ, from Th1 cells, enhances the cytotoxicity of natural killer cells. Cytokines secreted by Th1 cells promote differentiation of pCTL to allo-specific CTL, which lyse donor target cells. IgG antibodies assist cytotoxicity from macrophages and natural killer cells. In general Type 2 (not Type 1) cytokines are important for B-cell differentiation.

Transplantation

A. Recognition of self-class II MHC /microbial peptide complex

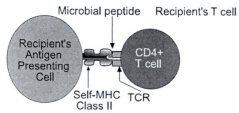

Typical antigen

B. Direct Recognition of Graft: Allo-Class II MHC

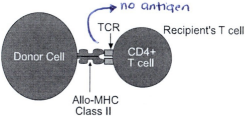

→ no antigen

Recognition of graft

C. Indirect Recognition of Graft: Self-Class II MHC/Allo-Class II MHC Peptide Complex

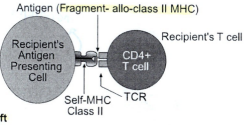

Recognition of graft

Fig. 17.12. CD4+ allo-recognition compared with microbial antigen recognition. CD4+ T cells recognize antigen presented by self-class II MHC. They can recognize allo-class II MHC *directly* if allo-class II MHC mimics self-class II MHC plus antigen. Donor class II MHC expressing cells include dendritic cells, B-cells, mononuclear phagocytes, and vascular endothelium. CD4+ T cells may also recognize fragments of shed allo-class II MHC presented by self-class II MHC on host cells (**indirect recognition**).

Role of CD8+ T cells in graft rejection

CD8+ T cells, differentiating to CTL in the presence of Th1-derived IL-2, are important in graft destruction. Detailed analysis of CD8+ CTL indicates that most CTLs recognize allo-class I MHC directly, i.e., that allo-class I MHC mimics foreign antigen/self-class I MHC (Fig. 17.13). Some CD8+ T cells are activated following recognition of self-class I MHC with donor-derived peptide. The mechanism(s) involved are not clear, though it is known that "empty" class I MHC on a cell surface can be "pulsed" with soluble peptide. Thus so-called INDIRECT allo-recognition can be documented for CD8+ T cells, though it is likely of much less

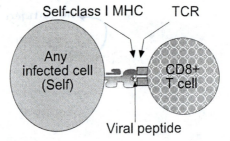

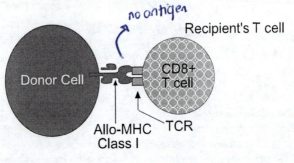

Fig. 17.13. CD8+ allo-recognition versus viral peptide recognition. CD8+ T cells recognize antigen (viral peptide) presented by infected cells expressing self-class I MHC. CD8+ T cells recognize allo-class I MHC directly if allo-class I MHC mimics self-class I MHC plus antigen. Most donor cells are targeted because all nucleated cells express class I MHC.

importance than for CD4+ T cells. It has been documented both experimentally and clinically that vigorous graft rejection occurs in the total absence of CD8+ T cells, but in the presence of CD4+ T cells, presumably following the activation of the nonspecific mechanisms referred to earlier.

Role of B cells
Because B-cell activation generally requires CD4+ T-cell mediated immune responses, it is difficult to demonstrate a unique role for antibodies in graft destruction. The presence of PREFORMED antibodies will initiate complement mediated tissue destruction minutes to hours after transplantation in so-called hyperacute rejection. Preformed antibodies to allografts often exist in multiparous women and in individuals who have rejected a first organ graft.

In the case of xenografts (e.g., pig grafts into humans) preformed, natural, circulating human antibodies recognize (cross react) with antigens expressed by the porcine blood vessels present in the graft. The predominant xenoantibody reactivity is one directed against the α1,3 galactosyl linkage of porcine carbohydrate antigens. Human cells lack an α1,3 galactosyl transferase, and this antigenic epitope does not exist in humans, so no tolerance to it is established. Exposure of the immune system during development to this antigen (on endogenous flora of the intestinal tract) induces high levels of anti-α1,3 galactose antibodies in all humans. When these human antibodies bind to porcine antigens they form immune complexes on the blood vessel wall. Because human complement proteins are always in circulation, the classic complement pathway is activated, leading to complement activation on endothelial cells lining graft blood vessels, activation of the coagulation cascade, thrombosis and graft loss.

Tissue Differences in Clinical Transplantation

Successful clinical transplantation of the following tissues/organs has become quite routine.

Corneal transplants occur in immunologically privileged sites and survive without immunosuppressive drug, because the foreign antigens expressed by the graft are not "seen" by host cells (except under inflammatory conditions, where local tissue permeability changes).

Heart transplants are standard clinical treatment for end organ failure following a number of insults (cardiomyopathies, chronic congestive heart failure, ischemic damage); 88% of patients survive at least one year posttransplantation. One problem with heart transplants is the high incidence of atherosclerotic disease in the recipients (including within the donor heart) occurring in the years following successful transplantation. This represents either an effect of the drugs used to avoid rejection and/or the long-term immune effects of subclinical rejection episodes.

Liver transplants are resistant to rejection once any early acute rejection episodes pass, and long-term graft survival is similar for both well-matched and unmatched tissues, with 80% of patients surviving at least one year. Both clinical and experimental data suggest that the presence of an allogeneic liver graft facilitates survival of another organ graft from the same donor. One explanation offered for this phenomenon is that the liver induces long-term tolerance because it is itself a lymphohematopoietic organ and stem cells from the donor liver migrate and "seed" recipient lymphoid tissues, inducing functional chimerism. Understanding the immunology of this phenomenon holds hope for progress in transplantation in general.

Kidney transplant survival after one year is approximately 90%, even for cadaveric kidney grafts (slightly higher rates are seen for living related grafts). Given an endless supply of organs, this, rather than continuous dialysis, is the primary treatment for renal failure. Nevertheless patients continue to take immunosuppressive drugs for the rest of their lives, producing, as it does for all transplant patients, significant side effects (drug toxicity; increased risk of infectious disease; increased incidence of malignancy). Since clinical kidney transplantation has been practiced over the longest period of time (30 years) changes in chronic survival of these grafts over this time can be measured. These data show unequivocally that while acute graft loss has slowed considerably (one year survival now approaches 90%, compared with less than 50% 20 years ago), the rate of chronic graft failure is relatively unchanged. These results highlight the urgent need for improved understanding of the (immuno)biology of chronic rejection.

Pancreas transplants are appealing for the treatment of diabetes and, combined with kidney grafts, for diabetic renal failure. Combined pancreas/kidney grafts survive well, with success rates comparable to that of kidneys alone. Isolated pancreas tissue may be given as a single cell suspension (islet grafts). Preliminary studies suggest these may survive optimally (and return the patients to normoglycemia) if given into the portal vein. The biological significance of the superior results following infusion into the liver bed remains unclear.

Bone transplants have been used to provide an inert "scaffold" for patients to bridge the time to replace allogeneic tissue with host bone matrix. Since bone grafts are avascular immune rejection is generally not a problem.

Bone marrow transplants are used to treat a variety of anemias, leukemias and lymphomas. Some problems are relatively unique to bone marrow transplantation. Rejection of allogeneic donor stem cells by immunocompetent hosts (host vs graft rejection) remains a problem, as in the case of solid organ grafts, which is treated using immunosuppressive drugs. The graft tissue is itself a source of lymphohematopoietic cells, capable of generating its own, donor-derived, immune system, which can recognize the host as foreign, resulting in the development of **graft-versus-host-disease** (GvHD). Other organ grafts where GvHD can also become a problem include the intestine and liver. This is easiest understood in terms of evidence that the liver represents an excellent adult source of hematopoietic stem cells, while intestinal transplantation also involves simultaneous transplantation of donor mesenteric lymphoid tissue and the Peyer's patch glands lining the intestinal wall.

GRAFT-VERSUS-HOST DISEASE

In graft-versus-host disease (GvHD) donor T cells present in the graft initiate rejection of all host tissue. Donor CD8+ and/or CD4+ T cells are activated when they interact with host cells expressing class I and/or class II MHC. Recipients of bone marrow transplants are themselves immunologically compromised and unable to initiate a counter attack. Skin sloughing, diarrhea, inflammation of the lungs, liver and kidneys are common problems associated with this disease, reflecting the end result of chronic inflammatory attacks on these organs/tissues, with altered tissue permeability, cell and fluid migration (Chapter 10).

This crucial role of T cells implied that T-cell depletion of the donor graft would eliminate GvHD. In practice, however, while removal of all donor T cells diminished GvHD, it concomitantly decreased engraftment of the donor bone marrow. Cytokines, often donor-T-cell-derived, are required for bone marrow engraftment. Accordingly, general practice now is to deplete donor T cells from the marrow prior to transplantation and simultaneously infuse patients with cytokines (IL-3 and GM-CSF) believed to "speed up" restoration of the lymphohematopoietic system from donor stem cells. Other sources of stem cells besides bone marrow are also under investigation, including cytokine-expanded CD34+ peripheral blood stem cells, and cord blood CD34+ cells. Banking of stem cells (rather like blood banking) has been initiated to provide an HLA-typed source of material for patients in urgent need.

Bone marrow transplantation is often the treatment of choice for leukemia/lymphoma. In such cases an added benefit of the presence of residual donor T cells in the bone marrow inoculum was a killing effect these cells had directed at residual host cancer cells, a so-called **graft vs leukemia effect** (GvL). When clinicians were most aggressive in eliminating T cells to avoid GvHD, the beneficial effect of GvL was also lost. Understanding the nature of the cells involved in GvHD and GvL is important, because if they do recognize distinct antigenic determinants there is hope that we may eventually be able to eliminate GvHD but preserve a GvL effect.

IMMUNOSUPPRESSION IN TRANSPLANTATION

Nonspecific immunosuppression

The immunosuppression required for effective long-term survival of any given graft differs between individuals. Nevertheless, high doses of immunosuppressive drugs generally lead to significant adverse effects, including an increased susceptibility to infectious disease, development of lymphoid/skin malignancies, and toxicity from the drugs themselves. These drugs are used clinically: Cyclosporin A (CsA); prednisone; azathioprine; FK506; rapamycin; and anti-CD3 and anti-CD4 antibodies.

Cyclosporin A and FK506 block the transcription and production of IL-2 by CD4+Th1 cells. They bind calcineurin in the cytoplasm and interfere with delivery of the IL-2 gene-activating stimulus to the nucleus.

Rapamycin inhibits a later stage in IL-2 gene transcription and synergizes, in immunosuppression, with FK506 or CsA.

Prednisone is a nonspecific anti-inflammatory agent, suppressing activation of macrophages and release of IFNγ. Rejection is inhibited at the antigen processing/presentation stage.

Azathioprine, an antimetabolite, is an analog of 6-mercatopurine. It inhibits purine metabolism and blocks cell division (and clonal expansion of activated cells).

Anti-CD3 antibodies suppress the activity of all T cells. Interaction of T-cell surface CD3 with anti-CD3 can cause an early, transient, activation of T cells before down regulation of CD3 expression occurs. Anti-CD3 is a murine antibody, and patients frequently generate an immune response to it, making further treatments less effective.

Anti-CD4 antibody treatment is coming into clinical practice to treat graft rejection, following many years of successful experimental trials.

Specific immunosuppression (tolerance)

This remains an unrealized goal for human transplantation. One of the seminal early observations in clinical transplantation was that prior exposure to donor antigens surprisingly led to prolonged survival of grafted organs, particularly in renal graft recipients pre-exposed to antigen in the form of blood transfusions. Transplantation was initially avoided in these individuals because of the fear of increased rejection (immunological memory). However, clinical experience showed grafts in these patients often fared better, not worse, than grafts to nontransfused individuals. These data form the basis of one of the few protocols currently used to produce donor-specific tolerance, the pretransplant (or peritransplant) transfusion protocols. Here the recipient receives *deliberate infusions* of donor cells (blood and/or bone marrow), in addition to the organ allograft.

Many hypotheses were used to explain the increased survival following transfusion. One suggests that pretransplant transfusion actually activates cells involved in allorejection, and that the immunosuppressive drugs given with the allograft eliminate these clonally activated T cells, producing operational tolerance of the graft. Alternatively, pretransplant transfusion may induce specific (or even nonspecific) "suppressor cells" capable of inhibiting graft rejection processes. Yet another model suggests that following transfusion preferential activation of CD4+ Th2 cells occurs, producing IL-10 (or IL-13) which suppresses the activation of CD4+ Th1 cells that secrete IL-2 and IFNγ, both of which are increased during rejection episodes. This notion that graft rejection is correlated with CD4+Th1 activation, and graft survival with CD4+Th2 activation, remains highly controversial.

Debate continues concerning the role of and/or need for persistent donor hematopoietic chimerism in graft recipients to produce long-term graft survival. Data from several groups suggests tolerance occurs to organ allografts only in cases where donor-derived dendritic cells migrate out from the donor organ, repopulate lymphoid tissues of the host, and persist. If tolerance is a passive process, dependent merely upon persistent donor antigen *per se*, it should occur simply from persistent presentation of allo-MHC itself on the grafted tissue. However, if tolerance is an active process, associated with, e.g., recipient CD4+Th2 activation, one might expect that persisting donor bone marrow-derived antigen presenting cells might be needed for tolerance maintenance. This proposal underlies some of the newer trials incorporating the introduction of small numbers of donor bone marrow cells to recipients of solid organs. This has also been used to explain why the liver, a known source of hematopoietic cells, might be so adept at promoting not only its own survival, but that of other (cotransplanted) organs.

Summary

In transplantation cells/tissue from one individual (a donor) are given to a second individual (a recipient). Transplants are classified according to the genetic disparity between donor and recipient (**isografts**: no genetic difference; **allografts**, transplants within a species; **xenografts**, transplants across a species barrier), and by the degree of immunological rejection they provoke. The latter is divided by time and the immunological mechanisms involved into **hyperacute rejection** (minutes to hours; antibody and complement mediated); **acute rejection** (weeks to months; T-cell mediated); and **chronic rejection** (months to years; mechanism(s) unclear).

The genetic disparity between donor and recipient helps predict the outcome of allografts, because genes of the **major histocompatibility complex** (MHC) encode the molecules that induce the most vigorous rejection episodes. "Tissue-typing" pretransplantation is an attempt to minimize MHC disparity between donor and recipient, using **serological, mixed lymphocyte typing reactions**, and (newer) **molecular typing** techniques. It is becoming increasingly clear that donor/recipient disparity at other genes, encoding so-called **minor histocompatibility antigens** (MiHs), sometimes produce as profound a rejection episode as differences at MHC loci.

Rejection is generally a function of the T-cell arm of the immune response, though bystander cells, especially macrophages, are often recruited following release of mediators (cytokines, etc.) from activated CD4+ T cells. CD4+ T cells assist the differentiation of other cytolytic effector CD8+ T cells, which lyse graft cells directly. A high frequency of T cells can recognize foreign MHC molecules, far greater than that number recognizing so-called nominal antigen. The manner in which these T cells "see" allo-MHC, whether **DIRECTLY** (without processing of MHC molecules as antigen, and presentation on antigen presenting cells) or **INDIRECTLY** (following such processing) dictates the nature, number and type of T cells activated, and often the severity of rejection. In unique circumstances (preimmunized recipients or recipients of grafts across a species barrier, xenotransplantation) antibody responses are important.

Following transplantation recipients receive long term nonspecific immunosuppressive drugs to prevent rejection. These treatments often cause significant side effects, including drug-related toxicity and an increased susceptibility to infection and malignancy. Protocols that induce graft-specific tolerance without the need for long-term nonspecific immunosuppression would be ideal. One uses donor specific pretransplant transfusion, though the mechanism(s) by which tolerance induction is achieved remain unclear.

Development of chimerism (coexistence of donor and host hematopoietic cells in the same host) may be essential for long-term tolerance, and probably occurs frequently after bone marrow transplantation. In this case the early period following transplantation is often also associated with a reaction of donor immune cells against the host (a graft-versus-host reaction), rather than the normal host antigraft reaction. When bone marrow transplantation is used in treatment of malignancy (leukemia/lymphoma), an anti-host reaction can be beneficial, a so-called graft-versus-leukemia effect. Balancing the outcome of all of these reactions is a major problem following bone marrow transplantation.

CLINICAL CASES AND DISCUSSION

Clinical Case #33
Gary is a 21-year-old boy with severe Crohn's disease. Multiple previous surgeries have resulted in home IV feeding for 6 months. He asked to be a candidate for an intestinal transplant program at the University Hospital and received a small intestinal transplant 4 weeks ago. He is given standard immunosuppressive treatment including cyclosporin A and FK506. He has gained weight, but has a diffuse "weeping" rash over his body, abdominal cramps and a fever for 5 days.

Questions and Discussion: Case # 33
1. Six key features we need to bear in mind in discussing this case are:
   - Young male
   - Immunosuppressive therapy
   - One month post intestinal transplant
   - Diffuse "weeping" rash
   - Fever of 5 days duration
   - Abdominal cramps
2. *An early complication of transplantation is acute graft rejection. The time frame of 4 weeks is right for* **acute rejection.** *How does this occur?*
   The **degree of MHC incompatibility between donor and host is critical.** MHC antigens are products of HLA-A, -B, and -C loci (class I MHC), and HLA-DP, -DQ, -DR loci (class II MHC). MHC differences between the donor and recipient are minimized by *pretransplant "matching"* of donor/recipient.
3. *The initial step in acute rejection is the recognition of the allogeneic graft as foreign by host CD4+ and CD8+ T cells. How do these cells recognize foreign MHC?*
   Approximately 1%-2% of the total T-cell population is reactive with any one allo-MHC antigen, whereas only 1 in 10,000 to 1 in 1,000,000 T cells of

the total T-cell population is reactive to a **nominal** protein antigen. One explanation suggests that allo-MHC (with or without peptide) mimics self-MHC plus (unspecified) antigen. CD4+ T cells recognize allo class II MHC, while CD8+ T cells recognize allo class I MHC.

4. *Explain the role of each class of T cells in allogeneic graft rejection.*
   Activated host CD4+T cells release Type 1 cytokines which contribute to nonspecific inflammatory processes (e.g., IFNγ/TNF) and IL-2 which is a growth factor for T cells expressing IL-2 receptors. IL-2 is also required for differentiation of naive CD8+ T cells to mature CTL, causing direct cytotoxicity to graft cells.

5. *Acute rejection causes nonspecific symptoms (e.g., the fever here) as well as physiological "failure" of the graft (leading, in kidney grafts, to rising serum creatinine; in intestinal grafts, to weight loss, cramping etc.). What is an immunological basis for cramping and fever?*
   Cramping could be caused by nonspecific mediators induced by cytokines produced by activated CD4 cells (e.g., activation of mast cells to release histamine). Activated CD4+ T cells secrete Type 1 cytokines (including IFNγ and TNF) that further activate macrophages to secrete IL-1. IL-1 can act on the hypothalamus to induce fever.

6. *Acute rejection episodes are treated by increasing nonspecific immunosuppression. The side-effects of immunosuppression often cause significant problems. What are some of these?*
   Increased infection, drug toxicity and increased evidence of malignancy.

7. *The incidence of malignancy is relatively restricted to two types. What are they?*
   Lymphomas and skin malignancies.

8. *Infection could cause this fever, particularly since he is on immunosuppressive therapy. What infections are prominent early after transplantation?*
   Viral infections (serum Ig levels do not fall, but functional T-cell activity is compromised!). Cytomegalovirus (CMV) infections are particularly prominent.

9. *What drug toxicity complicates immunosuppressive therapy?*
   Hypersensitivity reactions are possibilities, but are rare because the drugs themselves are immunosuppressive. Organ toxicity is common, e.g., renal toxicity and neurotoxicity are common with cyclosporin A and FK506.

10. *Gary has some (not all) of these findings (fever, intestinal cramping, loss of weight). What remains unexplained, and what is a possible cause?*
    The rash remains unexplained. Elevated permeability of blood vessels following cytokine release by CD4+ T cells would account for the "weeping rash", the cramps, and fever.

11. *In intestinal transplantation DONOR lymphoid tissue is transplanted as part of the intestinal graft. The intestine is a source of some 50% of the total body lymphoid pool. What is a problem in this type of transplantation?*
    Graft-vs-host disease (GvHD) is a significant problem.

12. Would GvHD present with cramping, fever, rash, and intestinal cramps?
   In GvHD massive cytokine production (from both activated host and donor CD4 cells) occurs, a so-called **cytokine storm.** This accounts for the "weeping rash" (elevated permeability of vessels following cytokine release) and the cramps (and fever).
13. What are treatment options?
   i   Increased (or different) immunosuppression, but beware of infection and/or malignancy.
   ii Graft removal. You must weigh the pros/cons of different treatments.
14. How could graft failure be measured directly?
   We need some specific assay for intestinal function (like serum creatinine for the kidney). The kidney normally filters creatinine from the blood, and failure to do so, producing rising serum creatinine, is a useful surrogate marker for declining kidney function from all causes. Measuring the absorptive function of the intestine is a good approach here.

Clinical Case #34

Adriana is 4 years postcardiac transplantation for cardiomyopathy that developed after receiving chemotherapy (adriamycin) for breast cancer. Routine annual endomyocardial biopsies, the last 6 months ago, were read as normal, with no signs of rejection. There has been no change in her antirejection therapy for the last 2 years; she is on prednisone and cyclosporin A. Her son found her at home quite confused and with a droop on the left side of her face/mouth. Routine blood work, including measurement of cardiac muscle enzymes, physical exam, and electrocardiogram (to check the heart) is normal. How do you proceed?

Questions and Discussion: Case #34
1. List the six likely key features we need to bear in mind in discussing this case.
   Mature female
   Heart graft
   Stable on anti-rejection therapy
   Blood work is normal, including cardiac muscle enzymes
   Cardiogram is normal
   Physical exam is normal
2. Is this a case of hyperacute or acute rejection? How do these differ immunologically and in treatment?
   Hyperacute rejection occurs in the immediate aftermath of transplantation and is antibody and complement mediated. It requires immediate graft removal. Acute rejection occurs weeks to months after transplantation, involves (T) cell mediated organ damage and is treated by increasing immunosuppressive   treatment.
3. In addition to the time, what other evidence makes acute rejection unlikely?
   Acute rejection involves organ damage, following CD4 and/or CD8 mediated "attack". Think of organ-specific "markers" for the damage. For the

heart, the EKG (cardiogram), and measurement of specific cardiac muscle enzymes would assess killing (lysis) of heart cells, with release into the serum of cardiac muscle enzymes. This patient has a normal cardiogram and normal cardiac muscle enzymes. [In kidney grafts, you would measure creatinine.]
4. *Could this be a case of chronic rejection? How would this manifest?*
Chronic rejection correlates with release of nonspecific growth factor-like mediators (e.g., fibroblast growth factor, endothelial growth factor etc.) and is an insidious fibrosing/proliferative reaction, relatively refractory to immunosuppressive treatment. A fibrotic heart is a poor pump, resulting in poor oxygenation of tissues. This might cause generalized neurological deficits (e.g., Adriana's confusion).
5. *In the absence of acute, hyperacute, or chronic rejection, what about the side effects of the treatment she received for her transplant. Immunosuppressed individuals are susceptible to?*
   a. Malignancy (lymphomas and skin cancer)
   b. Infection (especially viral); antibody levels are generally unaffected.
   c. Toxicity directly and indirectly from the drugs themselves.
6. *How could a malignancy, lymphoma or skin cancer, manifest as confusion? How would you investigate?*
Immunosuppression impairs tumor surveillance, so a secondary metastasis (to the brain) from her original breast cancer would be a concern in this lady, as would a new central nervous system lymphoma (Chapter 16). You should order a CT scan.
7. *Assume that the tests/examination from #6 are normal, is there evidence for infection? What viral infections are seen in immunosuppressed transplant patients? How would you detect them?*
Nothing suggests infection here, and even her blood work is normal. Two viral infections common in immunosuppressed transplant patients can present this way, cytomegalovirus (CMV) and herpes simplex virus (HSV). Serological titers of the virus might be measured (look for IgM (a new response) in a person known to be seronegative before transplantation; or elevated IgG, if previously positive). Alternatively, monitor a "response to treatment" or biopsy tissue.
8. *Assuming all tests are negative we are left with drug toxicity. What are toxic side effects of cyclosporin A and prednisone?*
Cyclosporin A is nephrotoxic (damages the kidney) and neurotoxic (damaging nervous tissue). Neurotoxicity is more evident in peripheral nerves (peripheral neuropathy) than in the central nervous system. Prednisone increases atherosclerotic disease, both in grafted organs (here the heart) and elsewhere (e.g., the brain). Narrowing of blood vessels puts people at risk for increased clots (emboli) to the heart (a heart attack) and the brain (a stroke). The latter is the most likely problem for this unfortunate lady.

TEST YOURSELF

Multiple Choice Questions

1. A patient on your transplant service is enrolled in a study designed to investigate levels of cytokines produced during various stages of transplantation/acceptance/rejection. A patient showing elevated levels of IL-2 in the grafted organ would likely be undergoing:
   a. "A healing in" process associated with a graft acceptance
   b. Graft rejection
   c. Cytotoxic reaction to immunosuppressive drugs
   d. Infection
   e. None of the above
2. XL received a kidney graft from her sister 6 years ago but lost the graft to rejection. This morning she underwent a further transplant from a younger brother. Ninety minutes following surgery she suffers severe cramps in the abdomen, is febrile, and looks quite unwell. She might be suffering from:
   a. Chronic rejection
   b. Acute graft rejection
   c. Cytotoxic T-cell mediated graft damage
   d. Hyperacute graft rejection
   e. Surgical sepsis
3. Appropriate treatment for the patient in question 2 would be:
   a. Anti-T cell antibodies
   b. Immunosuppression
   c. Removal of the graft
   d. Analgesia
   e. Anti-pyretics (anti-fever drugs)
4. You are running a tissue-typing laboratory and are faced with matching a potential kidney transplant recipient with one of several unrelated donors. Serology indicates 5/6 MHC matches. Which of the following would be the MOST judicious course of action?
   a. Proceed with transplantation, with no immunosuppression
   b. Proceed with transplantation, using cyclosporin and prednisone
   c. Await further matching data from PCR (6 hours)
   d. Await further matching from MLR (72 hours)
5. A child receives a bone marrow transplant from an HLA identical sibling. After successful engraftment, 3 weeks later the child has diarrhea and a rash on the palms and soles of the feet, spreading to the trunk, with jaundice. Administration of an anti-T cell serum plus cyclosporine produces improvement. The most likely cause is?
   a. Inadequate numbers of donor cells were transfused
   b. Donor lymphocytes are reacting with antigens on the recipient's cells
   c. Present symptoms are the long term effects of original drug ingestion
   d. There is a superimposed viral infection (CMV)
   e. There has been a failure of the graft to take

Answer: *1b ; 2d ; 3c ; 4c; 5b*

Short Answer Questions
1. Distinguish between autograft, isograft, allograft and xenograft.
2. Name three pieces of evidence for immune rejection of allografts.
3. What are the various potential phases of graft rejection and how does one treat them clinically?
4. What chromosomal locus (i) codes for the major gene(s) involved in human graft rejection and how do we routinely test for human histocompatibility antigens?
5. What unique problems surround the use of bone marrow transplants?

Index

A

Acquired immunodeficiency syndrome (AIDS) 222
Active immunization 241, 258
Acute rejection 106, 373, 391
Adaptive immunity 2
Addressin 134
Adhesion molecules 34, 134, 169
Adjuvants 3, 24, 244, 258, 282
Affinity 71
Affinity maturation 157
Allelic exclusion 132
Alloantigens 107
Allografts 368, 391
Allotransplant 107
Allotypes 69, 70
Alpha-fetoprotein (AFP) 342
Alternative pathway 20, 32
Alternative pathway C5 convertase (C3bBbC3b) 89
Anaphylatoxins 32, 93, 194
Anergy 169
Ankylosing spondylitis 295
Anti-CD4 antibody treatment 390
Anti-idiotypic antibodies 72
Antibody 3, 11, 20, 69
Antibody-mediated cellular cytotoxicity (ADCC) 45
Antigen 22
Antigen presenting cells (APC) 10, 51, 169
Antigen-dependent B-cell differentiation 12, 153
Antigenic determinant 22
Apo-1 184
Apoptosis 134, 182
Aspergillus 227
Autografts 368
Autoimmunity 290
Azathioprine 390

B

B lymphocytes 11, 52, 130, 131
β1 integrin family 198
β2 integrin chain 205
β2 integrin family 198
β7 integrin family 198
β7/CD28; CD40/CD40 ligand 155
Bacillus Calmette-Guerin (BCG) 120
Basophils 10, 32
BCR 134
Bence Jones proteins 330, 354
Beta chain 198
Beta human chorionic gonadotropin, (β-HCG) 342
Bone marrow transplants 388
Borrelia burgdorferi 212
Bradykinin 99, 191
Btk kinase 161

C

C1 esterase inhibitor (C1 INH) 101
C2b 95
C3a 93
C3b 93
C4a 93
C5a 93
C5b 95
Candida albicans 227
Candidiasis 229
Carcinoembryonic antigen (CEA) 342
Carrier effect 24
CCR5 52, 222
CD1 64
CD19 161
CD2 177
CD4 11, 52, 182
CD40 161
CD40 ligand 161
CD40/CD40 ligand interaction 155

CD45 161, 180
CD79a/b heterodimer 160
CD79a/CD79b 130
CD8 52, 182
CD8+ T cells 52
CD8+ T cells or cytotoxic
  T lymphocytes (CTL) 12, 177
CD95 184
Chagas disease 257
Chediak-Higashi syndrome 324
Chemokine receptor 52
Chemokines 3, 22, 31, 34
Chemotactic molecules 34
Chemotaxis 93
Chronic granulomatous disease
  (CGD) 42, 205, 324
Chronic mucocutaneous candidiasis
  231, 319
Chronic rejection 107, 373
Class I MHC molecules 53, 182
Class II MHC molecules 10, 53, 61,
  182
Classical complement pathway 20,
  89, 93
Clonal expansion 5
Clone 5
Codominant expression 56
Cold agglutinin disease 296
Combinatorial diversity 131
Common variable
  hypogammaglobulinemia 322
Common/terminal pathway 20
Complement system 20, 31, 32, 86
Complementary determining regions,
  CDRs 72
Constant region 69
Corneal transplants 387
Costimulatory molecules 52
Crohn's colitis 281
Cross reactivity 293
Cryptococcus neoformans 229
CTL 177
CTLA-4 182
Cutaneous basophil hypersensitivity
  282
CXCR4 52
Cyclosporin A 389
Cytokines 3, 10, 31, 111
Cytomegalovirus (CMV) 60

D

Death by neglect 14, 143
Decay accelerating factor (DAF) 327
Delayed type hypersensitivity reaction
  (DTH) 226, 281
Dendritic cell 52, 169
Determinant group 22
Di George's syndrome 319
Diapedesis 34, 202
Diversity 130

E

E-selectin 198
Edema 191
Enzyme-linked immunosorbent
  assays (ELISA) 77
Eosinophil cationic protein (ECP) 11,
  45
Eosinophil chemotactic factor of
  anaphylaxis (ECF-11)
Eosinophils 10, 45
Epitope 4, 5
Epstein-Barr virus (EBV) 59
Experimental allergic encephalitis
  301

F

F(ab) 71
Fab2 71
Factor B 89
Factor D 89
Factor XI 195
Factor XII 195
Family kinases 161
Farmer's lung 276
Fas ligand 182
Fas receptor 182
Fc 71
FcγR 43, 52
FcγRIIB 163
FK506 389
Follicle associated epithelium (FAE)
  18
Follicles 155
Furuncles 212

G

Galectin 9 340
Gelatinase B 202
Germinal centers 15, 155
Gonorrhea 214
Graft rejection 368, 371
Graft-vs-leukemia effect 388
Graft-versus-host-disease (GvHD) 367, 370, 388
Granuloma 281
Guanine exchange protein (GEF) 161
Guillain-Barre disease 255

H

Haemagglutinin 256
Hageman factor (Factor XII) 280
Hairy cell leukemia 329
Hapten 3, 24
Hashimoto's thyroiditis 290, 299
Heart transplants 387
Heavy chain variable region 69, 130, 132
Hematopoiesis 12
Hereditary angioedema (HAE) 101, 327
Herpes simplex virus (HSV) 58
High endothelial venules (HEV) 134, 146
Histamine 11, 32, 193
Human immunodeficiency virus (HIV) 223
Human leukocyte antigens (HLA) 55, 368
HvG 367, 370
Hybridomas 77
Hydrogen peroxide 38
Hydroxyl radical 38
Hyper IgM syndrome 159, 166
Hyperacute rejection 107, 371, 391
Hypersensitivity reactions 266
Hypochlorite 38
Hypogammaglobulinemia 159

I

ICAM (1-3) 177
Idiotype 69, 72
Ig 70
IgA 70
IgD 70
IgE 70
IgG 70
IgM 70
IL-1 201
IL-1 receptor antagonist 247
IL-10 203
IL-4 203
IL-8 201
Immune complex 89
Immunodeficiency disorders 315
Immunogen 22
Immunoglobulin A (IgA) 72
Immunoglobulin D (IgD) 73
Immunoglobulin deficiency with increased IgM 322
Immunoglobulin E (IgE) 76
Immunoglobulin G (IgG) 76
Immunoglobulin M (IgM) 77
Immunoglobulins 11, 20, 69
Inflammation 191
Innate immune system 2, 31
Insulin-dependent diabetes mellitus 296
Integrins 146, 196, 198
Interferon gamma (IFNγ) 329
Invariant chain, (Ii) 61
Isografts 368, 391
Isotype switching 155
ITAM 161, 180
ITIMs 163

J

J chain 72
Janus tyrosine kinases (JAKs) 111
Jones Mote Reaction 281
Junctional diversity 132

Index

K

Kallikrein 99, 194
Keratinocytes 281
Kidney transplant 388
Killer inhibitory receptors (KIR) 42
Kininogen 99

L

L-selectin 146, 184, 198
Lactoferrin 214
Langerhans cells 281
Lepromatous leprosy 281
Leukocyte adhesion deficiency (LAD) 205, 324
Leukocyte rolling 196
Leukotrienes 11
LFA-1 146, 177
LFA-3 177
Light chain variable region 131
Light chains 69
Lipopolysaccharide (LPS) 24, 25, 164
Liver transplants 387
Lyme's disease 212
Lymph nodes 14
Lysosomal enzymes 34
Lysosomes 38
Lysozyme 4, 214

M

Macrophages 9, 32, 52
MAGE-1 to -3 258, 340
Major basic protein (MBP) 11, 45
Major histocompatibility complex (MHC) 52, 368, 391
Mantoux 226
Marginate 34
Mast cells 10, 32, 194
Matrix metalloproteinases 146, 201
Mature naive B cells 134
MCP-1 201
MelanaA/MART-1 340
Membrane attack complex (MAC) 89, 93
Memory cells 3, 157, 184
Microglobulin 56
MIg 130, 160

Minor histocompatibility antigens (MiHs) 391
Minor histocompatibility proteins 368
MIP-1a 222
MIP-1b 222
Mitogens 24
MMP-2 202
MMP-9 202
Molecular mimicry 293
Molecular typing 391
Monoclonal antibodies 77
Monocyte 9
Multiple germline genes 131
Multiple myeloma 330
Multiple sclerosis 299, 301
Mycobacterium bovis 120
Mycobacterium leprae 281
Mycobacterium tuberculosis 226, 281
Mycoses 227
Myeloma 354

N

NADPH oxidase 38
Natural killer (NK) cells 2, 10, 31, 42
Negative selection 14, 143
Neissseria gonorrhea 214
Neuraminidase 256
Neutrophils 9, 32
Nitric oxide (NO) 40
Nitric oxide synthase 41
NOD mice 306
NY-ESO-1 340

O

Oligoclonal 24
Opportunistic 227
Opsonin-mediated 34
Opsonins 34, 214

P

P-selectin 198
Pancreas transplants 388
Paroxysmal nocturnal haemoglobinuria (PNH) 102, 327

Index

Passive immunization 241, 258
Perforin 45
Periarteriolar lymphatic sheath (PALS) 16
Pernicious anemia 296
Phagocytes (macrophages and neutrophils) 2, 9
Phagocytic vacuole 38
Phagocytosis 9
Phagosome 34, 38
Phosphatases 163
Phospholipase Cγ (PL-Cγ) 161, 180
Phytohemagglutinin (PHA) 25
Plasma cells 11
Plasmodium falciparum 257
Platelet activating factor (PAF) 11
Pluripotent stem cells 12
Pneumococcal polysaccharide 24, 164
Poison ivy dermatitis 281
Pokeweed mitogen (PWM) 25
Polyclonal 77
Polymorphism 55, 368
Positive selection 14, 143, 146
PPD 281
Pre-BCR 134
Prednisone 390
Prekallikrein 195
Primary follicles 15, 155
Primary immune response 52, 159
Primary immune tissues 3, 12
Primary immunodeficiency disorders 315
Primary response 5
Primitive pattern recognition receptors, PPRR 31, 34
Progelatinase B 202
Programmed cell death 182
Properdin 89
Proteosome 56

R

RAG-1 131
RAG-2 131
RANTES 201, 222
Rapamycin 390
Reactive nitrogen intermediates (RNIs) 34, 40
Reactive oxygen intermediate (ROI) 34, 38
Receptor-mediated cytotoxicity 43
Recipient 179
Reticular dysgenesis 317
Rheumatoid arthritis 290

S

Sarcoidosis 281
SDF-1 (stromal cell-derived factor 1) 222
Secondary follicles 15, 155
Secondary immune response 159
Secondary immune tissues 3, 12
Secondary immunodeficiency disorders 327
Secretory component 72
Selectins 196
Selective IgA deficiency 165, 322
Self tolerance 290
Serological, mixed lymphocyte typing reactions 391
Severe combined immunodeficiency (SCID) 316
SH2 (Src homology 2) domain/ 161, 180
SH3 (Src homology 3) domain 161, 180
Shigella dysenteriae 227
Sites of inflammation 202
Somatic mutation 157
Somatic recombination 131
Specificity 70
Spermine 4
Spleen 16
Staphylococcus aureus 212
STAT proteins 113
Streptococcus pneumoniae 214, 217
Sub-classes 69
Superoxide 38
Switch recombination 157
Syk 161
Systemic lupus erythematosus (SLE) 278, 290

T

T cell receptors (TCR) 11
T helper (Th) cells 11
T independent (T-indep) antigens 163
T lymphocytes 11
T-dependent antigens 3, 22, 24
Target cells 12, 52
Terminal complement pathway 93
Terminal deoxynucleotidyl transferase (Tdt) 132
Thrombi 107
TNF 201
Tolerance 290
Tolerance induction 13
TRAF (tumor necrosis factor associated factors) 161
Transient hypogammaglobulinemia of infancy 165
Transporter of antigen processing (TAP) 57
Trypanosoma cruzi 257
Tuberculoid leprosy 280
Tuberculosis 226
Tumor associated antigens (TAAs) 342
Tumor specific antigens (TSAs) 340
Tumor specific transplantation antigens (TSTA) 340
TYK2 111
Type I T-independent antigen 24, 164
Type II T-independent antigen 24, 164

V

Vaccination 241, 244, 258
Variable region 69

W

Waldenström's macroglobulinemia 330
White pulp 16

X

X-linked agammaglobulinemia (XLA) 161, 320
Xenotransplant 103, 107, 368, 391

Z

ZAP 70 kinase 180